Endocrine Problems in Cancer

Endocrine Problems in Cancer

Molecular Basis and Clinical Management

Editors

Roland T. Jung, MA, MD, MRCP

*Consultant Physician, Specialist in Endocrinology and
Diabetes, Ninewells Hospital, Dundee
Honorary Senior Lecturer in Medicine,
University of Dundee*

and

Karol Sikora, MA, MRCP, FRCR, PhD

*Director, Ludwig Institute for Cancer Research, Cambridge
Honorary Consultant in Radiotherapy and Oncology
Addenbrooke's and Huntingdon Hospitals, Cambridge*

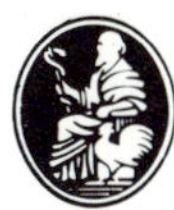

HEINEMANN MEDICAL BOOKS LTD
LONDON

First published in 1984 by William Heinemann Medical Books Ltd,
23, Bedford Square, London

ISBN: 0-433-30277-1

Photosetting by Thomson Press (India) Limited, New Delhi and
Printed in Great Britain by The Alden Press Oxford.

Contents

List of Contributors

Peter H. Baylis, BSc, MD, FRCP
  Consultant Physician, Royal Victoria Infirmary, Newcastle upon Tyne
  Senior Lecturer in Medicine, University of Newcastle, UK
Harvey S. Besterman, BSc, MRCP
  Senior Registrar in Endocrinology, St. Bartholomew's Hospital, London,
  UK
Adrian J.L. Clark, BSc, MRCP
  Visiting Research Fellow, Laboratory of Molecular Biology, National
  Cancer Institute, Bethesda, USA
Charles Coombes, MD, PhD, MRCP
  Clinical Scientist, Ludwig Institute for Cancer Research. Honorary
  Consultant Physician, Royal Marsden Hospital, London, UK
Michael W.J. Davie, MD, MRCP
  Consultant Physician and Director of Research, Robert Jones and Agnes
  Hunt Orthopaedic Hospital, Oswestry, Shropshire, UK
Martin Gore, MRCP
  Clinical Research Fellow, Ludwig Institute for Cancer Research,
  London. Honorary Senior Registrar in Medicine, Royal Marsden
  Hospital, London, UK
Roland T. Jung, MA, MD, MRCP
  Consultant Physician, Specialist in Endocrinology and Diabetes,
  Ninewells Hospital, Dundee. Honorary Senior Lecturer in Medicine,
  University of Dundee, UK
John A. Lynn, MD, FRCS
  Consultant Surgeon in Endocrinology, Hammersmith Hospital, London,
  UK
R. Timothy D. Oliver, MD, MRCP
  Senior Lecturer in Genito-urinary Oncology to the Institute of Urology,
  The London and St. Bartholomew's Hospitals Medical Colleges, UK
Piers N. Plowman, MA, MD, MRCP, FRCR
  Consultant in Radiotherapy and Oncology, The Hospital for Sick
  Children, Great Ormond Street, and St. Bartholomew's Hospital,
  London, UK

Bruce A.J. Ponder, MA, PhD, MRCP
  Cancer Research Campaign Fellow, Institute of Cancer Research. Honorary Consultant Physician, Royal Marsden Hospital, London, UK
Richard J. Pye, MA, MD, MRCP
  Consultant Dermatologist, Addenbrooke's Hospital, Cambridge, UK
John Rhodes, PhD
  Senior Scientist, Department of Experimental Immunobiology, The Wellcome Laboratories, Langley Court, Beckenham, Kent, UK
Martin O. Savage, MA, MD, MRCP
  Consultant Paediatric Endocrinologist, St. Bartholomew's Hospital, London. Consultant Paediatrician, Queen Elizabeth Hospital for Children, London, UK
Karol Sikora, MA, MRCP, FRCR, PhD
  Director, Ludwig Institute for Cancer Research, Cambridge. Honorary Consultant in Radiotherapy and Oncology, Addenbrooke's and Huntingdon Hospitals, Cambridge, UK
L. Otto Uttenthal, MA, DPhil, MRCP
  Research Fellow, Endocrine Unit, Hammersmith Hospital, London, UK
Jonathan H. Waxman, BSc, MRCP
  ICRF Research Fellow, The Department of Medical Oncology, St. Bartholomew's Hospital, London, UK
Michael C. White, MD, MRCP
  Senior Registrar in Endocrinology, Royal Victoria Infirmary, Newcastle upon Tyne, UK

Preface

Endocrine problems requiring clinical intervention occur in many patients with cancer. To the oncologist, general physician and endocrinologist they form an important part of clinical practice. The advent of aggressive surgery, radiotherapy and chemotherapy to successfully treat a variety of tumour types has increased the importance and awareness of supportive care in the management of cancer patients.

There are several ways in which endocrinology impinges on oncology. First, there are the classic endocrine diseases; Cushing's syndrome, Conn's syndrome and the various pituitary syndromes. These are due to benign tumours and are well described in many endocrine text books. The second meeting point of endocrinology and oncology are the endocrine and metabolic problems that can arise due either to the production of hormones by neoplastic cells, or by the interference of normal physiological systems by malignant cells. The aim of this book is to review this second subject, an area where endocrine expertise and intervention is vital for the management of the cancer patient.

The authors are clinicians who have experience in the management of the physiological problems and have been asked to emphasise the clinical aspects of the diagnosis and management of the endocrine problems described. This book is not concerned with the endocrine manipulation of tumours. The book begins by considering the biological basis of cancer, its secreted products and their relationship to the genetics of the cell and the individual. The metabolism of the cell is then discussed followed by a consideration of the individual clinical endocrine syndromes that occur. Their physiological basis and the diagnostic approach is described and then the management outlined in detail, so that the book provides practical advice.

We hope that this book will be a useful guide to those involved in the treatment of cancer.

Roland T. Jung, Dundee
Karol Sikora, Cambridge

Chapter 1

Karol Sikora

Molecular Biology of Cancer

INTRODUCTION

One in five of the population currently dies from cancer. Over 90% of these deaths are caused by one of the common solid tumours arising in organs such as lung, colon and breast. Over the last twenty years there have been tremendous advances in treating some of the rarer tumour types such as leukaemias, lymphomas and teratoma (Report of the Advisory Committee on Cancer Registration, 1983). The reasons for this advance are complex and not due solely to the advent of any single therapy. Perhaps the biggest advance in these relatively rare tumours has been the increased under-standing in their biology and response to different therapies at different stages in their natural history. No such advance has been seen in treating patients with common solid tumours, despite the huge investment of time, money and resources of many nations. There are currently three problems in treating these patients.

The first is the assessment of the size and site of the primary tumour and its metastases. It is impossible, using current techniques, to reliably detect tumour masses less than 1 cm in diameter. As can be seen from Fig. 1.1, this represents a mass of some 10^9 cells. After excision of the primary carcinoma in a woman with breast cancer, the chances of metastatic disease remaining are around 40%. Despite the advent of sophisticated scanning techniques, the local therapy carried out in this group of patients is inadequate because of the occult metastases. It is for this reason that so much controversy surrounds the management of early breast cancer (Bluming, 1982). A different problem in assessment comes in carcinoma of the bronchus. The opacity seen on a chest x-ray represents the effects of the tumour in causing bronchial obstruction with distal collapse of lung alveoli, rather than the tumour itself. Small changes in tumour size after radiotherapy or chem-otherapy may result in disproportionate x-ray responses, making assess-ment of different treatment regimens difficult. If better ways become available to assess both the initial tumour load and its response to therapy this would have significant benefit by aiding decisions in treatment.

A second problem is the lack of effective systemic therapies for many

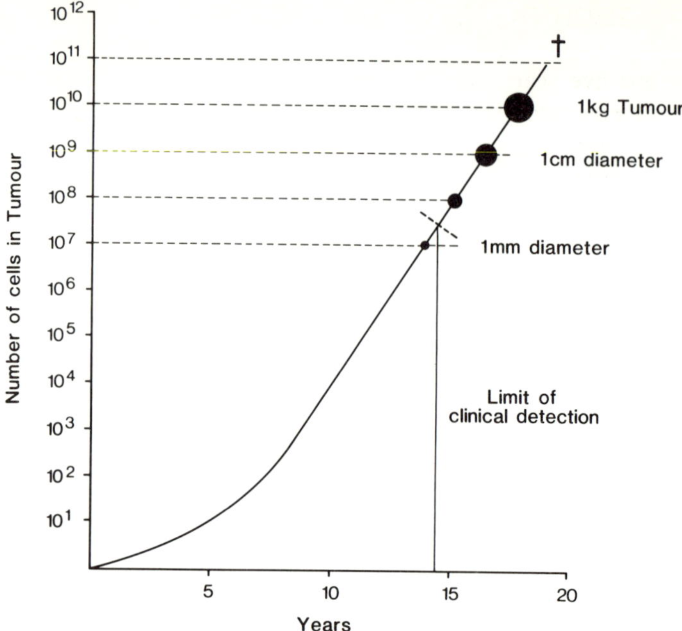

Fig. 1.1. *Hypothetical growth of a primary cancer.*

cancers. Combinations of surgery and radiotherapy, when used judiciously, are often effective in eradicating even the largest of primary neoplasms. The problem comes from recurrences at the edge of the treated volume and the distant metastases. Only the addition of systemic therapy can deal with these problems. Although chemotherapy is surprisingly effective in obtaining regressions of many solid tumours, drug resistance emerges quickly. Several studies have shown that, despite these regressions, little benefit occurs in terms of increased survival in breast and lung cancer (Powles *et al*, 1980).

The third problem is perhaps the key to the whole enigma of cancer. There are few specific, selective methods with which to attack the malignant cell. Chemotherapy, as presently used, is reminiscent of the treatment of infectious diseases in the pre-antibiotic era of the 1930s. There are a range of powerful cytotoxic drugs, but these are often unable to discriminate adequately between the malignant cell and its normal counterpart. By learning more about the molecular biology of the cancer cell, new biological systems can be identified that we can tamper with pharmacologically. Hormones have powerful effects on cancer cells and can also be produced by them. By increasing the understanding of the interaction between hormones and malignant disease, new therapeutic strategies can be developed for certain tumours.

TECHNIQUES OF MOLECULAR BIOLOGY

Over the last five years some remarkable techniques have been developed which allow a fresh look to be taken at some of the problems outlined above. Their increasing application in many laboratories has resulted in an information explosion, hopefully with far reaching impact.

The Gene

Genetic information in normal and diseased cells is coded by the sequence of nucleotides within the DNA of the cell's nucleus. Genes have two functions. The first is to replicate themselves precisely. The complementary base pairing of adenine–thymine and guanine–cytosine provides the specificity required to produce identical copies of each of the single strands of a segment of DNA. Deoxyribonucleic acid replication is a complex process, requiring the presence of several enzymes and cofactors. The most important of these is DNA polymerase which induces the polymerisation of

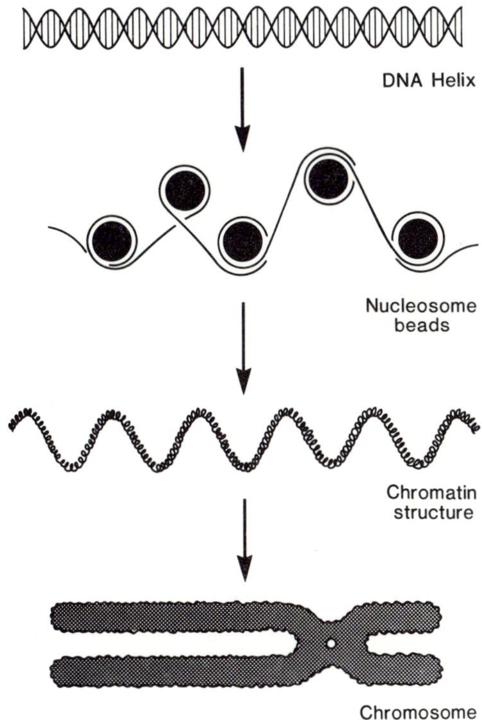

Fig. 1.2. *Chromatin structure demonstrates the remarkable packaging of DNA within chromosomes.*

the deoxyribonucleoside triphosphates. In addition to the synthesis machinery there are also 'proof reading' mechanisms to ensure fidelity of reproduction (Lindahl, 1982). These are vital functions to maintain the stability of the genome. The second function of the gene is to produce messenger RNA (mRNA); a process called transcription. The mRNA, in turn, produces protein by its translocation on ribosomes.

Deoxyribonucleic acid in mammalian cells is arranged in a complex structure, coupled to a set of proteins; these are the histone and non-histone proteins (Fig. 1.2). These proteins structure DNA into packets called nucleosomes which are, in turn, coiled up to form the chromosome (McGhee and Felsenfield, 1980). Most of the DNA in a human cell is not involved in information transfer directly. It has been estimated that there are 3×10^9 base pairs in a human cell's genome, with only 10^6 being transcribed at any one time into functional messenger RNA. Some of the apparently redundant sequences are involved in holding the expressed sequences in the correct position for transcription and its associated control mechanisms. Some sequences may represent genetic junk, acquired through the millenia of evolution and locked in by the continual process of replication. These pieces of DNA may be preserved purely by maintaining a correct sequence for self-preservation — so-called 'selfish DNA' (Orgel and Crick, 1980). There are four techniques vital in elucidating the biology of genes in health and disease: restriction enzyme digestion, gene cloning, DNA sequencing and nucleic acid hybridisation. These techniques are the essential ingredients of the recombinant DNA technology (Abelson and Butz, 1980).

Restriction Enzymes

Many bacteria make enzymes which can cleave DNA at defined sites. Such enzymes recognise specific sequences four to six nucleotides in length and make a cut. These enzymes protect bacteria from phage infection by destroying injected phage DNA which contains the sequences recognised. Over 200 restriction enzymes have now been isolated, and can be used to identify specific sequences in any piece of DNA (Smith, 1979). By using a combination of different restriction enzymes, followed by the separation of the resultant fragments, by electrophoresis on agarose gels, pieces of DNA can be compared (restriction mapping). Simple restriction enzyme digestion followed by electrophoresis, is able to discriminate between DNA from patients with sickle cell anaemia and their normal relatives (Orkin *et al.*, 1982).

Gene Cloning

Fragments of DNA can be amplified by inserting them into a plasmid or bacteriophage vector, and growing such vectors in their bacterial hosts—a

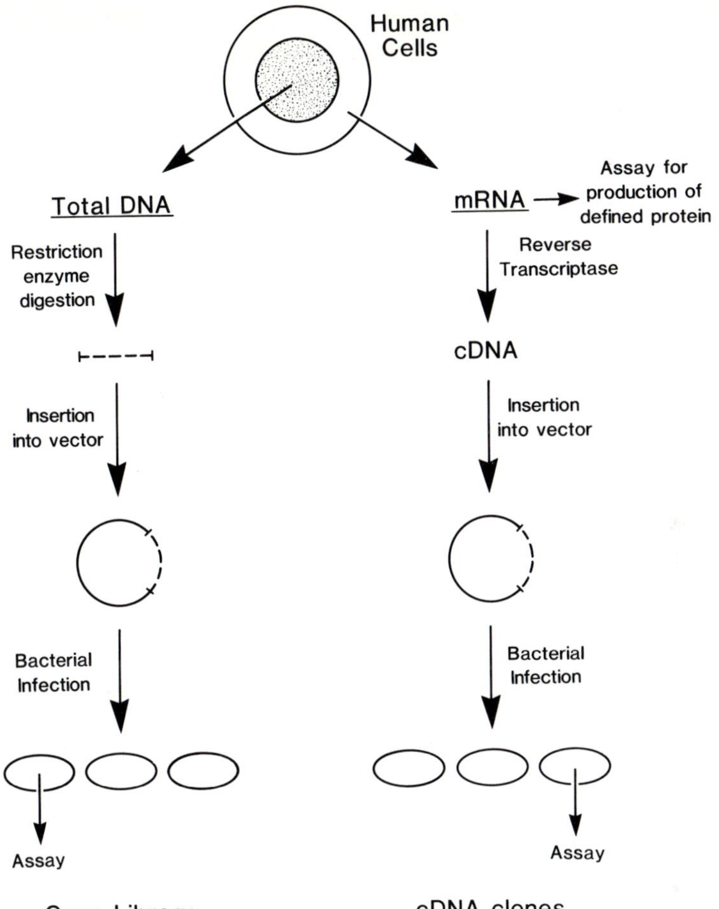

Fig. 1.3. *Gene cloning by preparation of a gene library and by reverse transcription of mRNA for a defined protein.*

process called gene cloning. A variety of tricks are used to increase the chances of obtaining the correct clones. These include the use of antibiotic resistance markers in the vector. A marker for tetracycline resistance within the site for insertion of the piece of DNA to be cloned will allow the recombinant vectors to be identified by their sensitivity to tetracycline. After selection of bacterial clones containing the vector, large amounts of DNA can be collected and isolated by restriction enzymes. A gene library consists of a large number of different clones, isolated by taking restriction fragments of a complex piece of DNA; for example, the entire human genome (Cohen, 1980). If large enough, such libraries will contain all the genes present in the DNA from which they were derived. The problem is how to index them for function. Some, of course, will be those involved in mRNA production; other clones in the library will have control function, and yet others will be genetic junk. An alternative strategy is to begin the cloning process by selecting only those DNA sequences that are transcribed into mRNA. Messenger RNA is extracted by using an affinity column composed of cellulose linked to oligo-deoxythymidine (oligo-dT). The oligo-dT binds to the poly-adenylated chains that mark the end of functional messages. Messenger RNA can be copied using the enzyme reverse transcriptase to produce cDNA ('c' stands for complementary). Single stranded cDNA molecules can be converted into double stranded DNA by DNA polymerase, inserted into vectors, and cloned (Fig. 1.3). Using such techniques the human genes for several protein hormones such as insulin, somatostatin and growth hormone have been cloned (Gilbert and Villa Komaroff, 1980). Furthermore, by modifying the vector so that it can transcribe functional message with its bacterial host, production of its protein can be induced in the bacteria. Genetically engineered human insulin is now made in this way.

DNA Sequencing

The nucleotide sequence of cloned DNA fragments can be determined simply and quickly (Sanger, 1981). There are now some 200 human genes whose complete nucleotide sequence has been determined. The application of minicomputers has become an essential part in the matching of overlapping DNA sequences, obtained by analysing many clones from a single long piece of DNA. One method is shown in Fig. 1.4. It is now easier to sequence the amino acids in a protein by first sequencing its gene and using the genetic code as a dictionary to work back to the protein sequence.

Hybridisation Techniques

Once a purified piece of DNA has been isolated by cloning, the presence of complementary sequences can be detected in any other DNA source using hybridisation techniques. Deoxyribonucleic acid is denatured by heating or increasing the pH. The strands fall apart, but by slowly cooling or bringing the pH back to neutral they renature or hybridise. Under appropriate conditions, hybridisation can be made base pair specific—i.e. adenine combining with thymine; guanine with cytosine. By making a piece of cloned DNA radioactive—using ^{32}P, for example—probes can be obtained which will identify specific sequences in mixtures of restriction fragments separated by electrophoresis. Let us say we have a cloned probe for insulin, produced by making cDNA from mRNA obtained from pancreatic islet cells. If we now take a restriction enzyme digest of total human DNA and run this on an agarose gel the insulin gene will be located in one or more of

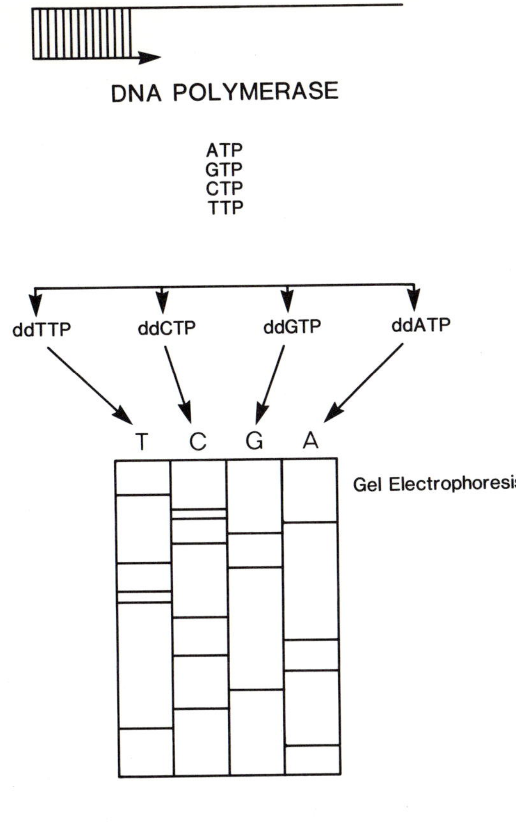

Fig. 1.4. *Deoxyribonucleic acid sequencing using the dideoxynucleotide method. The dideoxynucleotide stops chain elongation at the position of the relevant nucleotide.*

the fragments. By using a nitrocellulose filter we can make a replica of the gel by simple blotting. The blot can be denatured by heating (to make the DNA single stranded). The radioactive probe is now added under renaturing conditions, and after a suitable time any excess probe washed off the filter. The position of the probe, and hence the insulin sequences in the original DNA sample, can be identified by autoradiography (laying a photographic film onto the filter to detect the position of the radioactivity). This technique is often called Southern blotting, after its inventor Ed Southern (Southern, 1975) (Fig. 1.5). Hybridisation can also be carried out to RNA immobilised on filters—Northern blotting (Hood *et al.*, 1975). Specific DNA sequences can be localised within chromosomes using *in situ* hybridisation (Harper *et al.*, 1983). Here, the radioactive probe is added directly to squashed, fixed chromosomes whose DNA has been denatured by exposure to high pH.

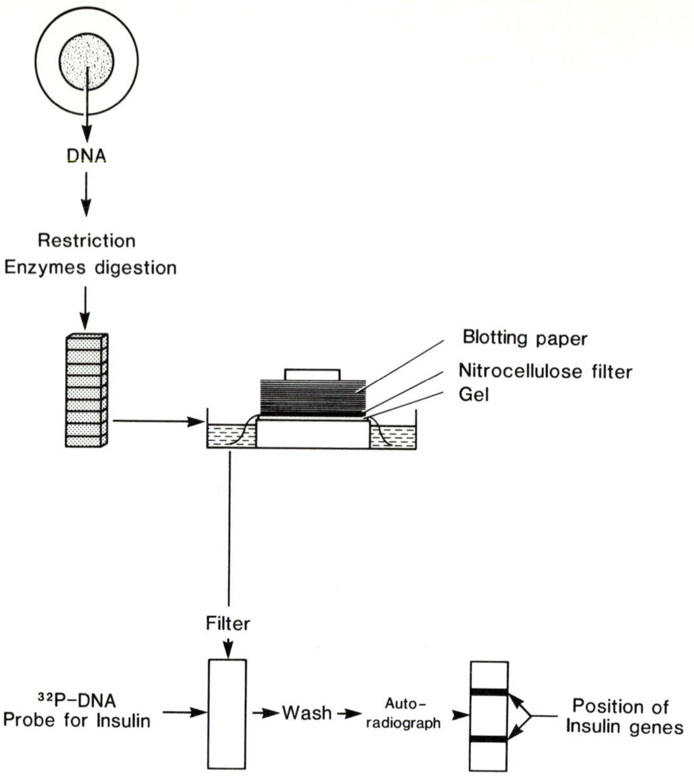

Fig. 1.5. *Detection of insulin genes in restriction enzyme digest of total human DNA using a* ^{32}P *labelled cDNA insulin probe and Southern blot.*

Using this technique, the precise chromosomal location of a number of genes has now been determined.

Messenger RNA

The process of transcription—the production of functional messenger RNA—is a key to understanding the changes that occur when a normal cell becomes malignant. In mammalian cells, three RNA polymerases appear to be involved in the process of transcription. A specific DNA sequence—the promoter—signals where RNA synthesis is to begin, the polymerase then moves along the DNA strand producing RNA in a 5′ to 3′ direction. A further specific DNA sequence provides the termination signal, causing the RNA to be released together with the polymerase enzyme (Rosenberg and Court, 1979). There are many unanswered questions about transcription in eucaryotic cells, mainly due to the complex organisation of DNA within nucleosomes. Furthermore, the primary messenger produced is modified before emerging through the nuclear membrane in several ways. The first modifications occur at either ends of the new message. At the 5′ end a 7-methyl guanosine residue is linked via a triphosphate. This cap will provide a binding site for the ribosomal proteins, enabling the message to be locked into the ribosome (Perry, 1981). At the 3′ end a further enzyme, poly A-polymerase, adds 100–200 residues of adenylic acid. The signal for this polymerase molecule to operate is provided by the short sequence AATAAA found 50–60 nucleotides upstream from the site of adenylation. The primary transcript, modified both at its 5′ and 3′ ends, is now processed. This entails the removal of large chunks of RNA sequence from the centre of the molecule which are not required for protein synthesis (Chambon, 1981). Such RNA splicing uses a series of enzymes and ribonucleoprotein to remove the non-coding, intervening sequences or introns. The existence of a splicing apparatus at first sight seems a wasteful use of a cell's resources. However, its main advantage is genetic flexibility. Changes in the splicing patterns can occur during differentiation allowing several different related proteins to be produced from a single piece of genome (Gruss *et al.*, 1979).

Proteins

The complex machinery of the ribosome translates the sequence encoded in mRNA into the amino acids found in proteins. New techniques have been devised recently with which to characterise the small numbers of diverse proteins found within a cell. These include new electrophoretic techniques such as two-dimensional gels—separating first on the basis of charge and secondly on the basis of molecular size (O'Farrell, 1975). In addition, monoclonal antibodies have provided tools of remarkable specificity to identify these end products of gene expression. Molecular biology now has the methods to look at each stage in the production of a protein and its subsequent post-translational modification by cleavage and glycosylation. We can now examine how this technology can be used to look at the differences between cancer cells and their normal counterparts.

DIFFERENTIATION

One of the remarkable features of a multicellular organism are the differences in structure and function found between cells in different tissues. The reasons for this differentiation must reside in the accumulation of different sets of proteins. Each cell possesses the same DNA content; but in differentiation genes are expressed in varying amounts. Although the control of gene expression is well understood in bacteria, in eucaryotes the co-ordination of the complex series of switches that occur in producing a muscle or brain cell remain a mystery. There are, however, three significant observations that concern the oncologist.

First, a fully differentiated cell nucleus can revert under certain circumstances to its less differentiated ancestor. Perhaps the best example is the insertion of a fully differentiated frog cell nucleus from intestinal epithelial cells into a frog egg whose nucleus has been removed. A normal tadpole will result, indicating that the fully differentiated nucleus possessed all the information required for the production of tissues of all differentiation types (Gurdon, 1968). Other examples include the repair of limbs by invertebrates, and the strange differentiation patterns seen in teratocarcinoma in man. Although certain gene blocks are normally switched on during the process of differentiation, reversion to a less differentiated state is clearly possible.

The second observation is that control of gene expression in eucaryotes is at the level of transcription. The best evidence for this comes from comparing mRNA populations in different tissues, using hybridisation techniques. Totally different populations are found, indicating that differentiation results in the production of different sets of mRNA molecules (Browder, 1980). In cancer, there is a reversion to a more primitive, or less differentiated mRNA pattern.

A third finding of importance is that differentiation results from the planned switching-on of gene blocks by gene regulatory proteins in a co-ordinated manner. The best experimental example of this comes from the homeotic mutations found in Drosophila—the fruit fly (Morata and Lawrence, 1977). Here, certain point mutations can cause a leg to be made, instead of an antenna. This mutation occurs in a major control site, which triggers the set of genes to produce limb proteins instead of antenna proteins. The bizarre differentiation states found in human teratocarcinoma and its benign counterpart, teratoma, are further examples of control in differentiation by combinatorial gene regulation (Mintz and Illmensee, 1975).

CANCER CELLS

Cancer cells differ from their normal counterparts by their ability to grow, divide and invade, without the normal restraining forces operating. In many ways, cancer cells resemble undifferentiated cells, which during normal embryogenesis exhibit similar properties. We can obtain a partial understanding of the reasons behind the changes by applying the techniques outlined above to examine cancer cells.

Cell Surface

The immune system has been used for many years to identify molecules on the surface of tumour cells that differ in quantity from those present on normal cells. Although there is considerable evidence that the immune system is able to recognise tumour cells, the complexity of the interaction has so far precluded detailed analysis. The advent of monoclonal antibodies (MCAs) and lines of cloned T-lymphocytes with defined specificity (Sikora and Smedley, 1982), now allow the immune system to be dissected into its individual components. We can use MCAs to detect circulating tumour markers precisely, and to target radioactive isotopes to tumour cells in patients (Smedley *et al.*, 1983).

Extensive studies are now being pursued to see if drugs, toxins, or high specific activity radionucleides can be coupled to MCAs to effect tumour destruction in patients. The selectivity is supplied by the monoclonal antibody, whilst the drug or toxin provides the killing mechanism. The availability of human MCAs may produce exciting clinical results. Work is also beginning on the use of cloned cytotoxic T-cell lines grown up in large number and given to patients with a variety of tumour types. In this way, the normal immune process occurring within the body can be augmented specifically.

Perhaps more important in the long term is the use of these precise tools to identify differences between tumour cells and normal cells that can be exploited in other ways. By defining molecules in the cell surface using immunological tools, we can then use gene cloning to understand fully the reasons for these differences.

The Cytoskeleton

The behaviour of a cell is determined not only by its surface properties but also by the cytoplasmic network of microfilaments in microtubules that form the cytoskeleton. This cytoskeleton influences a cell's shape, motility, adhesion and division; properties that are known to change with transformation. Cytoskeletal disruption is a common observation in malignant cells, although its cause remains unknown. The construction of human genomic DNA probes for cytoskeletal proteins, such as tropomyosin, provides a starting point to examine the reasons for this disruption (MacLeod and Talbot, 1983). Cloned genes for these proteins can be inserted into transformed cells and the effects of behaviour in the recipient cells studied. Specific cytoskeletal defects in malignant cells can be analysed and mechanisms to reduce these defects determined.

The Genome

Although the cell surface and cytoskeleton are altered in malignancy, the ultimate source of any change during the development of cancer must reside in the genome. Genetic rearrangements can now be studied directly in DNA extracted from biopsy samples of human tumours. Restriction enzymes which cleave DNA at specific sites can map changes occurring within any gene for which a probe is available. Using the hybridisation techniques described above, rearrangements, deletions and additions to the genome in a cancer cell can be determined. Certain segments of DNA have been found to have oncogenic potential in the transfection assay (Weinberg, 1982). In this assay DNA is prepared from human tumour cells, precipitated with calcium phosphate and incubated with a mouse fibroblast cell line. These fibroblasts normally grow as confluent monolayers in a culture. After exposure to oncogene-containing DNA, these cells may exhibit features of malignancy, such as the ability to form clumps of cells and grow in soft agar. Subsequent analysis has shown that in the process of transfection, donor DNA is taken up into the nuclei of the fibroblast cells and incorporated there. By combining the techniques of genetic engineering and the transfection assay, oncogenes from human tumours can now be isolated and characterised (Hamlyn and Sikora, 1983). Oncogenes from several tumour cell lines have been cloned and their nucleotide sequence analysed. Little is known about the products of these cellular oncogenes which must in turn be the triggers for malignancy. If we could find ways to control their function by drugs or other agents, then we might discover novel systems for treating cancer.

CELL COMMUNICATION

So far, we have considered how the information in the gene is converted into the differentiation pattern of a cell. In addition, elaborate communication systems exist to keep different tissues informed of events occurring at distant sites. Such communication systems are clearly essential for the survival of any multicellular organism.

Cell communication occurs at three levels (Fig. 1.6). The first is the gap junction. This is a tightly bonded region occurring in the plasma membranes of two adjacent cells, which permits the transmission of ion fluxes and other cytoplasmic signals (Staehelin and Hull, 1978). This is clearly only important in communication between adjacent cells; for example, in an epithelium lining the small intestine. A second and poorly documented method of communication is by the interaction of molecules attached to the cell surface. When cells bearing such interacting molecules meet, a defined response occurs. Such effects are difficult to investigate experimentally, as the surface bound molecules are in low concentration and difficult to solubilise. Finally, cells communicate by the secretion of chemicals. Specialised neurotransmitters such as acetylcholine are released locally and mediate their effects at concentrations of 10^{-4} M within the enclosed environment of a synaptic junction. Substances such as histamine and prostaglandins also interact locally at relatively high concentration. Finally, there are hormones which on secretion can bring about their actions at great distances from their cell of origin. Such molecules must operate at high dilution in the order of 10^{-8} M. Their chemical nature varies—peptides,

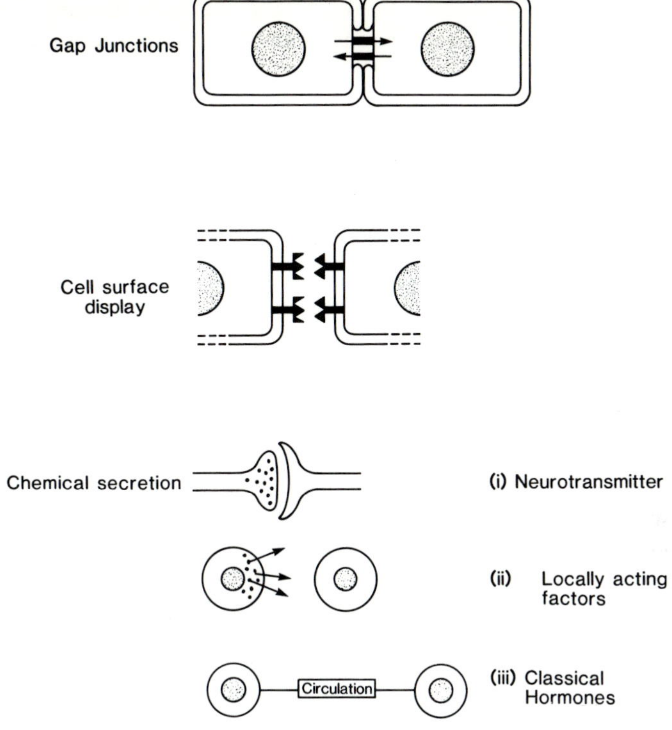

Fig. 1.6. *Cell communication methods.*

proteins, glycoproteins, steroids and modified amino acids all function as hormones binding to receptors with affinity constants of greater than 10^{-8} litre/mole.

Hormone Receptors

Receptors for hormones are present either in the target cell surface in the case of hydrophilic hormones (which are unable to traverse lipid membranes), or within the cytoplasm for the steroid hormones which are lipid soluble (Fig. 1.7). The interaction of a hormone with its receptor initiates a chain of events within the target cell, altering the rate of synthesis of existing proteins and starting the synthesis of new proteins. Cell surface receptors do this by triggering enzyme activation. Examples include the effects of adrenaline on adenylate cyclase, and epidermal growth factor on protein kinase. Alternatively, ion flux into the cell can increase. The entry of calcium into the cell's cytoplasm, with the resultant effects on the calcium binding intracellular protein, calmodulin, causes widespread changes in target cells (Klee *et al.*, 1980).

Lipid-soluble and hence membrane-crossing hormones cause allos-

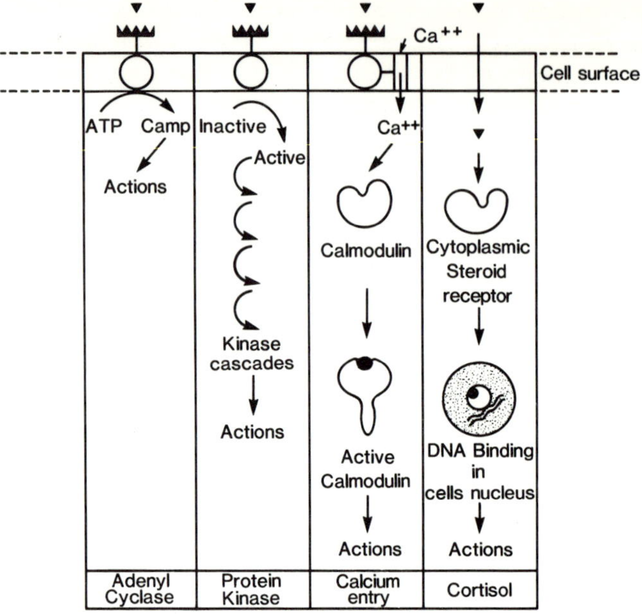

Fig. 1.7. *Hormone receptor mechanisms.*

teric changes in cytoplasmic receptor proteins. The complex of hormone plus its cytoplasmic receptor, binds specifically to defined DNA sequences within the cell so switching on gene blocks. The DNA sequences to which complexes of cortisol and its cytoplasmic receptor can bind specifically have now been isolated and cloned (Payvar *et al.*, 1981).

Hormones, growth control and cancer

Cancer cells, like their normal equivalents, retain methods of communication. In some cases this involves locally acting factors, whilst in others the more familiar endocrine systems operate. As cancer is a disorder of cell growth and communication, it is pertinent to examine the relationship between tumour development and the hormones involved in maintaining the normal cells from which the malignancy was derived. The growth of certain normal tissues is clearly hormonally controlled. Examples include the adrenal cortex and ACTH; the breast and oestrogens; the placenta and progesterones; and erythrocyte precursors and their response to erythropoietin. A variety of disease states exist where abnormal proliferation of cells within an organ occurs in response to the abnormally high secretion of a hormone. This does not, however, result in malignant transformation but rather benign hyperplasia. There are a number of much less well understood hormonal systems which operate at a local level to control the structure of epithelia, neural tissue and probably all cells. These growth factors are peptides which operate by binding to cell surface receptors and activating protein kinases (Carpenter and Cohen, 1979). These enzymes phosphorylate tyrosine, serine and threonine of a variety of intracellular enzymes—a process that stimulates growth. Protein phosphorylation patterns vary during differentiation and may well control the biochemical content of a cell at any given time, and hence its functional properties. Particularly intriguing, is the observation that certain oncogenes code for protein kinases (Groffen *et al.*, 1983). By changing the phosphorylation pattern of proteins in a cell it is possible to confer the properties of malignancy—growth and division with no control by the host.

Hormone receptors and cancer cells

Cancer cells have been shown to possess both surface and intracellular receptors appropriate to their cell of origin. However, these receptors may be lost or modified. It is possible that the new patterns of growth seen in the emergence of a tumour have, as their primary cause, a change in structure of a receptor involved in growth control. For example, if a growth factor receptor becomes modified in a cell in such a way that it becomes locked in the 'on' position—in the conformation normally found after binding to its ligand—then the cell's growth machinery will be in permanent action. Such a change might occur by mutation in a growth factor receptor gene. The consequence of this mutation would be survival advantage for the cell within a tissue and the emergence of a clone of tumour cells. Many investigators are currently looking at such mechanisms as possible initiators of malignancy.

Hormonal effects on cancer cells

Although cancer cells are growing outside the normal control processes of the host many are still responsive to the effects of circulating hormones. The best example is breast cancer. Dramatic regressions of large volumes of metastatic tumour are sometimes seen by changing the endocrine status of the patient. Such changes can be brought about by ablation of endocrine organs—ovaries, adrenals and pituitary—or by the addition of various hormones—oestrogens, anti-oestrogens, progestogens, androgens and corticosteroids. No unifying hypothesis exists to explain the complex interrelationships between the growth of breast cancer cells and their hormonal environment. Although the presence of receptors is necessary if a cancer cell is to respond to hormonal therapy, the methods involved in their detection are relatively crude and are not always predictive. Several tumours may, under certain circumstances, show growth inhibition in the presence of hormones. Lymphomas may respond to corticosteroids alone, especially when of the nodular poorly differentiated type histology—a tumour of B-lymphocytes. About 10% of renal cell adenocarcinomas and cancers of the uterine endometrium will show regression after the administration of a progestogen. As we learn more about individual tissue specific growth factors, more pathways for hormonal intervention will be uncovered.

PRODUCTION OF HORMONES BY CANCER CELLS

Cancer cells produce a variety of communication molecules. Some of these are involved in maintenance of growth of the tumour. We know little about the chemical nature of these locally acting substances. Tissue culture model systems are available to examine the importance of locally produced and acting factors. Malignant cells established in culture grow fastest when surrounded by each other. The growth of a single cell in isolation is often difficult to achieve, requiring stringent tissue culture medium contents. To the clinician it is the production of physiologically active hormones by tumours that is most significant.

1. Tumours derived from hormone-producing tissues

A variety of tumours, both benign and malignant, arise from tissues normally associated with hormone production. The state of differentiation required to produce large amounts of a hormone by such specialised cells is maintained after malignant transformation. A certain proportion of such tumours lose the ability to produce hormones—a feature seen in the more aggressively growing type of endocrine tumour. This loss of hormone production presumably streamlines the cell for rapid growth.

2. Tumours derived from tissues not normally associated with hormone production

Classical endocrinology associates the production of certain hormones to the main glandular structures. However, a variety of endocrine producing cells are scattered throughout the body which may become malignant. Cells of the amine precursor uptake and decarboxylase (APUD) system (Chapter 11) are an example, with their ability to produce a variety of peptide hormones. The distinction between abnormal hormone production by cells normally associated with such products but in an unusual site, e.g. small cell lung cancer, and truly ectopic synthesis by tumours arising from cells not normally involved in hormonal production is often difficult. The molecular mechanisms involved in true ectopic hormone synthesis are fascinating. The derepression of genes coding for hormones is only part of the widespread genetic changes that occur during the evolution of cancer, but one of the easiest to measure. In subsequent chapters the various endocrine syndromes caused by abnormal hormone production by tumours will be considered, the molecular mechanisms involved outlined, and their clinical management discussed.

REFERENCES

Abelson J., Butz E. (1980). Recombinant DNA. *Science*; **209**: 1317–438.

Bluming A.Z. (1982). Treatment of primary breast cancer without mastectomy. *Am. J. Med*; **72**: 820–8.

Browder L. (1980). *Developmental Biology*. Philadelphia: Saunders.

Carpenter G., Cohen S. (1979). Epidermal growth factor. *Ann. Rev. Biochem*; **48**: 193–216.

Chambon P. (1981). Split genes. *Sci. Am*; **244**: 60–71.

Cohen S.N. (1980). The manipulation of genes. *Sci. Am*; **243**: 102–107.

Gilbert W., Villa Komaroff L. (1980). Useful proteins from recombinant bacteria. *Sci. Am*; **242**: 74–94.

Groffen J., Heister Kamp N., Reynolds F.H., Stephenson J.R. (1983). Homology between phosphothyrosine acceptor site of human c-abl and viral oncogene products. *Nature*; **304**: 167–9.

Gruss P., Lai C.J., Dhar R., Khoury G. (1979). Splicing as a requirement for biogenesis of functional 163 mRNA of SV40 virus. *Proc. Natl. Acad. Sci*; **76**: 4317–21.

Gurdon J.B. (1968). Transplanted nuclei and cell differentiation. *Sci. Am*; **219**: 24–35.

Hamlyn P.H., Sikora K. (1983). Oncogenes. *Lancet*; **2**: 326–30.

Harper M.E., Simon M.I., Gallo R.C., Wong-Staal F. (1983). Chromosomal sublocalisation of human c-myb and c-fes cellular onc genes. *Nature*; **304**: 169–71.

Hood L.E., Wilson J.H., Wood W.B. (1975). *Molecular Biology of Eukaryotic Cells*. Meula Park Ca: Benjamin Cummings.

Klee C.B., Crouch T.H., Richman P.G. (1980). Calmodulin. *Ann. Rev. Biochem*; **49**: 489–515.

Lindahl T. (1982). DNA repair enzymes. *Ann. Rev. Biochem*; **51**: 61–88.

MacLeod A.R., Talbot K. (1983). A processed gene defining a gene family encoding a human non-muscle tropomyosin. *J. Mol. Biol*; **167**: 523–37.

McGhee J.D., Felsenfield G. (1980). Nucleosome structure. *Ann. Rev. Biochem*, **49**: 1115–6.

Mintz B., Illmensee K. (1975). Normal genetically mosaic mice produced from malignant teratocarcinoma cells. *Proc. Natl. Acad. Sci*; **72**: 3585–9.

Morata G., Lawrence P.A. (1977). Homeotic genes, compartments and cell determination in drosophila. *Nature*; **265**: 211–16.

O'Farrell P.H. (1975). High resolution, two-dimensional electrophoresis of proteins. *J. Biol. Chem*; **250**: 4007–21.

Orgel L.E., Crick F.H.C. (1980). Selfish DNA: The ultimate parasite. *Nature*; **284**: 604–607.

Orkin S.H., Little P.F., Kazazian H.H., Boehm C.D. (1982). 'Improved detection of the sickle mutation by DNA analysis. *N. Eng. J. Med*; **307**: 32–6.

Payvar F., Wrange O., Okret S., Gustafsson J.A., Yamamoto K.R. (1981). Purified glucocorticoid receptors bind selectively *in vitro* to a cloned DNA fragment whose transcription is regulated by glucocorticoids *in vitro*. *Proc. Natl. Acad. Sci*; **78**: 6628–32.

Perry R.P. (1981). RNA processing comes of age. *J. Cell Biol*; **91**: 28–38.

Powles T.J., Coombes R.C., Smith I.E., Mary Jones J., Ford H.T., Gazet J.C. (1980). Failure of chemotherapy to prolong survival in a group of patients with metastatic breast cancer. *Lancet*; **1**: 580–2.

Report of the Advisory Committee on Cancer Registration (1983). Office of Population Censuses and Surveys: HMSO.

Rosenberg M., Court D. (1979). Regulatory sequences involved in the promotion and termination of RNA transcription. *Ann. Rev. Genet*; **13**: 319–53.

Sanger F. (1981). Determination of nucleotide sequences in DNA. *Science*; **214**: 1205–10.

Sikora K., Smedley H. (1982). Clinical potential of monoclonal antibodies. *Cancer Surveys*; **1**: 521–41.

Smedley H., Finan P., Ritson A., Wraight P., Sikora K. (1983). Localisation of metastatic carcinoma by a radiolabelled monoclonal antibody. *Br. J. Cancer*; **47**: 253–9.

Smith H.O. (1979). Nucleotide sequence specificity of restriction endonucleoses. *Science*; **205**: 455–62.

Southern E.M. (1975). Detection of specific sequences among DNA fragments separated by gel electrophoresis. *J. Mol. Biol*; **98**: 503–17.

Staehelin L.A., Hull B.E. (1978). Junctions between living cells. *Sci. Am*; **238**: 141–52.

Weinberg R.A. (1982). Use of transfection to analyse genetic information and indignant transformation. *Biochem. Biophys. Acta*; **651**: 25–35.

Chapter 2

Martin Gore and Charles Coombes

Endocrine Markers in Cancer

INTRODUCTION

Since the introduction of radioimmunoassays for hormones there has been increasing interest in the possibility of using hormones as tumour markers. Hormone levels can be used diagnostically to follow the success or otherwise of treatment and, if treatment has been initially successful, to diagnose early otherwise occult recurrence. Other potential uses of hormones as markers are listed in Table 2.1. No hormone is 'cancer specific' but, as will be seen, some are able to fulfill at least one of the requirements of a useful tumour marker.

Many problems beset the use of endocrine markers in cancer (Table 2.2), but the major drawback is the variability of the assays used both in specificity and sensitivity. This particularly applies to hormones that are secreted ectopically, since they may be present in a variety of molecular forms (high molecular weight precursors or low molecular weight fragments), and these forms may differ from one another and from the native hormone in both immunoreactivity and bioactivity. Interpretation of the assays is made difficult by the use of unsuitable controls to determine the true upper limit of 'normal', since plasma from ill patients often leads to inhibition of binding of hormone to antibody. This tends to over-estimate

TABLE 2.1

Clinical Application of Hormones as Tumour Markers

---

1. Differential diagnosis of tumours.
2. Monitoring therapy.
3. Localisation of hormone-secreting tumours by venous sampling.
4. Screening 'at risk' populations, particularly those with familial endocrine syndromes.
5. Early detection of recurrence.

TABLE 2.2

Factors Limiting the Value of Hormones as Markers

1. Insensitivity and non-specificity of radioimmunoassay.
2. Heterogeneity of circulating hormones.
3. Pulsatile or intermittent secretion.
4. Rapid degradation of released hormone.
5. Lack of stoichiometric relationship between hormone level and tumour mass.
6. Heterogeneity of cellular constituents of the tumour.

the number of patients who have ectopic hormone-producing tumours. Great care must therefore be taken in evaluating reports of ectopic hormone production without any data on tissue extraction of the hormone and subsequent chromatographic studies.

Further problems are listed in Table 2.2. Secretion of hormones can often be intermittent; frequently the hormone is variably degraded in plasma, giving misleading results. Often, metastatic foci secrete hormones to a different extent within the same patient. Thus, plasma hormone concentrations can fall to within normal limits after excision of a metastatic focus, but this does not necessarily indicate that other occult foci do not exist.

This chapter will deal with the use of both 'eutopic' (appropriate hormone derived from a tumour of an endocrine organ, Table 2.3) and 'ectopic' (hormone production from a tumour originating in an organ that does not normally secrete the hormone) hormones as tumour markers, and their role in clinical management.

TABLE 2.3

'Appropriate' Hormones Used as Markers of Endocrine Tumours

Hormone	*Tumour*
1. Growth hormone	Pituitary chromophobe adenoma
2. Prolactin	Pituitary prolactinoma
3. ACTH	Pituitary basophilic adenoma
4. Human chorionic gonadotrophin	Choriocarcinoma: hydatidiform mole
5. Insulin Gastrin Vasoactive intestinal polypeptide (VIP) Glucagon Somatostatin	Pancreatic tumours
6. Calcitonin	Medullary thyroid carcinoma

MECHANISMS OF HUMORAL SYNDROMES

Although it is possible that transformed cells alter their genetic phenotype and acquire the *de novo* ability to produce hormones, some workers now assert that many of the 'so-called ectopic syndromes' occur in patients with tumours derived from various cellular constituents of normal tissues that usually have the ability to produce these hormones. Such cells may comprise a minority population in the normal tissue, hence their functional properties are difficult to determine by tissue extraction or other techniques. Examples of this are small cell lung cancers secreting calcitonin, and/or adenocortico-trophic hormone (ACTH) that possibly arises from the bronchial Kulchitsky cells. Thus, as radioimmunoassays and immunocytochemical methods become more sensitive so these hormones have been detected in normal tissue extracts. Extensive searches in various tumours previously thought not to have the morphological characteristics of endocrine cells reveal cells with endocrine characteristics often only visible ultrastructurally (Pearse and Polak, 1978).

A classification of ectopic hormone-producing tumours has been suggested by Imura (1980) (Table 2.4). He has grouped the cancer-associated syndromes into three separate categories, the first consisting of tumours that possibly arise from neuroectodermal cells with 'APUD' characteristics (APUD standing for Amine Precursor Uptake and Decarboxylation

TABLE 2.4

A Classification of Ectopic Hormone-producing Tumours and their Clinical Features

Group	Hormones	Tumours	Clinical features
I	ACTH, LPH, α-MSH	Bronchial carcinoma (oat cell)	Hyperadrenocorticism
	CRF	Bronchial carcinoma, carcinoid	Hyperadrenocorticism
	CLIP, β-endorphin	Thymoma, islet cell carcinoma, medullary carcinoma (oat cell)	Hyperpigmentation
	Vasopressin, oxytocin	Bronchial carcinoma (oat cell)	Inappropriate antidiuresis (SIADH)
	Neurophysin		
	GHRH	Bronchial carcinoma, carcinoid	Acromegaly
	Somatostatin	Bronchial carcinoma, medullary carcinoma	Asymptomatic
	Calcitonin	Bronchial carcinoma, carcinoid breast carcinoma	Asymptomatic

contd.

                                    Endocrine Problems in Cancer

TABLE 2.4 (*Contd.*)

Group	Hormones	Tumours	Clinical features
	Gastrin	Ovarian tumour, bronchial carcinoma	Peptic ulceration
	Vasoactive intestinal polypeptide	Bronchial carcinoma	Watery diarrhoea
	Insulin	Pancreatic carcinoma, carcinoid	Asymptomatic
	Glucagon	Bronchial carcinoma, carcinoid	Asymptomatic
II a)	PTH	Renal carcinoma, hepatoma, bronchial carcinoma	Hypercalcaemia
b)	GH	Bronchial carcinoma, gastric carcinoma	Osteoarthropathy
	Prolactin	Bronchial carcinoma, renal carcinoma	Gynaecomastia
c)	HCG	Bronchial carcinoma, hepatoma	Gynaecomastia, precocious puberty
	HCS	Bronchial carcinoma, hepatoma	Gynaecomastia
III	Erythropoietin	Hepatoma	Erythrocytosis
	Cerebrospinal fluid	Bronchial carcinoma, melanoma	Granulocytosis
	Non-suppressible insulin-like activity (NSILA)	Mesothelial tumours, hepatoma	Hypoglycaemia

(Pearse, 1968)). Tumours falling into this category include oat cell, islet cell, medullary thyroid and thymic carcinomas, and carcinoid tumours. The second group, usually tumours of mesodermal and endodermal origin, are associated with hypercalcaemia, ectopic production of growth hormone (GH) or human chorionic gonadotrophin (HCG); none of these hormones fit into the APUD theory. The third category consists of other tumours associated with humoral syndromes but for which mediators have yet to be characterised.

The incidence of ectopic hormone production is difficult to gauge, but one review (Bondy, 1981) disclosed that in an unselected series of patients with lung cancer 50% had either evidence of ectopic ACTH, calcitonin or HCG production. This is almost certainly not the case for other endocrine tumours such as breast cancer, but it gives some idea of the frequency within a single cancer.

Human Chorionic Gonadotrophin (HCG)

Human chorionic gonadotrophin is a hormone of approximately 45 000 daltons secreted by the syncytiotrophoblast of the normal placenta. It shares an alpha subunit in common with the gonadotrophin- and thyroid-stimulating hormones; the beta subunit is, however, specific to HCG. Tumour extracts of patients with 'endocrine' HCG-secreting tumours often contain a large molecular weight species of α-HCG in addition to β-HCG and the whole HCG molecule.

The use of HCG in gestational trophoblastic disease (GTD)

During normal pregnancy, HCG levels peak at approximately 60 days and reach a nadir at 18 weeks. During the first hundred days of pregnancy there is a wide range however, but after this time a serum HCG greater than 200 iu/ml is suggestive of molar pregnancy (Braunstein, 1979).

The initial plasma HCG has prognostic value; thus β-HCG levels greater than 70 iu/ml indicate a poor prognosis (Hertz *et al.*, 1961). In addition, the presence of excessive cerebrospinal fluid HCG indicates cerebral metastases and is also a prognostic indicator (Hammond *et al.*, 1973). Changes in serum HCG parallel the clinical course of GTD and a stoichiometric relationship exists between the HCG titre and tumour burden (Bagshawe, 1969).

Human chorionic gonadotrophin measurements should be continued indefinitely—initially at two-monthly intervals after complete clinical remission and subsequently every six months.

A further application is following evacuation of a molar pregnancy. Human chorionic gonadotrophin levels will fall for up to 40 weeks and the consensus appears to be that if the blood level continues to fall, no therapy is required.

Testicular tumours

Serum HCG is elevated in approximately one-third of patients with testicular teratomas at presentation (Raghavan *et al.*, 1979). Furthermore, occasionally, some patients previously diagnosed as having a seminoma can have high levels of HCG. Immunohistochemical studies of tissue sections of these patients' tumours often reveal HCG-containing cells. Human chorionic gonadotrophin measurements should be combined with AFP estimations, since 60% of patients have high AFP levels (Kohn *et al.*, 1976).

Serial HCG measurement can be used to monitor therapy but discordance is occasionally seen. Thus, recurrence of metastatic disease sometimes occurs without a concomitant rise in HCG. Clearly in these cases chemo-therapy appears to be effective in preferentially eradicating the HCG-secreting cells or inhibiting HCG synthesis. As with choriocarcinoma, the patients with high HCG appear to have a poor prognosis (Gerha-Lluch *et al.*, 1980).

Pituitary Hormones

The differential diagnosis of Cushing's syndrome is considerably facilitated by the radioimmunoassay for ACTH. It is estimated that 50–80% of patients with Cushing's syndrome have a pituitary-dependent tumour. Generally in these patients, the ACTH levels are lower than those with 'ectopic ACTH' production, and ACTH levels do not suppress with low-dose dexamethasone, but many do so with high doses. Adrenocorticotrophic hormone levels in patients with the ectopic syndrome do not suppress, even with high-dose dexamethasone. Basal ACTH levels in these cases often remain normal yet inappropriately elevated for the high serum cortisol. In contrast, 65% of patients with ectopic ACTH syndrome have values exceeding 200 ng/litre (Rees, 1977).

Adrenocorticotrophin

Yalow and Berson (1971) first discovered that tumours associated with Cushing's syndrome contained large amounts of ACTH with a molecular weight higher than 'normal' pituitary-derived ACTH. They subsequently found that such material could be trypsinised to yield normal molecular weight ACTH (Gerwirtz *et al.*, 1974).

To study the tumour-produced molecule further, tumour messenger RNA (mRNA) coding for this product has recently been obtained by Tsukada *et al.* (1981). Ribonucleic acid was isolated from a human ACTH-secreting thymic carcinoid as well as from a human pituitary and hybridised with a ^{32}P-labelled DNA complementary probe to the bovine ACTH precursor mRNA. The RNA from the tumour showed two hybridisation positive bands, whereas a single band was observed from the pituitary RNA. Both these forms of RNA were translated in the reticulocyte lysate cell-free protein synthesising system and the translation product appeared to contain both the ACTH and β-lipotropin precursors.

Lowry *et al.* (1976) purified ectopic ACTH from a malignant thymic carcinoid and showed that such ectopic ACTH lacked one amino acid at the N- and C-terminus, respectively. This could be explained by an abnormal endopeptidase being present and does not necessarily imply an abnormality in structure.

ACTH as a marker

Cushing's syndrome should always be considered in the patient who has cancer with hypertension, hypokalaemia, and mental disturbance. Differentiation from pituitary-dependent Cushing's syndrome, as mentioned above, is facilitated by the dexamethasone suppression test and the serum ACTH level. Using a conventional radioimmunoassay for ACTH, 53% of patients with lung cancer have been found to have raised plasma levels (Yalow *et al.*, 1977). In this latter study those with extensive disease showed elevated levels (57 out of 107 cases) more frequently than those in whom the disease was limited, i.e. disease confined to one hemithorax (11 out of 29 with elevated levels). Patients with adenocarcinoma of the bronchus showed lower ACTH values than those with other histological types of lung cancer.

The ACTH assay is of little value in mass screening, since a false elevation can occur in the absence of carcinoma. This can be reduced by sampling in the afternoon or by using the dexamethasone suppression test, as described above. However, many patients who are prone to develop lung cancer have chronic obstructive airways disease and this may itself result in an elavated plasma ACTH.

Concerning the value of ACTH in the post-diagnostic follow-up period, Yalow *et al.* (1979) have measured this hormone in a group of 50 patients pre-operatively, 19 of whom had ACTH levels greater than 300 ng/ml. Eleven out of nineteen showed significant decreases three months after surgery, but there are limitations to the use of ACTH as a monitor. Yalow *et al.* (1979) suggested that, in patients with lung cancer, much of the raised plasma ACTH is not derived from the tumour. Such elevations could be of pituitary origin or be derived from areas of bronchial squamous metaplasia. Accordingly, in some patients falls in ACTH levels may not indicate a response to treatment. Occasionally, as in the study by Jolivet *et al.* (1980), ACTH levels do not parallel disease activity. In this report a patient with Cushing's syndrome secondary to metastatic medullary carcinoma of the thyroid was studied. Cortisol levels were originally markedly elevated but returned to normal after total thyroidectomy. However, the cortisol level again rose with lymph node recurrence. Chemotherapy reduced these nodes to normal but the patient then developed further lymph node metastases in the absence of a further ACTH rise. Biopsy showed very few ACTH-containing cells in the tumour, implying that chemotherapy may have selectively killed the ACTH-producing components.

Selective venous catheterisation can help in differentiating between pituitary dependent and ectopic Cushing's syndrome, since occasionally both pituitary microadenomas and ectopic ACTH secreting tumours can be radiologically occult. Obviously this is important because specific therapy can now be directed against pituitary microadenomas. This approach can also assist in patients with recurrent symptoms but no overt tumour mass. However, with the advent of computerised axial tomography (CAT), selective venous catheterisation and sampling is seldom necessary now.

Tumours associated with Cushing's syndrome

Small cell lung cancer is the tumour most commonly associated, accounting for 60% of cases. The survival rates in small cell carcinoma of the lung do not seem to be related to increased plasma ACTH concentration (Abeloff *et al.*, 1981). Adrenocorticotrophic hormone secretion is common in other histological types of lung cancer; Yalow and co-workers (1979) found that 50% of patients with epidermoid carcinoma and 25% of those with adenocarcinoma also had raised ACTH levels, but as yet it is not known if this has any prognostic significance in patients with these tumours. It is important to note that elevated plasma ACTH levels have been found in one-third of patients with chronic obstructive airways disease but without any evidence of proven carcinoma (Aijazian *et al.*, 1975). The percentage of patients with carcinoma of the lung, of any histological type, that have demonstrable ACTH in their tissue is always much higher than the percentage of patients that have free ACTH in their plasma.

Other tumours have also been associated with ectopic ACTH secretion. Thymic and pancreatic tumours are associated with ectopic ACTH secretion in 10–12% of cases, and bronchial carcinoids in 4%. The remaining patients have either rare endocrine tumours, such as medullary carcinoma of the thyroid, or other solid tumours such as adenocarcinoma of the colon, prostate, kidney, ovary or uterus.

There has recently been some interest in β-lipotropin (β-LPH), because ACTH and β-LPH are synthesised in equimolar amounts. Beta-LPH is more stable than ACTH and therefore an essay for LPH might be regarded as an alternative to an ACTH assay. However, some workers have found that the molar ratio of LPH : ACTH had diagnostic significance, as patients with lung tumours that secrete ACTH have higher ratios than those with ACTH-secreting pituitary adenomas (Gray and Ratcliffe, 1979). However, high ratios are also found in other diseases and ratios reported by different laboratories are not consistent.

Prolactin

Prolactin adenomas

The major role of the radioimmunoassay for prolactin is in the diagnosis of pituitary prolactinomas. Prolactin levels in excess of 100 μg/litre (normal up to 15 μg/litre) almost always indicate the presence of a tumour. Levels from 15–100 μg/litre may also be indicative of a prolactinoma, but are often caused by drugs or other disorders that interfere with normal hypothalamic inhibition of prolactin secretion.

Unfortunately, neither suppressive nor stimulatory tests are able to differentiate between the different causes of hyperprolactinaemia. Although it was initially thought that bromocriptine may selectively suppress prolactin in patients with prolactinomas, this has subsequently been shown to be false. Similarly, both chlorpromazine and thyroid releasing hormone (TRH) increase prolactin secretion irrespective of the cause of hyper-prolactinaemia.

Serum prolactin can be used to evaluate ablative therapy of prolactin-secreting microadenomas. A rapid decline follows hypophysectomy but falls more slowly after radiation therapy. The number of patients developing pituitary recurrence is small following appropriate therapy, and it is not yet known whether a prolactin rise will antedate clinical recurrence.

Ectopic prolactin secretion

Patients with bronchogenic carcinoma sometimes have raised prolactin levels and this may be an indication of spread to the thoracic wall, since stimulation of the fourth, fifth and sixth intercostal nerves is known to release prolactin from the pituitary (Davis *et al.*, 1979).

Calcium-regulating Hormones

Use of the calcitonin radioimmunoassay in medullary thyroid carcinoma

Calcitonin is the hormone secreted by the C-cells (or parafollicular cells) of the thyroid gland. Medullary thyroid carcinoma originates from these cells and constitutes approximately 5–8% of surgically treated thyroid cancer.

Medullary thyroid carcinoma is either familial or sporadic. The former is often bilateral and multicentric and associated with phaeochromocytoma and parathyroid hyperplasia (multiple endocrine neoplastia type 2). Patients with this syndrome can have an abnormal phenotype characterised by a Marfanoid habitus, multiple mucosal neuroma and a more aggressive form of thyroid carcinoma.

The familial type is inherited with an autosomal dominant pattern of transmission. Since calcitonin secretion in the familial form is intermittent, basal levels are often within the normal range (Sizemore *et al.*, 1977), necessitating the use of a stimulation test to provoke secretion. These are either the pentagastrin test, in which 0·5 μg/kg of pentagastrin is injected over 5 seconds and samples taken over the ensuing 10 minutes (Hennessy *et al.*, 1974), or the calcium infusion test in which 2–4 μg/kg is given over 5 minutes. However, this latter method of stimulation only induces a minor degree of calcitonin secretion. The sporadic form is associated with hypercalcitoninaemia in more than 90% of cases (Deftos *et al.*, 1971).

It is important to confirm calcitonin levels outside the range 0·1–1 µg/litre, as often patients have been submitted to surgery with levels within this range and no tumour or even hyperplasia has been found.

It seems likely, however, that early operation of patients with the familial form of the disease who have hypercalcitoninaemia is important. Surgery in patients less than 10 years of age certainly seems to reduce recurrence rate. Serial measurements of calcitonin can be used following surgery to predict recurrence and often calcitonin levels rise in the absence of clinically-obvious disease, and in these cases selective venous catheterisation is needed to localise the metastasis.

Ectopic secretion of calcitonin

Hypercalcitoninaemia has been found to be associated with a variety of carcinomas—but there is no clear agreement how frequently this occurs. Different laboratories, using various reagents, seem to agree on the following points:

   a)   Carcinoma of endocrine origin, such as carcinoid tumours, have a high incidence of ectopic calcitonin production.
   b)   Lung carcinomas are capable of releasing calcitonin, and patients have high calcitonin levels irrespective of histological type (Coombes *et al.*, 1974; Ellison *et al.*, 1975). The incidence varies with radioim-munoassay and with the stage of the patient, but 10–70% have high levels.
   c)   The form of calcitonin released is heterogeneous and often the high molecular-weight material predominates (Coombes *et al.*, 1975; Becker *et al.*, 1978).

There is also no doubt that hypercalcitoninaemia occurs in association with other carcinomas such as breast carcinoma, but the origin of the hormone remains disputed. The frequency of skeletal metastases in these patients complicates the issue, since disturbances of calcium homeostasis could induce hypercalcitoninaemia.

In lung cancer, it has been suggested that there is a correlation between the fall of calcitonin and the result of systemic treatment (Silva *et al.*, 1973).

Parathyroid Hormone (PTH) and Hypercalcaemia

Incidence

Hypercalcaemia is a common accompaniment of malignant disease; in one recent series it accounted for 89 out of 166 cases of hypercalcaemia (Frisken *et al.*, 1981). The tumours most often associated with hypercalcaemia in this series were carcinoma of the bronchus (24 patients), breast (20 patients), renal (6 patients) and myeloma (7 patients). The remaining 32 patients had a variety of different tumours. There are two distinct types of hypercalcaemia in cancer patients: the first is exemplified in the patient with no evidence of bone metastases and who becomes normocalcaemic after removal of the primary tumour. The second type is when the patient has skeletal metastases and the hypercalcaemia is simply due to bone destruction. These patients have a normal or slightly elevated calcium accretion rate, low intestinal calcium absorption and an increased bone resorption rate (Coombes *et al.*, 1976*a*).

Markers in hypercalcaemia

Candidates for mediators of cancer-associated hypercalcaemia included osteolytic sterols, parathyroid hormone-like materials, prostaglandins and osteoclast-activating factor, but none of these materials have been conclusively shown to be responsible and none of them are consistently elevated in patients with hypercalcaemia.

Concerning the evidence for parathyroid hormones (PTH) as a mediator, the initial studies by Sherwood *et al.* (1967) using a bioassay for parathyroid hormone were followed by those of Benson *et al.* (1974) using a radioimmunoassay. These workers found inappropriately high levels of parathyroid hormone in many patients with cancer-associated hypercalcaemia and were able to find parathyroid hormone-like activity in tumour extracts. However, chromatography failed to show any material that was convincingly related to parathyroid hormone. Goltzman *et al.* (1981) developed a cytochemical assay for parathyroid hormone and assayed the serum of 33 patients with various malignancies. They found that, of 16 hypercalcaemic patients with elevated cyclic AMP secretion, ten had high cytochemical bioactivity. Nonetheless, the plasma bioactivity eluted on gel chromatography before the standard 1–84 amino acid parathyroid hormone, in contrast to the plasma of patients with primary hyperparathyroidism. Furthermore, prior incubation with parathyroid hormone antiserum only partially reduced the activity. These workers have postulated that there is a parathyroid hormone-like factor responsible for the high nephrogenous cyclic AMP observed in some patients with squamous lung and renal carcinomas, some of whom do not have bone metastases. No sequential studies have been carried out to indicate the value of this as a marker.

Powell *et al.* (1973) failed to find parathyroid hormone in the serum of patients nor did he find parathyroid hormone in the tumour extracts. However, prostaglandin metabolites were raised in the urine of some of these patients indicating a possible role for a prostaglandin-like factor. Although in some of these patients calcium fell to normal after prostaglandin synthesis inhibitors were administered, other workers have not been able to confirm this finding (Coombes *et al.*, 1976*b*).

The other major candidate for a tumour-produced osteolysin is the material described by Raisz's group. They initially found a material capable of causing osteolysis in phytohaemagglutinin-stimulated human peripheral blood leucocytes. Application of this material to bone resulted in the appearance of a large number of osteoclasts (Horton *et al.*, 1972), and it was thus termed 'osteoclast-activating factor' (OAF). Subsequently, these workers observed a similar activity in association with cell lines derived from six patients with Burkitt's lymphoma and myeloma, but the controls for these experiments were limited to acute leukaemic cells, normal lymphocytes, and HeLa cells. Molecular-sieve chromatography demonstrated a poorly-defined material existing over a wide range of molecular weights (Mundy *et al.*, 1974). However, no good data exist to indicate the clinical value of the measurement of OAF.

Differential diagnosis from primary hyperparathyroidism

Levels of PTH in hypercalcaemic patients with malignant disease tend to be lower than the levels in patients with primary hyperparathyroidism (Riggs *et al.*, 1971). There are now assays using human PTH and anti-human PTH, in contrast to previous assays based on bovine reagents which seem to have had a much lower detection rate of elevated PTH levels. Thus, in one study, 100% of patients with primary hyperparathyroidism were found to have elevated PTH levels when the human assay was used, whereas only 57% of patients had elevated levels using the bovine material (Papapoulos *et al.*, 1980).

A further possible aid in the differential diagnosis of primary hyperparathyroidism and cancer is to relate the serum immunoreactive parathyroid hormone to the serum calcium. Plasma parathyroid hormone is elevated in 80–90% of patients with primary hyperparathyroidism, but for a given serum calcium PTH is much higher than in the cases of cancer-associated hypercalcaemia, in whom the elevation is often slight and of doubtful significance (Coombes *et al.*, 1976*a*).

Antidiuretic Hormone (ADH)

Schwartz *et al.* (1957) described this syndrome in two patients who were found to have carcinoma of the lung, and hyponatraemia. Since this time it has become increasingly recognised as a cause of significant morbidity in patients with lung cancer. There are many causes of the syndrome of inappropriate secretion of ADH, and several tumours have been associated with raised ADH levels in their plasma (lung, pancreas, thymus, lymphosarcoma and bronchial carcinoid).

Nature of ectopic ADH

Concerning the nature of tumour-associated ADH, chromatographic studies have shown that the majority of tumours contain both vasopressin and 'nicotine-stimulated' neurophysin (NSN), the natural carrier protein for the neurohypophyseal hormones. A small amount of oxytocin is also detected in some tissues. On Sephadex G50 gel filtration the majority of immunoreactive NSN emerges at a molecular size of 10 000 daltons, and this is similar to the NSN extracted from human pituitary glands. In some tumour extracts a material with a molecular weight of 20 000 was discovered after exposure to dissociating agents and this may well be a common precursor to vasopressin and neurophysin (Yamaji *et al.*, 1981). Pentengill *et al.* (1977) have found that in one cell line, established from an anaplastic lung carcinoma, vasopressin was present in the cells and secreted into the culture medium but neither neurophysin nor oxytocin could be found. All this may be of greater relevance than is immediately apparent, since the specific neurophysin that is associated with vasopressin also rises after cigarette smoking, and vasopressin is known to be a promoter of carcinogenesis.

Value as a marker

An important factor to bear in mind when considering patients exhibiting the inappropriate ADH syndrome and cancer is that it is commonly caused by lung or brain metastases rather than ectopic production of ADH *per se*. Furthermore, interpretation of results is complicated by the fact that ADH is commonly degraded in the lungs and that patients with diseased lungs therefore, are more likely to have high plasma ADH levels. The syndrome can also be precipitated by treatment with vincristine and vinblastine or high-dose cyclophosphamide.

Gilby *et al.* (1976) showed that 34 out of 49 (69%) unselected patients with small cell carcinoma had abnormal water load tests. In 17 out of 49 cases, the syndrome of inappropriate ADH secretion (SIADH) was confirmed by observing raised plasma ADH with hypotonic plasma and concentrated urine. In the remaining 17 patients, the abnormal water load test was thought to be due to factors other than the ectopic secretion of ADH.

A radioimmunoassay has been developed to measure the neurophysin binding protein (Hamilton *et al.*, 1972). Extracts of tumours from patients with SIADH showed activity. North *et al.* (1980) employed a radioimmunoassay for ADH-associated neurophysins and found elevated plasma levels in 11 of 26 patients (42%). They followed six patients during the course of therapy and in five the level of ADH mirrored the clinical picture.

Gastrointestinal Hormones

Gastrin

A number of cases of gastrinoma have been detected by screening patients with peptic ulceration. Thus, of 709 patients referred for gastric secretory testing at the Mayo Clinic, 31 (2·9%) were found to have a gastrinoma (Malagelada *et al.*, 1982).

Diagnosis is difficult, because serum gastrin is often elevated ($>$ 0·3 µg/litre) in patients with duodenal or gastric ulceration due to other cases. In the Mayo Clinic study, for example, 93% of patients with a gastrinoma had a raised basal gastrin, but so did 10% of patients with new or recurrent peptic ulceration and 20% of those with functional symptoms.

The gastric acid output, both 'basal' and secretin or histamine stimulated, has also been examined and there is a suggestion that this can help in diagnosis (Modlin *et al.*, 1982).

Other causes of high serum gastrin levels such as pernicious anaemia, atrophic gastritis, short bowel syndrome, renal insufficiency and retained gastric antrum syndrome, are easy to distinguish from Zollinger–Ellison syndrome on clinical grounds. Antral G-cell hyperplasia may be distinguished from Zollinger–Ellison syndrome as there is a decrease in the gastrin level after secretin stimulation as opposed to the increase that is seen in gastrinomas. Others have suggested that gastrin may be a marker of the extent of disease, in that patients with a gastrin level greater than 1·5 µg/litre have lymph node involvement, whereas in those with a level greater than 8 µg/litre extensive liver metastases are likely (Marshall *et al.*, 1980).

Five- and ten-year survival rates are at 42% and 30%, respectively. Early diagnosis of gastrinoma, however, is extremely important, as a large percentage of the patients may die prematurely from the complications of peptic ulceration which can be prevented by adequate treatment. In the familial form of gastrinoma, which is associated with hyperparathyroidism, the diagnosis is particularly important, as a raised calcium may stimulate the growth of the tumour (Betts *et al.*, 1980).

Insulin

In the individual patient with a suspected insulin-secreting islet cell tumour, plasma insulin measurements are invaluable since elevated insulin levels indicate the presence of an insulinoma. Fasting blood sugar measurements are insufficient to make a diagnosis of insulinoma *per se*, but if the immunoreactive insulin : blood sugar ratio is measured after a 19 hour fast, then 100% of patients with insulinomas have an abnormal ratio (normal, 0·3) (Fajans and Floyd, 1979). A further diagnostic test is the proportion of pro-insulin to total immunoreactive insulin since pro-insulin is found only in small amounts in normal ($< 22\%$ of total immunoreactive insulin). Insulinomas, however, secrete excessive amounts of pro-insulin and in this situation it constitutes greater than 25% of total immunoreactive insulin in 85% of patients.

An important application of the insulin radioimmunoassay is venous sampling in the localisation of occult insulinomas. In contrast to the more aggressively metastatic gastrinomas or glucagonomas, insulinomas are often benign and are occasionally impalpable. To avoid total pancreatectomy, multiple plasma samples can be taken to indicate whether a proximal or distal pancreatectomy should be carried out.

Hypoglycaemia due to other causes

Despite occasional reports demonstrating increased insulin-like activity, evidence for ectopic insulin synthesis is lacking in most cases of non-pancreatic tumours (Skrabanek and Powell, 1978). Sarcomas are the commonest non-pancreatic tumours associated with hypoglycaemia, though other tumours such as hepatoma, adrenocortical and gastrointestinal carcinoma have also been shown to be associated with this phenomenon.

There are other factors that can lower blood sugar. Two decades ago, it was found that only 10% of serum insulin-like activity could be neutralised by anti-insulin antibodies. It was, therefore, termed non-suppressible insulin-like activity (NSILA). Subsequent studies have shown that this consists of at least six separate materials: insulin-like growth factors 1 and 2, somatomedin A, B and C, and 'multiplication-stimulating activity' (MSA). These are collectively termed the somatomedins and originate from the liver. Some are controlled by growth hormone, have molecular weights ranging from 7400–7700 daltons and have several amino acids in common with human pro-insulin. Most of these factors circulate bound to high molecular-weight proteins.

Megyesi and her co-workers (1974), using a radioreceptor assay, demonstrated increased non-suppressible insulin-like levels in 3 out of 7 patients with non-islet cell tumours. They have now extended this series and 40% have elevated NSILA levels. A fall in the NSILA levels to normal occurs after anti-tumour treatment in some patients.

No study has yet demonstrated an arterio-venous tumour gradient of NSILA, although elevated levels have been found in tumour extracts.

Other possible causes of hypoglycaemia, including over-utilisation of glucose by the tumours themselves, have been postulated. However, most measurements of glucose utilisation by tumours have not substantiated this claim. Destruction of the liver by metastases occasionally may result in hypoglycaemia. The authors have recently seen a patient with liver metastases due to breast cancer who became comatose due to hypoglycaemia.

Vasoactive intestinal peptide (VIP)

Vasoactive intestinal peptide is secreted primarily from the pancreas. The Verner–Morrison syndrome, i.e. watery diarrhoea, hypokalaemia, and raised plasma VIP levels, is usually associated with pancreatic lesions. Nearly half these tumours are malignant (Modlin and Bloom, 1978). Elevated VIP levels have also been found in association with phaeochromocytomas (Bloom, 1978). The value of VIP measurements is not confined to diagnosis since it can be used to monitor therapy. Vasoactive intestinal peptide levels have been found to fall within 10 minutes of successful surgery for VIPoma (Hoile *et al.*, 1979).

Glucagon

Glucagonomas are rare tumours arising from the α-cells of the pancreas. They cause a complicated clinical picture which usually includes diabetes, skin rashes, stomatitis and nail changes, and may be accompanied by anaemia, weight loss and a variety of gastrointestinal symptoms.

Glucagon is a good tumour marker in that although it is elevated in various conditions such as pancreatitis, cirrhosis, trauma, infection, and malabsorption, levels greater than $0.5\,\mu g$/litre are virtually diagnostic of a glucagon-secreting tumour. In this situation, glucagon is usually monomeric with a molecular weight of 3500 daltons. In some tumour-free relatives of patients with glucagonoma, hyperglucagonaemia is found. However, the hormone circulates as 'big glucagon' (molecular weight, 30 000 daltons) or 'proglucagon' (molecular weight, 9000 daltons).

A recent literature review (Stacpole, 1981) has revealed that most glucagonomas are already widespread at the time of diagnosis, and although treatment is rarely successful, a decrease in plasma glucagon level probably indicates a response to treatment.

Somatostatin

The nature of somatostatin has recently been investigated by Penman *et al.* (1980). Three patients, one with a thymic tumour and two with lung carcinomas, had lesions which contained large amounts of somatostatin and ACTH. Gel filtration chromatography showed the two lung tumour extracts contained predominantly somatostatin monomer (1600 daltons), while the thymic tumour contained a 3000–3500 daltons form, 77% of which was not converted to the 1600 somatostatin with reducing agents.

Plasma from these patients contained both the 1600 and 3000–3500 daltons somatostatins. It may be, therefore, that human tumours are capable of secreting a pro-somatostatin.

CONCLUSION

There is an undoubted use for endocrine markers in certain rare tumours, particularly HCG in choriocarcinoma and teratoma of the testis, and calcitonin measurements are essential in patients with medullary thyroid carcinoma and their relatives.

Patients with symptoms suggestive of the syndromes detailed above should be screened for the relevant ectopic hormone. However, these syndromes are rare and because of this the use of hormone measurements in monitoring therapy has not yet been elucidated.

REFERENCES

Abeloff M.D., Trump D.L., Baylin S.B. (1981). Ectopic adrenocorticotrophic (ACTH) syndrome and small cell carcinoma of the lung—Assessment of clinical implications in patient on combination chemotherapy. *Cancer*; **48**: 1082–7.

Aijazian L.F., Schneider B., Gewirtz G., Yalow R.S. (1975). Ectopic production of big ACTH in carcinoma of the lung: Its clinical usefulness as a biological marker. *Am. Rev. Respir. Dis*; **3**: 279–81.

Bagshawe K.D. Choriocarcinoma. (1969). *The Clinical Biology of the Trophoblast and its Tumours*. Baltimore: Williams & Williams.

Becker K.L., Snider R.H., Silva O.L., Moore, C.F. (1978). Calcitonin heterogeneity in lung cancer and medullary thyorid cancer. *Acta Endocrinol*; **87**: 88–99.

Benson R.C., Riggs B.L., Pickard B.M., Arnaud, C.D. (1974). Immunoreactive forms of circulating parathyroid hormone in primary and ectopic hyperparathyroidism. *J. Clin. Invest*; **54**: 175.

Betts J.B., O'Malley B.P., Rosenthal F.D. (1980). Hyperparathyroidism: A prerequisite for Zollinger–Ellison syndrome in multiple endocrine adenomatosis Type 1—Report of a further family and a review of the literature. *Quart. J. Med*; **49**: 69.

Bloom S.R. (1978). Vasoactive intestinal peptide, the major mediator of the WDHA (pancreatic cholera) syndrome: Value of measurement in diagnosis and treatment. *Amer. J. Digest. Dis*; **23**: 373.

Bloom S.R., Polak J.M. (1980). Glucagonomas, vipomas and somatostatinomas. *Clin. Endocrinol. Metab*; **9**: 285–99.

Bondy P.K. (1981). The pattern of ectopic hormone production in lung cancer. *Yale J. Biol. Med*; **54**: 181-5.

Braunstein G.D. (1979). Use of human chorionic gonadotrophin as a tumour marker in cancer. In *Immunodiagnosis of Cancer Part I*. (Herberman R.B., McIntire K.R. eds.) pp. 383–409. New York: Marcel Dekker Inc.

Coombes R.C., Hillyard C., Greenberg P.B., MacIntyre I. (1974). Plasma-immunoreactive-calcitonin in patients with non-thyroid tumours. *Lancet*; **1**: 1080–3.

Coombes R.C., Easty G.C., Detre S.I., *et al.* (1975). Secretion of immunoreactive calcitonin by human breast carcinomas. *Br. Med. J*; **4**: 197.

Coombes R.C., Ellison M.L., Easty G.C., Hillyard C.J., James R., Galante L., Girgis S., Heywood L., MacIntyre I., Neville A.M. (1976*a*). The ectopic secretion of calcitonin by lung and breast carcinomas. *Clin. Endocrinol*; **5**: Suppl. 387s–396s.

Coombes R.C., Ward M.K., Greenberg P.B., Hillyard C.J., Tulloch B.R., Morrison R., Joplin G.F. (1976*b*). Calcium metabolism in cancer: Studies using calcium isotopes and immunoassays for parathyroid hormone and calcitonin. *Cancer*; **38**: 2111–120.

Davis S., Proper S., May P.B. *et al* (1979). Elevated prolactin levels in bronchogenic carciroma. *Cancer*; **44**: 676.

Deftos L.J., Bury A.E., Habener J.F., Singer F.R., Potts J.T. Jr. (1971). *Metabolism*; **20**: 1129–37.

Ellison M., Woodhouse D., Hillyard C., Dowsett M., Coombes R.C., Gilbey E.D., Greenberg P.B., Neville A.M. (1975). Immunoreaction calcitonin production by human lung carcinoma cells in culture. *Brit. J. Cancer*; **32**: 373.

Fajans S.S., Floyd J.C. (1979). Diagnosis and medical management of insulinomas. *Ann. Rev. Med*; **30**: 313.

Frisken R.A., Heath D.A., Somers S., Bold A.M. (1981). Hypercalcaemia in hospital patients. Clinical and diagnostic aspects. *Lancet*; **1**: 202–207.

Gerha-Lluch J.R., Begent R.H.J., Bagshawe K.D. (1980). Tumour marker levels and prognosis in malignant teratoma of the testis. *Br. J. Cancer*, **42**: 850–5.

Gerwirtz G., Schneider B., Krieger D.T., Yalow, R.S. (1974). Big ACTH: Conversion to biologically active ACTH by trypsin. *J. Clin. Endocrinol. Metabol*; **38**: 227.

Gilby E.D., Bondy P.K., Forsling, M. (1976). Impaired water-load excretion in oat-cell lung cancer. *Br. J. Cancer*: **34**: 323.

Goltzman D., Stewart A.F., Broadus, A.E. (1981). Malignancy-associated hyper-calcemia: Evaluation with a cytochemical bioassay for parathyroid hormone. *J. Clin. Endocrinol. Metab*; **53**: 899.

Gray C.E., Ratcliffe J.G. (1979). Clinical evaluation of a radioimmunoassay for beta-MSH-related peptides (lipotrophins) in human plasma. *Clin Endocrinol*; **10**: 163.

Hamilton B.P.M., Upton G.V., Armatrude T.T. Jr. (1972). *J. Clin. Endocrinol. Metab*; **35**: 764–7.

Hammond C.B., Borchert L.G., Tyrey L., Creasman W.T., Parker R.T. (1973). *Am. J. Obst. Gynaecol*; **98**: 71–8,

Hennessy J.F., Wells S.A. Jr., Ontjen D.A., Cooper C.W. (1974). *J. Clin. Endocrinol. Metab*; **39**: 487–95.

Hertz R., Lewis J.L. Jr., Lipsett M.B. (1961). *Am. J. Obst. Gynaecol*; **82**: 631–7.

Hoile R.W. (1979). *Br. Med. J*; **1**: 487.

Horton J.E., Raisz L.G., Simmons H.A., Oppenheim J.J., Mergenhagen S.E. (1972). Bone resorbing activity in supernatant fluid from cultured human peripheral blood leukocytes. *Science*; **177**: 793–5.

Imura H. (1980). Ectopic hormone production viewed as an abnormality in regulation of gene expression. *Adv. Cancer Res*; **33**: 39–75.

Jolivet J., Beuregard H., Somma M., Band P.R. (1980). ACTH secreting medullary carcinoma of the thyroid: Monitoring of clinical course with calcitonin and cortisol assays and immunohistochemical studies. *Cancer*; **46**: 2667–70.

Kohn J., Orr A.H., McElwain T.J., Bentall M., Peckham M.J. (1976). *Lancet*; 433–6.

Lowry P.J., Rees L.H., Tomlin S., Gilkes G., Landon J. (1976). Chemical characteristics of ectopic ACTH purified from a malignant thymic carcinoid tumour. *J. Clin. Endocrinol. Metab*; **43**: 831–5.

Malagelada J-R., Glanzman S.L., Go V.L.W. (1982). Laboratory diagnosis of gastrinoma. II A prospective study of gastrin challenge tests. *Mayo. Clin. Proc*; **57**: 219–26.

Marshall J.B., Settles R.H. (1980). Zollinger–Ellison syndrome. *Postgraduate Medicine*; **68**(1): 38–50.

Megyesi K., Kahn C.R., Roth J., Gorden, P. (1974). Hypoglycaemia in association with intrapancreatic tumours: Demonstration of elevated plasma NSILA-5 by a new radioreceptor assay. *J. Clin. Endocrinol. Metab*; **47**: 1240.

Modlin I.M., Bloom S.R. (1978). VIPomas and the watery diarrhoea syndrome. *S. Afr. Med. J*; **54**: 53.

Modlin I.M., Jaffe B.M., Sank A., Albert D. (1982). The early diagnosis of gastrinoma. *Ann. Surg*; **196**: 5, 512–7.

Mundy G.R., Raisz L.G., Cooper R.A., Schecter G.P., Salmon S.E. (1974). Evidence for the secretion of an osteoclast stimulating factor in myeloma. *N. Eng. J. Med*; **291**: 1041.

North W.C., O'Donnell J.F., Rist K., Naurer L.H. (1980). Elevated human neurophysins (HNPs): A specific high incidence with small cell carcinoma. *J. Clin. Endocrinol. Metab*; **51**: 892.

Papapoulos S.E., Manning R.M., Hendy G.N. *et al.* (1980). Studies of circulating parathyroid hormone in man using a homologous amino-terminal specific immunoradiometric assay. *Clin. Endocrinol*; **13**: 57.

Pearse A.G.E. (1968). Common cytochemical and ultrastructural characteristics of cells producing polypeptide hormones (the APUD series) and their relevance to thyroid and ultimobranchial C cells and calcitonin. *Proc. Roy. Soc. B.*; **170**: 71–80.

Pearse A.G.E., Polak J.M. (1978). The diffuse neuroendocrine system and the APUD concept. In *Gut Hormones*. (Bloom S.R. ed.) pp. 33-9. New York: Churchill Livingstone.

Penman E., Wass J.A.H., Besser G.M., Rees L.H. (1980). Somatostatin secretion by lung and thymic tumours. *Clin. Endocrinol*; **13**: 613–20.

Pentengill O.S., Faulkner C.S., Wurster-Hill D.H., Maurer L.H., Sorensen G.D., Robinson A.G., Zimmerman E.A. (1977). Isolation and characterization of a hormone-producing cell line from human small cell anaplastic carcinoma of the lung. *J. Natl. Cancer. Inst*; **58**: 511–18.

Powell D., Singer F.R., Murray T.M., Minkin C., Potts J.T. (1973). Non-parathyroid humoral hypercalcaemia in patients with neoplastic diseases. *N. Engl. J. Med*; **287**: 176.

Raghavan D., Heyderman E., Peckham M.J., McElwain T.J., Kohn J., Orr A.H. (1979). *Tumour Markers: Input and Prospects*. (Boelsma E., Rjimke P.H. eds.) Elsvier/North Holland Biomedical Press.

Rees L.H. (1977). *Clinics in Endocrinology and Metabolism*; **6**: 137.

Riggs B.L., Arnaud C.D., Reynolds J.C., Smith L.H. (1971). Immunologic differentiation of primary hyperparathyroidism due to non-parathyroid cancer. *J. Clin. Invest*; **50**: 2079–83.

Schwartz W.B., Bennet W., Curelop S., Barter F.C. (1957). A syndrome of renal sodium loss and hyponatremia probably resulting from inappropriate secretion of antidiuretic hormone. *Am. J. Med*; **23**: 529–42.

Sherwood L.M., O'Riordan J.L.H., Aurback G.D., Potts J.T. Jr. (1967). Production of parathyroid hormone by non-parathyroid tumours. *J. Clin. Endocrinol. Metab*; **27**: 140.

Silva O.L., Becker K.L., Primack A., Doppman J., Snider R.H. (1973). Ectopic production of calcitonin. *Lancet*; **2**: 317.

Sizemore G.W., Carney J.A., Heath H. (1977). Epidemiology of medullary carcinoma of the thyroid gland: A 5-year experience (1971–1976). *Surg. Clin. North Am*; **57**: 633–45.

Skrabanek P., Powell D. (1978). Ectopic insulin and Occam's Razor: Reappraisal of the riddle of tumour hypoglycaemia. *Clin. Endocrinol*; **9**: 141–54.

Stacpole P.W. (1981). The glucagonoma syndrome: Clinical features, diagnosis and treatment. *Endocrine Res*; **2**: 347–61.

Tsukada T., Nakai Y., Jingami H., Imura H., Taii S., Nakanishi S., Numa S. (1981). Identification of the mRNA coding for the ACTH-β-lipotropin precursor in a human ectopic ACTH-producing tumor. *Biochem. Biophys. Res. Commun*; **98**: 535–40.

Yalow R.S., Berson S.A. (1971). Size heterogeneity of ACTH in plasma and in extracts of pituitary glands and ACTH-producing thymoma. *Biochem. Biophys. Res. Commun*; **44**: 439–45.

Yalow R.S., Wolf J., Lee L.E. (1977). Ectopic ACTH in bronchogenic carcinoma. *ASCO Abstr*; **18** C-42: 277.

Yalow R.S., Eastridge C.E., Higgins G. Jr., Wolf, J. (1979). Plasma and tumour ACTH in carcinoma of the lung. *Cancer*; **44**: 1789–92.

Yamaji T., Ishibashi M., Katayama, S. (1981). Nature of the immunoreactive neurophysins in ectopic vasopressin-producing oat cell carcinomas of the lung. Demonstration of a putative common precursor to vasopressin and neurophysin. *J. Clin. Invest*; **68**: 388–98.

Chapter 3

Bruce A.J. Ponder

Genetic Problems of Endocrine Significance

INTRODUCTION

Genetic Contribution to Cancer Incidence

Cancer has not generally been regarded as a disease with a major inherited component. Cancer syndromes in which an inherited influence is sufficiently strong to be clinically evident account for only a small minority of cancer incidence, and the endocrine tumours to be discussed in this chapter will necessarily be drawn from this small minority. It is as well to realise at the outset, however, that this view of the role of inherited factors in cancer incidence is almost certainly too restricted. The lack of obvious family clustering of most cancers is not, as has been supposed, evidence against the operation of inherited factors. Peto (1980) has pointed out that the presence in the population of a dominant 'cancer gene' which confers, for example, a 100-fold increased risk of a particular cancer in homozygotes and heterozygotes, and which has a frequency of 0·1, will result in 95% of the cancers occurring in the 19% of the population who are gene carriers. Even so, the relative risk in siblings of cancer patients will be only about 2·8-fold that in the general population, so that no familial clustering will be clinically evident. The same conclusion is reached for a wide variety of gene frequencies and relative risks, and for dominant or recessive genes. For cancers of endocrine organs, as for cancers at other sites, significant inherited predisposition may therefore exist outside the recognised inherited cancer syndromes. The implications of this, and the possible ways in which such predisposition may in the future be detected, are discussed in several recent reviews (Bodmer, 1982; Ponder, 1983).

The remainder of this chapter will be confined to inherited disorders likely to be referred to an endocrinologist in which a link with an increased risk of cancer is already clinically apparent. A classification of inherited disorders associated with an increased risk of cancer which is based on possible mechanisms of predisposition, is shown in Table 3.1. Inherited predisposition to tumours at each of the endocrine sites will be considered with reference to this classification.

TABLE 3.1
*Examples of Inherited Disorders Associated with an
Increased Risk of Cancer*

1. *Constitutional chromosomal abnormalities*
   Down's syndrome
   Klinefelter's syndrome
   Turner's syndrome
2. *Mendelian traits*
   a) 'Inherited cancer syndromes'
        Retinoblastoma
        Familial polyposis coli
        Multiple endocrine neoplasia syndromes
   b) Preneoplastic states
      i) DNA repair defects and chromosomal instability syndromes;
            xeroderma pigmentosum; Fanconi; Blooms;
            ataxia–telangiectasia
      ii) Disturbances of tissue organisation
            Hamartomatous syndromes: Cowden;
            Peutz–Jeghers; Neurofibromatosis
      iii) Immune deficiency syndromes
      iv) Metabolic variation:
            Albinism
            Aryl hydrocarbon hydroxylase induction
            Variations in oestrogen metabolism
3. *Multifactorial predisposition*
   Ethnic cancer differences
   Familial cancer aggregations

MULTIPLE ENDOCRINE NEOPLASIA TYPE I (MEN I; WERNER SYNDROME)

Multiple endocrine neoplasia type I is inherited as an autosomal dominant trait, and is classified (Table 3.1) with the 'inherited cancer syndromes'. The spectrum of involvement in a series of 85 patients (Ballard *et al.*, 1964) is shown in Table 3.2. Studies of families with Zollinger–Ellison syndrome (Freisen *et al.*, 1972), familial islet cell adenomatosis and diabetes (Tragl and Mayr, 1977) and familial hyperglucagonaemia (Boden and Owen, 1977) have been reported separately; in the latter family the index patient had a medullary thyroid carcinoma, suggesting a possible link with MEN II (*see* below; Fig. 3.1). Eight other such 'mixed' MEN I and MEN II patients were reviewed by Hansen *et al.* (1976). Tumours of the MEN I type have also been reported in association with neurofibromatosis (Hope and Mulvihill, 1981). Schwannomas and non-lymphoid thymomas have been described in patients with MEN I (Rimoin and Schimke, 1971).

TABLE 3.2

Spectrum of Involvement in 85 Patients with MEN I

Parathyroids (adenoma or chief cell hyperplasia affecting multiple glands; rarely malignant)	84%
Pancreatic islet cells (usually multiple; may involve β and non-β cells; may be malignant)	81%
Pituitary (functioning or non-functioning; rarely malignant)	65%
Adrenal cortex (hyperplasia, single or multiple adenomas; may be malignant)	38%
Thyroid (adenomas, colloid goitre, thyroiditis, thyrotoxicosis; one patient with carcinoma)	19%
Lipomas	12%
Carcinoid (foregut)	4%

It has been suggested (Schimke, 1977) that the common factor in this seemingly diverse set of tumours is that they arise from cells which are derived embryologically from neural crest; but the evidence for this is much weaker than for the components of the MEN II syndrome, described below. An alternative hypothesis is that some components of the syndrome are secondary to abnormal hormonal stimulation from primary pancreatic islet cell tumours (Vance *et al.*, 1972).

The clinical presentations depend upon the organs involved and whether the tumours are functioning. Frequent clinical presentations include those

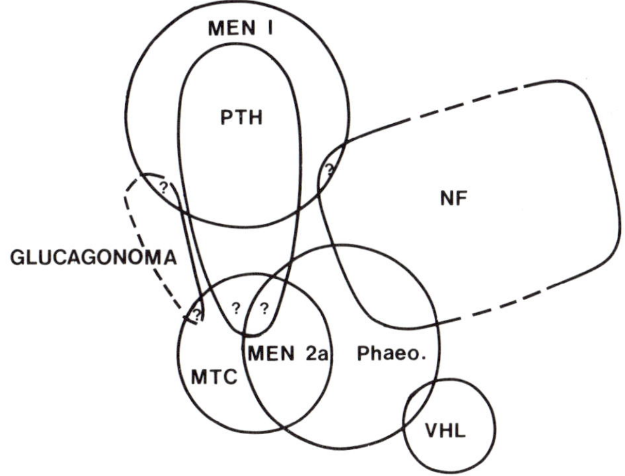

PTH = Parathyroid

NF = Neurofibromatosis

VHL = Von Hippel – Lindau syndrome

Fig. 3.1. *Venn diagram to illustrate postulated relationships between familial forms of some endocrine tumour syndromes.*

resulting from functioning islet cell tumours: Zollinger–Ellison syndrome (intractable peptic ulceration and unexplained diarrhoea) from gastrin-secreting non-β cell tumours (Freisen *et al.*, 1972); hyperglycaemia from insulinomas, and profuse watery diarrhoea from tumours secreting vasoactive intestinal peptides (VIP). Details can be found in standard endocrinological textbooks.

Each of these tumours can occur not only as part of the familial syndrome, but in sporadic form. The spectrum of tumours varies in different individuals with the familial form, as does the age at presentation. It is thus a complex problem to decide, when confronted with a patient in whom one of the tumours has been diagnosed, how energetically to set about screening that individual for the presence of the other possible tumours in the syndrome, and whether to screen other family members. There is no correct answer to this question. A careful family history is essential (but often neglected). The presence of multiple tumours at a single site or different sites in one individual should raise strong suspicion of a hereditary tumour, and a young age at onset (e.g. under 35 years) is also suggestive. It has been estimated that 10–20% of patients with apparently sporadic parathyroid tumours will have a familial syndrome (Jackson *et al.*, 1977; Boey *et al.*, 1975), and that about 50% of patients with Zollinger-Ellison syndrome have MEN I (Schimke, 1976). Without knowing how carefully the family history was checked before accepting the patient as 'sporadic', and how carefully familial involvement was sought subsequently, it is difficult to assess these figures; but they suggest that the possibility of familial involvement is such that the clinician should constantly bear it in mind. The question of screening will be discussed further in the final section.

MULTIPLE ENDOCRINE NEOPLASIA TYPE II (MEN II; SIPPLE'S SYNDROME)

Multiple endocrine neoplasia type II is also an autosomal dominant inherited cancer syndrome. It consists of medullary carcinoma of the thyroid (MTC), phaeochromocytoma, and in some patients, parathyroid adenomas (for reviews, *see* Wolfe and DeLellis, 1981; Williams, 1979). A rare variant, MEN IIB (Gorlin *et al.*, 1968; Dyck *et al.*, 1979; Gorlin and Vickers, 1971) comprises in addition some or all of the following: mucosal neuromas of the oral cavity and eyelids, thickened corneal nerve fibres (Riley and Robertson, 1981; Khalil and Lorenzetti, 1980), a characteristic facies, ganglioneuromatosis of the bowel and urinary tract (Carney and Hayles, 1977), various skeletal abnormalities (Rasmusson, 1980) and features of Marfan's syndrome. Although the classical description of MEN II is of families with both MTC and phaeochromocytoma, perhaps as many as 50% of families with MTC have no evidence of phaeochromocytoma, even after careful screening; familial MTC should therefore be recognised as a separate entity. It is possible also that the description of MEN II as autosomal dominant with high penetrance is an over-simplification. Data from Norway (Normann, 1977) and our own experience (unpublished) indicates that penetrance may sometimes be incomplete, in that family members who were clinically normal aged 65 or more have transmitted the gene; and in some families the phenotypic expression of the syndrome seems to differ in different branches. Unfortunately, much of this information is still at an anecdotal level, but has important implications for management of the families (*see* below).

Medullary carcinoma of the thyroid arises from the 'C' or parafollicular cells of the thyroid, which secrete calcitonin, and phaeochromocytomas arise from sympathetic neuroblasts in the adrenal medulla or in extra-adrenal sympathetic ganglia. Both these sets of cells, as well as the Schwann cells which form the mucosal neuromas, and the ganglion cells in the alimentary tract, are derived embryologically from neural crest. It is reasonable, therefore, to regard the syndrome as one affecting neural crest derivatives. Where the parathyroid involvement fits into this picture is less clear; the evidence that the parathyroid cells are derived from neural crest is not strong, yet parathyroid adenoma and hyperplasia are associated only with the familial form of MTC, and moreover with MEN IIA rather than IIB, which suggests a genetic basis to the involvement.

Medullary carcinoma of the thyroid accounts for about 7% of all thyroid tumours (Fletcher, 1970). It has been estimated that 20% of patients with MTC are of the familial type (Chong *et al.*, 1975; Jackson *et al.*, 1979; Sizemore *et al.*, 1980); but screening of the relatives of apparently sporadic cases has on occasion revealed unsuspected familial involvement, and this figure may well be a considerable under-estimate. For this reason, some authors advocate that families of all index patients with MTC should be offered screening (Baylin and Wells, 1981; Emmertsen *et al.*, 1980; Russell *et al.*, 1983). Apart from the stigmata of the MEN IIB phenotype, there are no clinical features which reliably distinguish patients with sporadic from those with familial tumours, although the familial tumours on average present at a younger age (Jackson *et al.*, 1979).

Medullary carcinoma of the thyroid commonly presents in one of two ways: most often, as a painless lump in the neck, sometimes of many years standing; less often as unexplained diarrhoea (Steinfeld *et al.*, 1973). About one-quarter of patients with extensive MTC have diarrhoea, which usually responds to removal of the tumour; the mechanism is unclear. The tumour tends to metastasise locally in the neck before distant spread to lungs, liver and bones; the course in different patients varies from extremely indolent to aggressive, with death from metastases within two years.

In the familial form, both MTC and phaeochromocytoma develop through a stage of multifocal hyperplasia to multiple small tumours (Wolfe

and DeLellis, 1981). The multifocal hyperplasia may represent the phenotypic expression of the inherited mutation, which requires a second,
somatic, mutation to transform the hyperplastic cell into a cancer cell
(Jackson *et al.*, 1979; Knudsen, 1977). This mode of development is of
practical importance for two reasons: (1) it provides a stage at which early
tumour can be detected and treated in individuals at risk, and (2) the
presence of multiple areas of C-cell adrenal medullary hyperplasia or
tumour in operation specimens may prove to be a reliable indication that the
patient has the familial form of the tumour, and that his family is therefore at
risk (Jackson *et al.*, 1979).

Screening for MTC rests on the detection of a raised plasma calcitonin,
indicating an expanded C-cell mass. The sensitivity which is required to
achieve sufficiently early diagnosis to give a high probability of cure by
thyroidectomy is a matter of debate, probably because different centres have
based their policy on experience of families with tumours of differing
aggressiveness. Correlations of calcitonin levels with operative findings
(Wells *et al.*, 1978, 1982) suggest that basal unstimulated calcitonin is not
sufficiently sensitive for screening, and a stimulation test should be used.
The alternatives are 30–50 ml vodka or whisky by mouth (Dymling *et al.*,
1976), intravenous pentagastrin (PG) 0·5 µg/kg, or a combination of PG
0·5 µg/kg and calcium (reviewed by Baylin and Wells, 1981). Each has its
advocates: the PG with calcium test is probably the most sensitive, but such
sensitivity may not be necessary; alcohol is more appealing but may have an
unacceptable incidence of false negative results. In our practice we have
used PG alone and found it acceptable to children and adults, and without
the disadvantage of alcohol for the majority of relatives who come to the
hospital for screening by car. The calcitonin levels which should prompt a
recommendation for thyroidectomy are also a matter of debate. In general,
groups in the USA follow a more aggressive policy (Wells *et al.*, 1978, 1982),
proceeding to surgery in known families on the basis of raised calcitonin
after stimulation only, compared with the policy to date in the UK, where
many surgeons prefer to delay until the basal (unstimulated) calcitonin is
clearly abnormal. These attitudes depend to some extent on the aggressiveness of the disease in the family members already diagnosed; some caution
also arises from the multiplicity of causes of a raised plasma calcitonin apart
from MTC, and the consequent risk of a false positive diagnosis (Becker
et al., 1982; *Lancet*, 1983).

Screening for the associated phaeochromocytomas can be carried out by
catecholamine measurements, adrenal imaging, and perhaps in the future by
radioisotope scanning with ^{125}I iodo-benzyl-guanidine (Sisson *et al.*, 1981).
It should be noted that phaeochromocytomas may sometimes secrete
immunoreactive calcitonin (Weinstein and Ide, 1980).

The surgical treatment of MTC is reviewed by Russell *et al.* (1983) and
Baylin and Wells (1981) and in Chapter 14 of this book. Patients not

uncommonly have persistent raised calcitonin levels after surgery, which show no tendency to rise over many years, and which may not be associated with evident metastatic disease. The explanation and the natural history remain obscure.

PHAEOCHROMOCYTOMA

Familial phaeochromocytoma may occur in a variety of forms other than MEN II syndrome (Moorhead *et al.*, 1965; Funyu *et al.*, 1973; Tank *et al.*, 1982) (Table 3.3). The proportion of patients presenting with apparently isolated phaeochromocytomas who have a familial tumour was estimated at 6% in a collection of over 500 patients (Hermann and Mornex, 1964) but, as with the components of MEN I syndrome, this may well be an under-estimate. Familial phaeochromocytomas are commonly bilateral; extra adrenal tumours are more common, but malignant behaviour is unusual, estimates ranging from 5 to 12% in adrenal tumours (Schimke, 1978; Mahoney and Harrison, 1977). Phaeochromocytomas in MEN II syndrome are reported to secrete more adrenaline than non-adrenaline, unlike other phaeochromocytomas (Sato *et al.*, 1975).

The incidence of neurofibromatosis (NF) in patients with phaeochromo-cytoma has been estimated between 5 and 25%; the incidence of phaeochromocytoma in patients presenting with NF is, however, considerably less (Hope and Mulvihill, 1981). Von Hippel-Lindau syndrome consists of cerebellar haemangioblastoma, other haemangiomas, hyper-nephroma, renal cysts, and phaeochromocytoma. Because of the haem-angiomata and cysts, this syndrome is generally classified as a hamartoma syndrome (Warkany, 1977); the underlying mechanism of tumour for-mation is obscure. Noonan's syndrome consists of phenotypic features resembling Turner's syndrome (Becker *et al.*, 1969; Kaplan *et al.*, 1968) (*see* below) in XY males; associated Schwann cell tumours and phaeochromo-cytomas have been described.

TABLE 3.3
*Phaeochromocytoma: Occurrence
in Familial Syndromes*

Non-familial (? > 90%)
Familial (autosomal dominant)
   Phaeochromocytoma only
   MEN IIA, MEN IIB
   Neurofibromatosis
   Von Hippel–Lindau syndrome
   Noonan's syndrome
   With carotid body tumours

ADRENAL CORTICAL TUMOURS

Apart from MEN I syndrome, adrenal cortical tumours have been described in a cancer family syndrome which consists of adrenal cortical carcinoma, breast cancer, sarcoma, leukaemia and brain tumour (Li and Fraumeni, 1975). They have also been recorded in Gardners syndrome (familial polyposis with multiple fibromatous tumours) and in children with hemihypertrophy (Haicken *et al.*, 1973) though not on a proven familial basis, and in the related Beckwith–Wiedemann syndrome (Beckwith, 1969; *see also* Bolande, 1977). Cushing's syndrome with adenomatous hyperplasia in three siblings and adrenal carcinoma in a fourth, without evidence as to the cause, has also been reported (Arce *et al.*, 1978).

PITUITARY

Familial occurrence of pituitary adenomas outside the MEN I syndrome is rare. Reports of acromegaly in families before growth hormone assays were available may possibly have resulted from confusion with dominantly inherited pachydermoperiostosis or with cerebral gigantism (Schimke, 1978). Two brothers with growth-hormone-producing pituitary tumours and acanthosis nigricans were described by Levin *et al.* (1974). Amenorrhoea and galactorrhoea have been described in a mother and daughter, both of whom had pituitary adenomas (Schimke, 1977), but these may have represented part of a MEN I syndrome. Pituitary tumours have been reported in single individuals with ganglioneuroma (Greenfield and Shelley, 1965) and with chemodectoma (quoted in Hansen *et al.*, 1976); both the latter tumours are thought to be of neural crest origin, but the associations may have been fortuitous.

THYROID (EXCLUDING MEDULLARY CARCINOMA)

Papillary carcinoma has been described in a medullary thyroid cancer family (Lamberg *et al.*, 1981), and we have a family (unpublished) in which the mother of three siblings with MTC had a papillary carcinoma.

As with pituitary tumours, it is not clear whether familial thyroid cancers occur outside the multiple endocrine neoplasia syndromes. Both papillary adenocarcinoma and Hurtle cell adenomas have been described in different sets of twins (Rohnson and Orr, 1955; Nagamachi, 1973), and the twins with papillary adenocarcinoma both subsequently developed bilateral breast cancer (Schimke, 1978). There may also be a significant association of thyroid adenoma with ovarian arrhenoblastoma in families (Jensen *et al.*, 1974). A mother and son with non-medullary thyroid cancer, diagnosed in the son at the age of 9 years, were reported by Nemec *et al.* (1975). Thyroid carcinoma occurred in two of four siblings affected by familial goitre and nerve deafness (Elman, 1958).

Thyroid adenoma and carcinoma occur as part of two hamartomatous syndromes: Gardner's syndrome and Cowden syndrome (reviewed in Gorlin, 1977).

PARATHYROID

A study of the families of 100 consecutive patients with parathyroid tumours revealed familial involvement in ten cases (Jackson *et al.*, 1977). In three, there was evidence of MEN I syndrome; and in two, of MEN II. The other five appeared to have familial hyperparathyroidism alone, but one cannot exclude that these were also part of families in which the other components of a multiple endocrine neoplasia syndrome had not been detected. In another series, of 119 patients with primary hyperparathyroidism, 17·5% were deemed to have evidence of MEN I (Boey *et al.*, 1975). The great majority of patients in these and other series appear to have had adenomas, but hyperplasia, adenomas and carcinomas may co-exist within a single individual and in members of a single family (Mallette *et al.*, 1974).

Malignant thyroid lesions were found in 11·4% of 272 cases with primary hyperparathyroidism, which was thought to be a significant association (Livolsi and Feind, 1976). The association is unexplained, and there was no evidence of an hereditary component. Kaplan *et al.* (1971) reported an increased incidence of a variety of common epithelial tumours in hyperparathyroid patients. This also is unexplained.

GONADAL DYSGENESIS

For a full account of neoplasia in disorders of abnormal sexual differentiation, the reader is urged to consult Simpson and Photopoulos (1976). What follows is a highly selective account of a complex subject.

In individuals with gonadal dysgenesis, the gonads are represented by streaks of connective tissue lacking germ cells. Only some of these individuals have the phenotype of Turner's syndrome (*see* below; Mulvihill *et al.*, 1975). Two forms are distinguished: (1) cytogenetic, associated with monosomy for the X chromosome (45,X) or structural rearrangements of the X or Y chromosomes; and (2) genetic, in which the gonadal dysgenesis is associated with an inherited mutant gene, but there is a normal female (46,XX) or male (46,XY) chromosome component.

The essential point in relation to risk of malignancy is that only in those individuals with a Y chromosome is the risk increased. Gonadal tumours, usually gonadoblastoma or dysgerminoma, develop in 10–15% of 45X/46XY patients with streak gonads, and in 20–30% of patients with 46XY gonadal dysgenesis. Familial and non-familial cases of XY gonadal dysgenesis have been reported; in 26 familial cases, 15 had a gonadal tumour, compared with 11 of 45 non-familial cases (Simpson and Photopoulos, 1976). Patients with gonadal dysgenesis who have a Y chromosome should be offered resection of the dysgenetic gonad soon after diagnosis.

TESTICULAR FEMINISATION

Testicular feminisation may be inherited either as an X-linked recessive or a male-limited autosomal dominant trait. 46XY individuals have bilateral testes (usually intra-abdominal), female external genitalia, a blindly ending vagina and no Müllerian structures. Normal female pubertal development occurs. In patients over the age of 30, there is a risk of gonadal neoplasia, usually seminoma. It is unclear whether this risk is greater than could be attributed to the cryptorchidism which is part of the syndrome.

SYNDROMES WITH CONSTITUTIONAL CHROMOSOMAL ABNORMALITY

The cultured lymphocytes of 3068 patients referred for radiotherapy for cancer in Edinburgh revealed no excess of constitutional chromosomal abnormalities over the prevalence in the general population, so that constitutional chromosomal abnormalities do not in general seem to contribute substantially to cancer incidence (O'Riordan *et al.*, 1972). In some individuals with 'inherited cancer syndromes' such as retinoblastoma and Wilm's tumour, however, such chromosomal abnormalities are present and consistently associated with the development of the tumour (Harnden and Herbert, 1982). In distinction to this, there are three examples of constitutional chromosomal abnormality (two involving the sex chromosomes) in which the chromosomal abnormality is associated with a syndrome of physical anomalies, plus a slightly increased risk of certain malignancies which falls well short of a consistent association.

Down's Syndrome (Trisomy 21)

There is an increased risk of acute leukaemia in children with Down's syndrome, of the order of 20 times that in the general population (Miller, 1970). The risk in any individual Down's syndrome patient is still, therefore, small. There is at present no convincing evidence of an increased risk of any other cancer.

Klinefelter's Syndrome

Males with at least one X and two Y chromosomes have Klinefelter's syndrome. Gonadal tumours are rare, although bilateral teratomas were reported in each of two 47,XXY siblings (Gustavson *et al.*, 1975). There is, however, a 20-fold increased risk of breast cancer over that in normal males (Harnden *et al.*, 1971; Scheike *et al.*, 1973); the risk of breast cancer in a male with Klinefelter's syndrome is about one-fifth that in normal females (Schimke *et al.*, 1973). A single case has been reported of a 47,XXY male who developed six primary neoplasms, five being malignant (Coley *et al.*, 1971).

Turner's Syndrome

Turner's syndrome is sometimes discussed as if synonymous with gonadal dysgenesis. This may be misleading. The principal risk of malignancy in gonadal dysgenesis is of dysgerminoma in the individuals who are outwardly normal in appearance, and who have a Y chromosome (*see* above). Turner's syndrome consists of dysgenetic gonads associated with a variety of congenital anomalies, including short stature, webbing of the neck, short metacarpals and coarctation of the aorta. Approximately 50% of these individuals have a 45,XO chromosome complement; others are mosaic 45,XO/46,XX or have structural rearrangements or deletions in one X chromosome. There is no excess risk of gonadal tumours in Turner's syndrome, but associations have been reported with various hamartomatous growths, and non-gonadal tumours, including some of neural crest origin (Wertelecki *et al.*, 1970; Pendergrass *et al.*, 1974).

SCREENING OF FAMILY MEMBERS AT RISK

The practical reason for a clinician to be interested in the possibility that a cancer is familial is the potential for early diagnosis and more successful treatment of second tumours in the index patient, and of tumours in apparently healthy family members. Tumours of the endocrine organs might appear to be particularly suitable for screening because, if they are functional, they may be detected at an early stage by their abnormal endocrine activity.

The basic requirement is to be able to specify the risk of the cancer in the individual in question, and to balance that against the particular costs of screening. These include the anxiety and uncertainty which the family may suffer, the logistics of screening possibly large numbers of family members at regular intervals over a long period (in MEN II, for example, it is recommended that screening be carried out yearly from about age 6 until well into adult life (Gagel *et al.*, 1982)) and the risk that the treatment may be inappropriate, either because the natural history of the tumour does not warrant it, or because of a false positive diagnosis.

In XY gonadal dysgenesis, for example, the problem is fairly straight-forward. Physical and chromosomal abnormalities indicate clearly who is at risk, and surgical removal of the dysgenetic gonad is an acceptable procedure to set against a 20–40% risk of malignant dysgerminoma. Despite the success of screening programmes in MEN II syndrome (Graze *et al.*, 1978; Wolfe and DeLellis, 1981; Emmertsen *et al.*, 1982), the decisions here are less clear-cut. The major problem (as with the other endocrine tumours described in this chapter) is that a large but unknown proportion of index patients with the tumour probably have a sporadic form, so that their families are not at risk and screening is unnecessary. Recognition of the families which are at risk and management of individuals within these families is complicated by the variable penetrance and natural history of the tumours which comprise the syndrome. To take one example, consider the pedigree shown in Fig. 3.2. The index patient presented aged 45 with a lump in the neck, which was found to be MTC. There was no evidence of phaeochromocytoma, and no family history suggestive of MTC or MEN II syndrome. The parents of the index case were dead and so could not be screened. What are the risks to his siblings and to their children? (In other words, is this case sporadic or familial?) Should the siblings be screened;

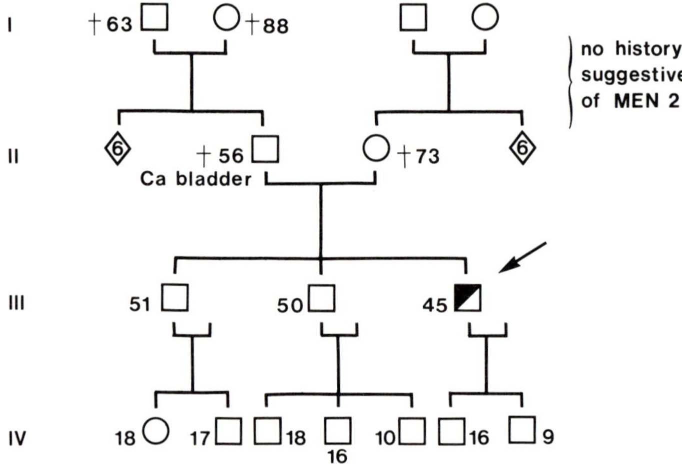

Fig. 3.2. *Pedigree of patient presenting with medullary thyroid carcinoma.*

and if the screening test is positive, how likely is this to be a true rather than false positive result? What should be the criteria for recommending thyroidectomy? The risks to the children of the index case are greater than to the siblings because: (1) the index case may be a new mutation to the familial syndrome (but the incidence of new mutations is unknown); and (2) they are younger, so that if they indeed carry the MTC gene, it is less likely to have already become clinically manifest. The case for screening them is therefore stronger; but it is a 20-year commitment which may require some emotional stamina from them and their parents.

So long as there is no readily identified phenotypic or genotypic marker of individuals at risk, and only imprecise data on the natural history of the tumours and the stage at which intervention is required, these questions will not have a 'correct' answer. That is not an argument against screening, but it does argue strongly that the implications of a screening programme should be thought through carefully beforehand.

ACKNOWLEDGEMENTS

B.A.J. Ponder holds a Career Development Award from the Cancer Research Campaign.

REFERENCES

Arce B., Licea M., Hung S., Padron R. (1978). Familial Cushings syndrome. *Acta Endoc*; **87**: 139–47.

Ballard H.S., Frame B., Hartsock R.J. (1964). Familial multiple endocrine neoplasia—peptic ulcer complex. *Medicine*; **43**: 481–516.

Baylin S.B., Wells S.A. (1981). Management of hereditary medullary thyroid carcinoma. *Clin Endocrin Metab*; **10**:367–78.

Becker C.E., Rosen S.W., Englemann K. (1969). Phaeochromocytoma and hyporesponsiveness to thyrotrophin in a 46,XY male with features of the Turner phenotype. *Ann. Intern. Med*; **70**: 325–33.

Becker K.L., Silva O.L., Snider R.H., Moore C.F., Geelhoed, G.W. (1982). The surgical implications of hypercalcitoninemia. *Surg. Gyn. Obst*; **154**: 897–908.

Beckwith J.B. (1969). Macroglossia, omphalocoele, adrenal cytomegaly, gigantism and hyperplastic visceromegaly. *Birth Defects*; **5**: 188–96.

Boden G., Owen O.E. (1977). Familial hyperglucagonemia—an autosomal dominant disorder. *N. Engl. J. Med*; **296**: 534–8.

Bodmer W.F. (1982). Cancer genetics. In *Cancer Surveys*, Vol. 1. pp. 1–15. Oxford University Press.

Boey J.H., Cooke T.J.C., Gilbert J.M., Sweeney E.C., Taylor S. (1975). Occurrence of other endocrine tumours in primary hyperparathyroidism. *Lancet*; **2**: 781–4.

Bolande R.P. (1977). Childhood tumours and their relationship to birth defects. In *Genetics of Human Cancer: Progress in Cancer Research and Therapy*, Vol. 3.

(Mulvihill J.J., Miller R.W., Fraumeni J.F., eds) pp. 43–75. New York: Raven Press.

Carney J.A., Hayles A.B. (1977). Alimentary manifestations of multiple endocrine neoplasia type 2b. *Mayo Clin. Proc*; **52**: 543–8.

Chong C.C., Beahrs O.H., Sizemore G.W., Woolner L.H. (1975). Medullary carcinoma of the thyroid gland. *Cancer*; **35**: 695–704.

Coley G.M., Otis R.D., Clark W.E. (1971). Multiple primary tumours including bilateral breast cancer in a man with Klinefelter's syndrome. *Cancer*; **27**: 1476–971.

Dyck P.J., Carney J.A., Sizemore G.W., Okazaki H., Brimijoin W.S., Lambert E.H. (1979). Multiple endocrine neoplasia type 2b: Phenotypic recognition, neurological features and their pathological basis. *Ann. Neurol*; **6**: 302–14.

Dymling J.F., Ljungberg O., Hillyard C.J., Greenberg P.B., Evans I.M.A., MacIntyre I. (1976). Whisky: A new provocative test for calcitonin secretion. *Acta Endoc*; **82**: 500–509.

Elman D.S. (1958). Familial association of nerve deafness with nodular goitre and thyroid carcinoma. *N. Engl. J. Med*; **259**: 219–23.

Emmertsen K., Nielsen H.E., Hansen H.H., Elbrond O., Mosekilde L. (1980). Screening for familial medullary thyroid carcinoma. *Dan. Med. Bull*; **27**: 262–5.

Emmertsen K., Elbrond O., Nielsen H.E. *et al.* (1982). Familial medullary thyroid carcinoma in multiple endocrine neoplasia (MEN) IIa: Diagnosis and problems in treatment. *Eur. J. Cancer Clin. Oncol*; **18**: 645–50.

Fletcher J.R. (1970). Medullary (solid) carcinoma of the thyroid gland. *Arch. Surg*; **100**: 257–66.

Freisen S.R., Schimke R.N., Pearse A.G.E. (1972). Genetic aspects of the Z-E syndrome. *Ann. Surg*; **176**: 370–83.

Funyu T., Shiraiwa Y., Nigawara K., Kudo S., Mikuni T. (1973). Familial phaeochromocytoma: Case report and review of the literature. *J. Urol*; **110**: 151–6.

Gagel R.F., Jackson C.E., Block M.A. *et al.* (1982). Age-related probability of development of hereditary medullary thyroid carcinoma. *J. Paediat*; **101**: 941–6.

Gorlin R.J. (1977). Monogenic disorders associated with neoplasia. In *Genetics of Human Cancer: Progress in Cancer Research and Therapy*, Vol. 3. (Mulvihill J.J., Miller R.W., Fraumeni J.F., eds.) pp. 169–78. New York: Raven Press.

Gorlin R.J., Vickers R.A. (1971). Multiple mucosal neuromas, phaeochromocytoma, medullary carcinoma of the thyroid and Marfanoid body build with muscle wasting: Re-examination of a syndrome of neural crest malmigration. *Birth Defects: Original Article Series* **VII**: 69–72.

Gorlin R.J., Sedano H.O., Vickers R.A., Cervenka J. (1968). Multiple mucosal neuromas, phaeochromocytoma and medullary carcinoma of the thyroid—a syndrome. *Cancer*; **22**: 293–9.

Graze K., Spiler I.J., Tashjian A.H. Jr. *et al.* (1978). Natural history of familial medullary thyroid carcinoma: Effect of a program for early diagnosis. *N. Engl. J. Med*; **299**: 980–5.

Greenfield L.J., Shelley W.M. (1965). The spectrum of neurogenic tumours of the sympathetic nervous system: Maturation and adrenergic function. *J. Natl. Cancer Inst*; **35**: 215–23.

Gustavson K.-H., Gamstrop I., Meurling S. (1975). Bilateral teratoma of testis in two brothers with 47,XXY Klinefelter's syndrome. *Clin. Genet*; **8**: 5–7.

Haicken B.N., Schulman N.H., Schneider K.M. (1973). Adrenal cortical carcinoma and congenital hemihypertrophy. *J. Paediat*; **83**: 284–5.

Hansen O.P., Hansen M., Hansen H.H., Rose B. (1976). Multiple endocrine adenomatosis of mixed type. *Acta Med. Scand*; **200**: 327–31.

Harnden D.G., Herbert A. (1982). Association of constitutional chromosome rearrangements with neoplasia. In *Cancer Surveys*, Vol. 1 (Bodmer W.F., ed) pp. 150–73. Oxford University Press.

Harnden D.G., Maclean N., Langlands A.O. (1971). Carcinoma of the breast and Klinefelter's syndrome. *J. Med. Genet*; **8**: 460–1.

Hermann H., Mornex R. (1964). *Human Tumours Secreting Catecholamines*. New York: MacMillan.

Hope D.C., Mulvihill J.J. (1981). Malignancy in neurofibromatosis. In *Advances in Neurology Vol 29: Neurofibromatosis* (Riccardi V.M., Mulvihill J.J., eds.) pp. 33–56. New York: Raven Press.

Jackson C.E., Frame, B., Block M.A. (1977). Prevalence of endocrine neoplasia syndromes in genetic studies of parathyroid tumours. In *Genetics of Human Cancer: Progress in Cancer Research and Therapy*, Vol. 3. (Mulvihill J.J., Miller R.W., Fraumeni J.F., eds.) pp. 205–208. New York: Raven Press.

Jackson C.E., Block M.A., Greenawald K., Tashjian A.H. (1979). The two-mutational event theory in medullary thyroid cancer. *Am. J. Hum. Genet*; **31**: 704–10.

Jensen R.D., Norris H.J., Fraumeni J.F. Jr. (1974). Familial arrhenoblastoma and thyroid adenomas. *Cancer*; **33**: 218–23.

Kaplan L., Katz A.D., Ben-Isaac C., Massoy S.G. (1971). Malignant neoplasms and parathyroid adenoma. *Cancer*; **28**: 401–407.

Kaplan M.S., Opitz J.M., Gosset F.R. (1968). Noonan's syndrome. *Am. J. Dis. Child*; **116**: 359–66.

Khalil M.K., Lorenzetti D.W.C. (1980). Eye manifestations in medullary carcinoma of the thyroid. *Brit. J. Ophthalmol*; **64**: 789–92.

Knudsen A.G. (1977). Genetics and etiology of human cancer. *Adv. Hum. Genet*; **8**: 1–16.

Lamberg B.-A., Reissel P., Stenman S. *et al.* (1981). Concurrent medullary and papillary thyroid carcinoma in the same thyroid lobe and in siblings. *Acta Med Scand*; **209**: 421–4.

Lancet (1983). Plasma calcitonin in medullary thyroid carcinoma (leading article). *Lancet*; **1**: 338–9.

Levin S.R., Hofeldt F.D., Becker N., Wilson C.B., Seymour R., Forshan P.H. (1974). Hypersomatotropism and acanthosis nigricans in two brothers. *Arch. Int. Med*; **134**: 365–7.

Li F.P., Fraumeni J.F. Jr. (1975). Familial breast cancer, soft-tissue sarcomas, and other neoplasms. *Ann. Intern. Med*; **83**: 833–4.

Livolsi V.A., Feind C.R. (1976). Parathyroid adenoma and non medullary thyroid carcinoma. *Cancer*; **38**: 1391–3.

Mahoney E.M., Harrison J.H. (1977). Malignant phaeochromocytoma: Clinical course and treatment. *J. Urol*; **118**: 225–9.

Mallette L.E., Bilezikian J.P., Ketcham A.S., Aurbach G.D. (1974). Parathyroid carcinoma in familial hyperparathyroidism. *Am. J. Med*; **57**: 642–8.

Miller R.W. (1970). Neoplasia and Down's syndrome. *Ann. N.Y. Acad Sci*; **171**: 637–44.

Moorhead E.G. II, Brennan M.J., Caldwell J.R., Averill W.C. (1965). Phaeochromocytoma: A familial tumour. A study of 11 cases. *Henry Ford Hosp. Med. Bull*; **13**: 467–77.

Mulvihill J.J. (1977). Genetic repertory of human neoplasia. In *Genetics of Human Cancer: Progress in Cancer Research and Therapy*, Vol. 3. (Mulvihill J.J., Miller R.W., Fraumeni J.F., eds.) pp. 137–43. New York: Raven Press.

Mulvihill J.J., Wade W.M., Miller R.W. (1975). Gonadoblastoma in dysgenetic gonads with a Y chromosome. *Lancet*; **1**: 863.

Nagamachi Y. (1973). Hurtle cell adenoma of the thyroid in identical twins with 13 year follow up. *Jap. J. Surg*; **3**: 212–17.

Nemec J., Soumar J., Zamrazil V., Pohunkova D., Motlik K., Mirejovsky P. (1975). Familial occurrence of differentiated (non-medullary) thyroid cancer. *Oncology*; **32**: 151–7.

Normann T. (1977). Medullary thyroid carcinoma in Norway. *Acta Path. Microbiol. Scand. A*; **85**: 775–86.

O'Riordan M.L., Langlands A.O., Hernden D.G. (1972). Further studies on the frequency of constitutional chromosome aberrations in patients with malignant disease. *Eur. J. Cancer*; **8**: 373–9.

Pendergrass T.W., Fraumeni J.F. Jr., Fagan E.L. (1974). Brain tumours in sibs, one with the Turner syndrome. *J. Paediatr*; **85**: 875–7.

Peto J. (1980). Genetic predisposition to cancer. In *Banbury Report No. 4: Cancer Incidence in Defined Populations*, pp. 203–13. New York: Cold Spring Harbor Laboratory.

Ponder B.A.J. (1983). Genetic predisposition to cancer. In *19th Symposium on Advanced Medicine*, Vol. 19. (Saunders K.B., ed.) pp. 216–29. London: Pitman.

Rasmusson B. (1980). Bone abnormalities in patients with medullary carcinoma of the thyroid. *Acta Radiologica Oncologica*; **19**: 461–5.

Riley F.C., Robertson D.M. (1981). Ocular histopathology in multiple endocrine neoplasia type 2b. *Am. J. Ophthalmol*; **91**: 57–64.

Rimoin D.L., Schimke R.N. (1971). *Genetic Disorders of the Endocrine Glands*. St. Louis, Mo.: Mosby.

Rohnson D.W., Orr T.G. (1955). Carcinoma of the thyroid and other diseases of the thyroid in identical twins. *Arch Surg*; **70**: 923–7.

Russell C.F., Van Heerden J.A., Sizemore G.W. *et al.* (1983). The surgical management of medullary thyroid carcinoma. *Ann. Surg*; **197**: 43–8.

Sato T, Kobayashi K., Miura Y., Sakura H., Yoshinaga K., Nakamura K. (1975). High epinephrine content in the adrenal tumours from Sipple's syndrome. *Tohoku J. Exp. Med*; **115**: 15–22.

Scheike O., Visfeld J., Peterson B. (1973). Male breast cancer III. Breast cancer in association with the Klinefelter syndrome. *Acta Pathol. Microbiol. Scand*; **81**: 352–4.

Schimke R.N. (1976). Multiple endocrine adenomatosis syndromes. *Adv. Intern. Med*; **21**: 249–65.

Schimke R.N. (1977). Tumours of the neural crest system. In *Genetics of Human Cancer: Progress in Cancer Research and Therapy*, Vol. 3. (Mulvihill J.J., Miller R.W., Fraumeni J.F., eds.) pp. 179–98. New York: Raven Press.

Schimke R.N. (1978). *Genetics and Cancer in Man*. Edinburgh: Churchill Livingstone.

Simpson J.L., Photopoulos G. (1976). The relationship of neoplasia to disorders of abnormal sexual differentiation. *Birth Defects*; **XII**: 15–50.

Sisson J.C., Frazer M.S., Valk T.W. *et al.* (1981). Scintigraphic localisation of phaeochromocytoma. *N. Engl. J. Med*; **305**: 12–17.

Sizemore G.W., Heath H. III, Carney J.A. (1980). Multiple endocrine neoplasia type 2. *Clin. Endoc. Metab*; **9**: 299–315.

Steinfeld C.M., Moertel C.G., Woolner L.B. (1973). Diarrhoea and medullary carcinoma of the thyroid. *Cancer*; **31**: 1237–9.

Tank E.S., Gelbard M.K., Blank B. (1982). Familial phaeochromocytomas. *J. Urol*; **128**: 1013–16.

Tragl K.-H., Mayr W.R. (1977). Familial islet-cell adenomatosis. *Lancet*; **2**: 426–8.

Vance J.E., Stoll R.W., Kitabchi A.E., Buchanan K.D., Hollander D., Williams R.H. (1972). Familial nesidioblastosis as the predominant manifestation of multiple endocrine adenomatosis. *Am. J. Med*; **52**: 211–57.

Warkany J. (1977). Phacomatosis, hamartoses, and neurocristopathies: A personal view. In *Genetics of Human Cancer: Progress in Cancer Research and Therapy*, Vol. 3. (Mulvihill J.J., Miller R.W., Fraumeni J.F. eds) pp. 199–204. New York: Raven Press.

Weinstein R.S., Ide L.F. (1980). Immunoreactive calcitonin in phaeochromocytomas. *Proc. Soc. Exp. Biol. Med*; **165**: 215–17.

Wells S.A., Baylin S.B., Gann D.S. *et al.* (1978). Medullary thyroid carcinoma: Relationship of method of diagnosis to pathological staging. *Ann. Surg*; **188**: 377–83.

Wells S.A., Baylin S.B., Johnsinde I.S. *et al.* (1982). Thyroid venous catheterisation in the early diagnosis of familial medullary thyroid carcinoma. *Ann. Surg*; **196**: 505–11.

Wertelecki W., Fraumeni J.F. Jr., Mulvihill J.J. (1970). Non-gonadal neoplasia in Turner's syndrome. *Cancer*; **26**: 485–8.

Williams E.D. (1979). Medullary carcinoma of the thyroid. In *Endocrinology*, Vol. 2. (De Groot *et al.*, eds.) pp. 777–92. New York: Grune and Stratton.

Wolfe H.J., DeLellis R.A. (1981). Familial medullary carcinoma and C cell hyperplasia. *Clin. Endoc. Metab*; **10**: 351–65.

Chapter 4

Roland T. Jung

Nutritional Support

In this survey of the role of nutritional support for the cancer patient, the major issues will be discussed on a question and answer basis so that each point can be emphasised. The science relating to the value of nutrition will be initially discussed and then the practical aspects will be given.

CANCER CACHEXIA—WHY DOES IT OCCUR?

Numerous studies have shown that malnutrition accompanies cancer (Schein *et al.*, 1975; Ohnuma and Holland, 1977) but the reasons for this are unclear, for many factors appear to be involved. Weight loss may be a consequence of a decrease in energy input and/or an increase in energy expenditure.

Energy Input

A reduction in energy intake may result from mechanical obstruction or a decrease in appetite.

Mechanical

In some patients with tumours of the mouth, oropharynx or upper gastrointestinal tract, actual physical obstruction, ileus, impaired digestion, reduced absorption of nutrients or a protein losing enteropathy may be involved. Several studies have attempted to determine whether chemotherapy can result in significant malabsorption. In one such study (Smith *et al.*, 1979) no evidence of malabsorption could be shown although gastrointestinal mucosal mitotic indices were diminished immediately after therapy, but apparently quickly recovered. Follow-up examinations did not show any cumulative effect of repeated chemotherapy in terms of significant malabsorption. Nevertheless, drugs that cause considerable desquamative mucositis may result in a diminished intake, as may the effects of radiation treatment on the gastrointestinal tract.

Appetite

A reduction in appetite often accompanies cancer but the mechanisms responsible remain poorly understood. Abnormalities in taste have been reported (De Wys, 1977) and, in a few, may be the consequence of deficiencies in zinc or other trace elements. In other studies, food preferences appear not to differ between controls and cancer patients although taste recognition thresholds may be increased in some with cancer (Settle *et al.*, 1979). Many antineoplastic drugs cause nausea, vomiting and anorexia, symptoms which usually abate after cessation of therapy. Improvement of the nutritional status of the patient has been reported to improve appetite, but evidently only in those seriously malnourished. Similarly, appetite may be enhanced by containment or reversal of the malignant process.

Energy Expenditure

Not all cancer patients, despite weight loss, have a significant decrease in energy intake. Warnold *et al.* (1978) in a study of ten weight losing cancer patients noted similar mean daily energy intakes compared to that of healthy control subjects. However, 24-hour energy expenditure, as well as the resting metabolic rate, were about 40% higher in those with cancer. Bozzetti *et al.* (1980) reported that the resting metabolic rate (RMR) was elevated above 20% in 60% of their patients with advanced cancer, and were also able to show a significant correlation ($p < 0.005$) between weight loss and the elevation of the RMR. They also showed that removal of the tumour reversed the weight loss and returned the RMR to normal levels. Other authors have also reported raised RMR in patients with advanced cancer, and a heightened energy expenditure appears to be a major factor in their weight loss. Appetite control must also be abnormal, for such an increase in energy expenditure should produce a rise in energy intake. It also implies that many of the adaptive mechanisms seen with semi-starvation in healthy man are impaired or overridden in anorexic patients with advanced cancer. To understand how this might occur, one has to appreciate the components making up the body's 24-hour energy expenditure, and the way in which the body adapts to altered energy requirements in a healthy subject.

Components

Energy expenditure in a healthy man has three major components, namely, the basal metabolic rate which accounts for 65% of energy output, physical activity (20%), and thermogenic increments (15%). The latter includes thermogenesis associated with maintaining body temperature, dietary-induced thermogenesis and thermogenesis associated with drugs (e.g.

TABLE 4.1

*Contribution to the Resting Metabolic Rate
(RMR) by the Major Organs in a Healthy
Resting Man*

Organ	RMR (%) (of total)
Liver and splanchnic bed	27
Brain	19
Kidneys	7
Heart	10
Skeletal muscle	18
Remainder	19

caffeine), smoking and stress. The basal metabolic rate is defined as the
energy output of an individual in a supine position, at least 12 hours after a
meal and at a thermoneutral (about 28°C) environmental temperature. This
is not easy to achieve, and so the term resting metabolic rate (RMR) is used
when the conditions are not met precisely.

The RMR represents the combustion of fuel sources required to supply
energy for the metabolic processes involved in maintaining the function and
integrity of cells and organs. These include protein, nucleic acid and lipid
synthesis, gluconeogenesis, transport processes and ion pumping. Table 4.1
summarises the contribution made by the various body organs to the RMR
in a healthy adult. The major substrates used as sources of energy in man are
glucose, fatty acids, ketone bodies, amino acids and lactate. It has been
estimated (Young, 1977) that a healthy adult man at rest utilises 140 g of
glucose, 20 g of lactate, oxidises 130 g of triglyceride and 75 g of amino acids
per day; the released energy supplies the mechanisms contributing to the
RMR (Table 4.2).

TABLE 4.2

Fuels for Individual Tissues in a Healthy Man

Major energy source	Tissue
Glucose	Blood cells, renal medulla, brain, skeletal muscle, intestinal mucosa
Free fatty acids	Liver, renal cortex, cardiac muscle, skeletal muscle (not in severe exercise)
Ketone bodies	Cardiac and skeletal muscle, brain, renal cortex

Adaptation to semi-starvation

In a healthy man a semi-starvation state results in a rapid decline in the RMR. This is initially due to changes in energy utilisation but later to a reduction in lean body mass (e.g. muscle). This fall in the RMR can be as much as 30% at 21 days of energy deprivation. Associated with this there is also a reduction in plasma noradrenaline (Jung *et al.*, 1979), glucose, insulin and serum triiodothyronine.

Mechanisms for an Elevated Energy Expenditure in Cancer

How does cancer override the normal adaptive mechanisms and produce a rise in the RMR? A number of mechanisms have been proposed.

Increased demand by the tumour

The tumour appears to ignore the adaptive and conservation mechanisms of the post-absorptive state at the expense of the host. Norton *et al.* (1980) studied substrate utilisation by a sarcoma of the limb in ten patients (five osteosarcoma and five soft tissue sarcoma) and compared this with substrate utilisation by the patient's other healthy limb. The tumour extracted five-fold more glucose than the control limb, and the amount extracted was proportional to the tumour size. The sarcomatous limb also released fewer amino acids, suggesting that they were being utilised in gluconeogenesis. They were also able to correlate the degree of glucose uptake by the tumorous limb with the amount of gluconeogenic amino acids in the arterial blood. This suggested that host muscle protein was being degraded and amino acids released to fuel gluconeogenesis. Others (Buzby *et al.*, 1980) have also shown in animal models that starvation increases depletion of the host without actually reducing tumour growth.

Substrate utilisation by the tumour could account for an increase in the host's RMR, but this is likely to be small. It has been calculated (Brennan, 1981) that only large tumours (above 1·4 kg) could consume such energy as to account for a 40% rise in the metabolic rate. Nevertheless, the tumour, in some way, alters the host's responses to varying energy input states, so that it receives energy and amino acids to fuel its growth. A hormonal influence has been proposed although no specific hormone has been identified. Recently, Brooks *et al.* (1981) have suggested that catecholamines may be elevated; this could account for the enhanced gluconeogenesis and possibly the impaired glucose tolerance and apparent insulin resistance of the host (Schein *et al.*, 1979).

Cori cycle

Others have searched for different reasons to explain the elevated energy expenditure in malignancy. Gold (1974) proposed that the increased rate of resynthesis of glucose in the liver from lactate (i.e. Cori cycle) produced by the tumour may enhance the host's energy expenditure. However, increased Cori cycle activity does not appear to account for a significant fraction of daily energy expenditure (Young, 1977), for if one assumes that 15% of the body's lactate is oxidised to carbon dioxide and water, and the rest is converted to glucose, then there is no need to supply ATP from external sources and hence no increase in energy expenditure.

Protein synthesis

Whole body protein synthesis approximates to 3–4 g per kilogram body weight per day or 200–300 g for a 70 kg subject. It has been estimated that 6 kJ (1·4 kcal) of energy is required to synthesise 1 g of protein. On this basis, protein turnover in the healthy adult would account for at least 25% of the RMR. In cancer patients, there does not appear to be any significant increase in protein synthesis or turnover (Norton *et al.*, 1980) to account for the raised RMR.

Futile cycles and ion pumping

Futile cycles are energy utilising pathways in which a reaction in one direction requires ATP while the reaction in the opposite direction is energetically spontaneous. Adenosine triphosphate is thus hydrolysed and energy wasted (*see* Fig. 4.1). This recycling may not be as wasteful as it appears if these cycles serve a role in metabolic regulation (Katz and Rognstad, 1976), and it is not thought likely that they could account for such energy wastage as to produce a 20–40% rise in the RMR.

Ion pumping to maintain electrochemical gradients requires energy but the amount of energy used has been disputed. Himms-Hagen (1976) and Clausen (1966) believe that energy utilised directly in sodium pumping is relatively small, possibly less than 10% of the RMR, and is unlikely to account for more than a small percentage of the rise in the RMR in cancerous patients.

Brown fat thermogenesis

Brown fat has been shown to be the tissue responsible in some animals for the thermogenesis associated with overfeeding and with cold adaptive thermogenesis. The mechanism responsible for the heat production appears to involve an uncoupling of oxidative phosphorylation with the production of heat from a proton shunting mechanism. A recent experiment (Brooks *et*

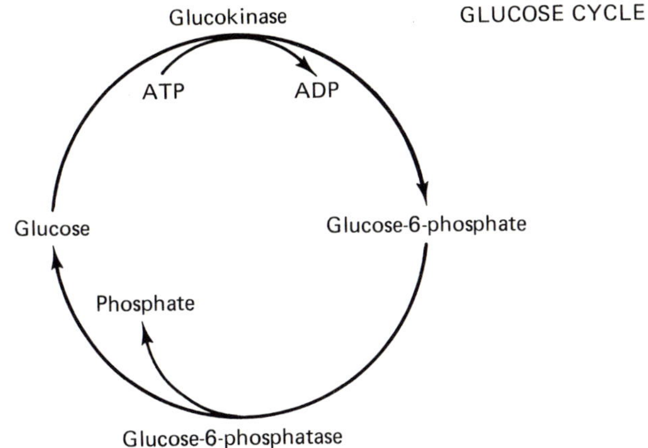

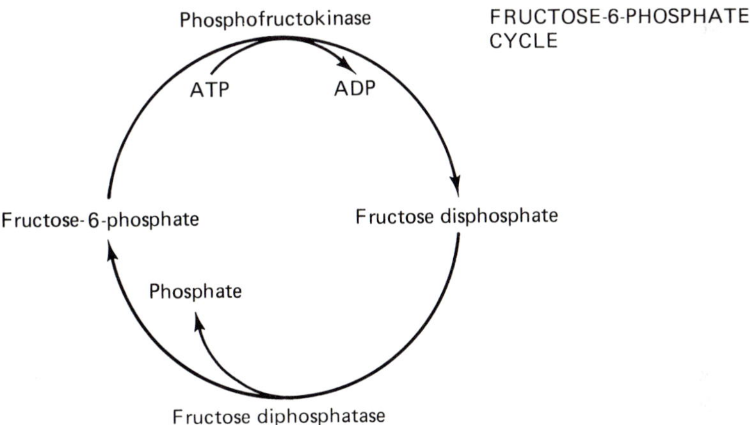

Fig. 4.1. *Two 'futile' cycles.*

al., 1981) involving the transplantation of human hypernephroma tissue into mice has shown that the mice lose about 40% of carcass weight and that this is associated with a 40% rise in metabolic rate. The rise in metabolic rate was blocked by a β-adrenergic blocking agent, indicating that it was catecholamine dependent. Injection of noradrenaline, a potent stimulator of non-shivering thermogenesis (NST), showed that NST was increased in the cancer-bearing animals. Although the total brown fat mass was not altered, guanosine diphosphate binding to brown adipose tissue mitochondria, an index of thermogenic capacity, was significantly increased in the tumour-bearing mice. This is a preliminary study but does suggest a possible role for brown fat thermogenesis in cancer cachexia. This awaits further study in man.

DOES HYPERALIMENTATION REVERSE THE NUTRITIONAL AND METABOLIC CONSEQUENCES OF CANCER?

The cancerous host shows profound metabolic consequences, namely, (a) defects in protein synthesis in the host's muscle (Lundholm *et al.*, 1976), and a negative nitrogen balance, (b) relative glucose intolerence by the host, (c) increase in lactic acid production (Holyroyde *et al.*, 1979), (d) enhanced gluconeogenesis from alanine, and (e) enhanced RMR.

The tumour itself has a higher protein synthesis rate than the host and a high energy utilisation rate, especially for glucose which is unaffected by adaptive changes secondary to the changes in the host's energy status. Hyperalimentation can reverse many of the abnormalities in the host. Hyperalimentation can increase the host's weight not just by fat accretion, but also by an increase in lean body mass as shown by an improvement in total body potassium and an increase in total body nitrogen turnover (Burt *et al.*, 1981). Gluconeogenesis is also suppressed by hyperalimentation, appetite is improved and a positive nitrogen balance can be achieved (Brennan, 1981). Reversal of anergy can occur with nutritional support alone (Daly *et al.*, 1980), although successful treatment of the tumour is often more effective.

DOES HYPERALIMENTATION STIMULATE TUMOUR GROWTH?

One criticism of parenteral and enteral feeding has been the suggestion that feeding the host also stimulates tumour growth. In animal models, it does appear that the tumour will grow more rapidly if nutritional support is provided in the absence of antineoplastic therapy. However, the growth of the tumour appears to maintain the usual ratio to the weight of the host and does not show an 'explosive' growth (Daly *et al.*, 1976). The type of food used to replete the animal may be important. Repletion of anorectic tumour-bearing mice by carbohydrates alone (Buzby *et al.*, 1980) neither improved the host nor stimulated tumour growth. Adequate amino acids alone improved host maintenance but also stimulated tumour growth. When carbohydrates and amino acids were given simultaneously the host improved but tumour growth was stimulated. However, repletion with isocaloric fat and isonitrogenous amino acids promoted the host, without tumour growth stimulation. This suggests that manipulation of the feed may have some value in the nutritional support of cancer patients, but this has yet to be shown.

The data for man does suggest that stimulation of tumour growth is not a regular finding with nutritional support. Copeland *et al.* (1979) could find no evidence of an increase of tumour growth in over 1000 patients given hyperalimentation. Shils (1979) has reported that in some patients tumour mass increased during hyperalimentation, but it was thought likely that the ratio of tumour mass to host weight remained constant. Such a stimulation of growth may, of course, have some benefit for therapy, since the actively dividing tumour is more likely to respond to radiation and chemotherapy than a slow growing tumour. It would seem prudent and possibly beneficial to combine nutritional support with anti-tumour therapy.

IS THE RESPONSE TO CANCER THERAPY IMPROVED BY ADJUNCT HYPERALIMENTATION?

The overall answer to this question appears to be in the negative. Serrou and his colleagues (1979), in a pilot study of 103 patients with advanced solid tumours, reported 'partial tumour responses' (no details were given) in 37% of patients receiving chemotherapy with nutritional support, compared to 10·5% in those receiving chemotherapy alone. Lanzotti *et al.* (1975) initially reported the results in 38 patients with bronchogenic carcinoma (oat cell excluded). The overall response rate, defined as a 50% or more reduction in tumour size, in those given nutritional support with chemotherapy was similar to those given chemotherapy alone. However, in those with a 'high' weight loss (i.e. greater than 6% loss in body weight), five out of ten patients given nutritional support responded to chemotherapy, as compared to a nil response in those given chemotherapy alone. An enlarged study by the same group (Lanzotti *et al.*, 1980) of 47 patients with non oat cell bronchogenic carcinoma also indicated no difference in survival in those given hyperalimentation with chemotherapy. Similarly, no significant difference in survival has been reported in prospective randomised studies of chemotherapy with or without nutritional support in lymphoma (Popp *et al.*, 1981), oat cell and squamous carcinoma of the lung (Issell *et al.*, 1978; Jordan *et al.*, 1981; Lanzotti *et al.*, 1980), metastatic colonic carcinoma (Nixon *et al.*, 1980), acute leukaemia (Coquin *et al.*, 1980), and sarcoma (Shamberger *et al.*, 1981).

The overall results of surgery for gastrointestinal tumours have generally shown no improvement with adjunct hyperalimentation (Moghissi *et al.*, 1977; Heatley *et al.*, 1979; Lim *et al.*, 1981), although one study did report a minimal benefit (Holter *et al.*, 1977). Similarly, with radiotherapy, survival times are not increased with nutritional support; this has been shown for pelvic (Valerio *et al.*, 1978), ovarian (Solassol and Joyeux, 1979) and other abdominal tumours (Bothe *et al.*, 1979) treated by radiotherapy.

DOES HYPERALIMENTATION REDUCE THE SIDE EFFECTS OF CANCER THERAPY?

The tolerance to chemotherapy, surgery and radiation has been studied with only a few reports of any improvement. Issell *et al.* (1978) in a study of 26 patients with squamous cell carcinoma of the lung treated by chemo-immunotherapy noted a significant decrease in nausea and vomiting in those given nutritional support. Jordan *et al.* (1981) also noted a minimal protection from the side effects of chemotherapy in those treated for adenocarcinoma of the lung with nutritional support. Studies of the effects of hyperalimentation in patients undergoing abdominal or pelvic radiotherapy have failed to show evidence that such patients could tolerate increased dosages (Valerio *et al.*, 1978). Some studies of the complications of surgery in oesophageal and gastric cancer have shown a decrease in patients receiving hyperalimentation (Heatley *et al.*, 1979; Lim *et al.*, 1981) who are adequately repleted. However, others have found no change in tolerance to chemotherapy, surgery or radiation, nor in operative mortality, morbidity, planned dose of chemotherapeutic agents or radiation, or haematopoietic toxicity (Holter and Fischer, 1977; Valerio *et al.*, 1978).

DOES HYPERALIMENTATION HAVE A ROLE IN PATIENTS WITH CANCER?

Its role appears to be as a nutritional support in the severely malnourished patient until he can recover from the side effects of antineoplastic therapy. Hyperalimentation will cure malnutrition, but not cancer. There is always the possibility that it may stimulate neoplastic growth, so it is prudent to combine it with active treatment of the cancer whether by surgery, radiation or chemotherapy.

HOW DOES ONE ASSESS THE PATIENT FOR SIGNS OF MALNUTRITION?

Table 4.3 summarises those tests which indicate the development of malnutrition. Weight can be a poor indicator of malnutrition, for if the patient has a low albumin, oedema can occur with weight increase. Mid-arm muscle circumference, or better still, muscle area, are the most useful indicators of nutritional depletion. Serum albumin is a slow reflector of nutritional status as it has a long half-life (several weeks). Transferrin is low in malnutrition but can be raised by a low iron status or severe infection.

TABLE 4.3

Evidence for Nutritional Depletion in a Patient with Cancer

Weight	
Recent weight loss	$> 10\%$
Body weight	$> 20\%$ below ideal
Fat reserves	
Triceps skinfold thickness (TST)	< 10 mm in males
	< 13 mm in females
Fat area (FA)	
$\left[\begin{array}{l} \text{FA} = \text{arm area} - \text{muscle area} \\ \text{Arm area} = \dfrac{\Pi}{4} \times \dfrac{(\text{arm circumference})}{\Pi} \end{array} \right]$	< 17 cm^2 in males
	< 30 cm^2 in females
Muscle Protein Reserves	
Mid-arm muscle circumference (MAMC)	< 25 cm in males
(MAMC = arm circumference = (TST))	< 20 cm in females
Muscle area (MA)	
$\text{MA} = \dfrac{\text{arm circumference} - \Pi(\text{TST})}{4\Pi}$	< 61 cm^2 in males
	< 38 cm^2 in females
Visceral protein reserves	
Serum albumin	< 35 g/litre
Serum albumin	< 1.7 g/litre
Thyroxine binding pre-albumin	< 25 mg/litre
Impaired immunology	
Lymphopenia	$< 1.2 \times 10^9$/litre
Skin allergy	
Vitamin and mineral depletion	
Vitamin C	Iron
Folate	Zinc
B$_{12}$	Calcium, Phosphate,
	Alkaline phosphatase
	Magnesium

Thyroxine binding pre-albumin (or retinol binding protein) is preferred as a measure of visceral protein reserves, for it responds rapidly to changes in the nutritional state because of its short half-life of 48 hours, is unchanged by iron status and does not increase with infections (Shetty *et al.*, 1979). Thyroxine binding pre-albumin is also useful to monitor whether nutritional repletion is adequate, for it rises some 10 to 14 days before the serum albumin begins to show an increase.

HOW DOES ONE DESIGN A SUITABLE NUTRITIONAL REGIMEN?

The oral route is to be preferred if the gastrointestinal tract is functional. If the patient's appetite is poor and supplementary feeds (e.g. Complan) are insufficient, then it may be necessary to feed via a thin bore tube inserted through the nostril, via the oesophagus into the stomach. This is comfortable for the patient who is able to eat normally if required. The feed is dripped continually through the tube over 24 hours. Diarrhoea can be prevented by a slow build up of the feed strength over 72 hours, and by the use of isotonic, lactose-free preparations.

If the gastrointestinal tract is impaired, needs to be rested, or the patient has nausea or vomiting, then parenteral nutrition will be required (Grant, 1980). This is best given via a subclavicular tunnelled catheter, inserted under aseptic conditions. Table 4.4 gives the general requirements for intravenous nutrition. Many centres are now able to mix all but the fat in a

TABLE 4.4

General Ground Rules Governing the Requirements for Parenteral Nutrition

1. Adequate hydration.
2. Correct PCV to 45% by giving blood or packed cells.
3. Keep serum albumin greater than 30 g/litre by giving albumin or plasma until nutritional repletion increases albumin synthesis.
4. Assess nitrogen requirements from 24-hour urinary urea and plasma urea rise. Minimum requirement is about 0·3 g nitrogen/kg ideal weight/24 h.
5. Give non-protein calories at kilocalories per nitrogen ratio of 150–200 to 1. Divide energy as equally fat and glucose. Do not use ethanol, sorbitol, fructose, or xylitol as an energy source.
6. Nitrogen and energy should be given together, for this results in a better nitrogen balance than that achieved when nitrogen and energy are given separately.
7. Give nutrition evenly over 24 hours.
8. Sodium as required; 50 mmol sodium per 24 hours plus additional requirements due to extra losses.
9. Chloride; about 100 mmol/24 h.
10. Potassium to nitrogen ratio of 5 mmol potassium per 1 g nitrogen.
11. Magnesium to nitrogen ratio of 0·5 mmol magnesium per 1 g nitrogen.
12. Phosphate given as 10 mmol per 1000 kcal (4·2 MJ) glucose or 1–2 mmol per gram nitrogen infused.
13. Calcium of about 5 mmol per 24 hours.
14. Essential fatty acids are necessary if no fat emulsion is used; 500 ml of 20% Intralipid twice per week.
15. Essential trace elements (e.g. one ampoule Addamel (KabiVitrum) per day).
16. Essential vitamins.

3 litre plastic bag made up in the pharmacy. Recently, KabiVitrum has indicated that Intralipid may also be added to their amino acid mixture, Vamin, in a 3 litre bag. Other centres utilise a Y-tube system, with the amino acids being given at the same time as the energy; the drip tubes are united near the catheter insertion.

There is much literature on ways of assessing nutritional requirements. Cancer patients can show marked variation in requirements from week to week, and so some easy way of roughly assessing requirement is necessary. One method involves the measurement of both the plasma urea and the 24-hour urine urea excretion. The requirements are calculated as follows:

$$\text{Urine nitrogen loss (g)} = \frac{\text{mmol urinary urea}/24\,\text{h}}{35 \cdot 7}$$

$$\text{Total nitrogen loss (g)} = \text{Urine nitrogen loss} + 2\,\text{g for insensible losses}$$

To promote anabolism, one adds on 2 or 3 g. So,

$$\text{Nitrogen input (g)} = \frac{\text{mmol urinary urea}/24\,\text{h}}{37 \cdot 5} + 5$$

For example, if urine urea is 357 mmol/24 h, then:

$$\text{Nitrogen input required} = \frac{357}{35 \cdot 7} + 5 = 15\,\text{g}$$

$$\text{Protein input (g)} = 6 \cdot 25 \times \text{nitrogen required (g)}$$

The requirement of non-protein energy can be calculated roughly as follows:

	Energy (kcal)	:	*Nitrogen (g)*
Non-catabolic or mild depletion	180	:	1
Catabolic or severe depletion	150	:	1
Severely hypercatabolic	120	:	1

If the patient is in renal failure and urea is rising then the rise in plasma urea over 24 hours is added to the nitrogen requirements. For example,

24-h urinary urea	= 357 mmol
9 a.m. plasma urea on Day 1	= 10 mmol
9 a.m. plasma urea on Day 2	= 13 mmol

Therefore:

$$\text{Nitrogen input (g)} = \frac{357}{35 \cdot 7} + 5 + (13 - 10)$$

$$\text{Nitrogen input} = 18\,\text{g}$$

$$\text{Protein input} = 18 \times 6 \cdot 25 = 112 \cdot 5\,\text{g}$$

The energy required at a ratio of 150 : 1 will be 2700 kcal, given as fat and carbohydrates of equal caloric ratio. Such a rise in plasma urea would necessitate dialysis if the above feed was given, but many consider this preferable to severe dietary restriction in the face of continuing catabolism.

The patient should be regularly monitored (e.g. electrolytes, thyroid binding, pre-albumin) to assess whether the nutritional support is adequate and, if not, should be re-assessed and adjusted.

REFERENCES

Bothe A. Jr., Valerio D., Bistrian B.R., Blackburn G.L. (1979). Randomised controlled trial of hospital nutritional support during abdominal radiotherapy. *Parent. Ent. Nut*; **3**: 292 (abstract).

Bozzetti F., Pagnoni A.M., Del Vecchio M. (1980). Excessive caloric expenditure as a cause of malnutrition in patients with cancer. *Sug. Gynaecol. Obst*; **150**: 229–34.

Brennan M.F. (1981). Total parenteral nutrition in the cancer patient. *N. Engl. J. Med*; **305**: 375–82.

Brooks S.L., Neville A.M., Rothwell N.J., Stock M.J., Wilson S. (1981). Sympathetic activation of brown adipose tissue thermogenesis in cachexia. *Biosci. Rep*; **1**: 509–17.

Burt M.E., Steen T.P., Schwade J.G., Brennan M.F. (1981). Effect of total parenteral nutrition on protein metabolism in man. *Am. J. Clin. Nut*; **34**: 628 (abstract).

Buzby G.P., Mullen J.L. Stein T.P., Miller E.E., Hobbs C.L., Rosato E.F. (1980). Host-tumour interaction and nutrient supply. *Cancer*; **45**: 2940–8.

Clausen T. (1966). The relationship between the transport of glucose and cations across cell membranes in isolated tissues. II Effects of K^+ free medium, ouabain and insulin upon the fate of glucose in rat diaphragm. *Biochim. Biophy. Acta*; **120**: 361–8.

Copeland E.M. III, Daly J.M., Ota D.M., Dudrick S.J. (1979). Nutrition, cancer and intravenous hyperalimentation. *Cancer*; **43**: 2108–16.

Coquin J.Y., Maraninchi D., Gastaut J.A., Carcassonne Y. (1980). Parenteral nutrition in chemotherapy of acute leukaemia: Preliminary results. *J. Parent. Ent. Nut*; **4**: 437 (abstract).

Daly J.M., Dudrick S.J., Copeland E.M. III (1980). Intravenous hyperalimentation: Effect on delayed cutaneous hypersensitivity in cancer patients. *Ann. Surg*; **192**: 587–92.

De Wys W.D. (1977). Anorexia in cancer patients. *Cancer Res*; **37**: 2354–8.

Gold J. (1974). Cancer cachexia and gluconeogenesis. *Ann. N. Y. Acad. Sci*; **230**: 103–10.

Grant J.P. (1980). *Handbook of Total Parenteral Nutrition*. New York: W.B. Saunders.

Heatley R.V., Williams R.H.P., Lewis M.H. (1979). Pre-operative intravenous feeding: A controlled trial. *Postgrad. Med. J*; **55**: 541–5.

Himms-Hagen J. (1976). Cellular thermogenesis. *Ann. Rev. Physiol*; **38**: 315–51.

Holter A.R., Fischer J.E. (1977). The effects of perioperative hyperalimentation on complications in patients with carcinoma and weight loss. *J. Surg. Res*; **23**: 31–4.

Holter A.R., Rosen H.M., Fischer J.E. (1977). The effect of hyperalimentation on major surgery in patients with malignant disease: A prospective study. *Acta Chir. Scand*; (Suppl.) **466**: 86–7.

Holyroyde C.P., Axelrod R.S., Skutches C.L., Haffac P.P., Reichard G.A. (1979). Lactate metabolism in patients with metastatic colorectal cancer. *Cancer Res*; **39**: 4900–4.

Issell B.F., Valdivieso M., Zaren H.A. *et al.* (1978). Protection against chemotherapy toxicity by IV hyperalimentation. *Cancer Treat. Rep*; **62**: 1139–43.

Jordan W.M., Valdivieso M., Frankmann C. *et al.* (1981). Treatment of advanced adenocarcinoma of the lung with florafier, doxorubicin, cyclophosphamide and cisplatin and intensive IV hyperalimentation. *Cancer Treat. Rep*; **65**: 197-205.

Jung R.T., Shetty P.S., Barrand M., Callingham B.A., James W.P.T. (1979). The role of catecholamines in the hypertensive response to dieting. *Br. Med. J*; **1**: 12–13.

Katz J. Rognstad R. (1976). Futile cycles in the metabolism of glucose. *Curr. Topics Cell. Reg*; **10**: 237–89.

Lanzotti V.J., Copeland E.M. III, George S.L., Dudrick S.J., Samuels M.L. (1975). Cancer chemotherapeutic response and intravenous hyperalimentation. *Cancer Chem. Rep*; Part 1, **59**: 437–9.

Lanzotti V.J., Copeland E.M. III, Bhuchar V., Wesley M., Corriere J., Dudrick S.J. (1980). A randomised trial of total parenteral nutrition with chemotherapy for non-oat cell lung cancer. *Proc. AACR, ASCO*; **21**: 337 (abstract).

Lim S.T.K., Choa R.G., Lam K.H., Wong J., Ong G.B. (1981). Total parenteral nutrition versus gastrostomy in the preoperative preparation of patients with carcinoma of the oesophagus. *Br. J. Surg*; **68**: 69–72.

Lundholm K., Bylund A.C., Holm J., Schersten T. (1976). Skeletal muscle metabolism in patients with malignant tumor. *Europ. J. Cancer*; **12**: 465–73.

Moghissi K., Hornshaw J., Teasdale P.R., Dawes E.A. (1977). Parenteral nutrition in carcinoma of the oesophagus treated by surgery: Nitrogen balance and clinical studies. *Br. J. Surg*; **64**: 125–8.

Nixon D., Moffitt S., Ansley J. *et al.* (1980). Central intravenous hyperalimentation as an adjunct to chemotherapy in advanced colon cancer. *Proc. AACR, ASCO*; **21**: 173 (abstract).

Norton J.A., Burt M.E., Brennan M.F. (1980). In vivo utilisation of substrate by human sarcoma-bearing limbs. *Cancer*; **45**: 2934–9.

Ohnuma T., Holland J.F. (1977). Nutritional consequences of cancer chemotherapy and immunotherapy. *Cancer Res*; **37**: 2395–406.

Popp M.B., Fisher R.I., Wesley R., Aamodt R., Brennan M.F. (1981). A prospective randomised study of adjuvant parenteral nutrition in the treatment of advanced diffuse lymphoma: Influence on survival. *Surgery*; **90**: 195–205.

Schein P.S., MacDonald J.S., Waters C. *et al.* (1975). Nutritional complications of cancer and its treatment. *Sem. Oncol*; **2**: 337–47.

Schein P.S., Kisner D., Haller D., Blecher M., Hamosh M. (1979). Cachexia of malignancy. Potential role of insulin in nutritional management. *Cancer*; **43** (Suppl.): 2070–6.

Serrou B., Joyeux H., Dubous J.B., Favier C., Solassol C. (1979). Pilot study of peripheral intravenous nutrition in patients bearing solid tumors. A simple and valuable adjunct to chemotherapy. *Proc. AACR, ASCO*; **20**: 305 (abstract).

Settle R.G., Quinn M.R., Brand J.G., Kare M.R., Mullen J.L., Brown R. (1979).

Gustatory evaluation of cancer patients. In *Nutrition and Cancer*. (Van Eys J., Seelig M.S., Nichols B., eds.) pp. 171–85. New York: Medical and Scientific Books.

Shamberger R.C., Brennan M.F., Goodgame J.T. Jr., Lowry S.F., Maher M.M., Pizzo P.A. (1981). Effect of total parenteral nutrition on metabolic parameters of patients undergoing ablative chemotherapy. *Proc. AACR, ASCO*; **22**: 420 (abstract).

Shetty P.S., Watrasiewicz K.E., Jung R.T., James W.P.T. (1979). Rapid turnover transport proteins: An index of subclinical protein-energy malnutrition. *Lancet*; **2**: 230–2.

Shils M.E. (1979). Principles of nutritional therapy. *Cancer*; **43**: 2093–102.

Smith F., Kisner D., Wideslite L., Schein P. (1979). Chemotherapeutic alteration of small intestinal morphology and function. *J. Clin. Gastro*; **1**: 203–7.

Solassol C., Joyeux H. (1979). Artificial gut with complete nutritive mixtures as a major adjuvant therapy in cancer patients. *Acta Chir. Scand.* (Suppl.); **494**: 186–7.

Valerio D., Overett L., Malcolm A., Blackburn G.L. (1978). Nutritional support for cancer patients receiving abdominal and pelvic radiotherapy: A randomised prospective clinical experiment of intravenous versus oral feeding. *Surg. Forum*; **29**: 145–8.

Warnold I., Lundholm K., Schersten T. (1978). Energy balance and body composition in cancer patients. *Cancer Res*; **38**: 1801–7.

Young V.R. (1977). Energy metabolism and requirements in the cancer patients. *Cancer Res*; **37**: 2336–47.

Chapter 5

Adrian J. L. Clark

Glucose Homeostasis

INTRODUCTION

The maintenance of a normal blood glucose is arguably the most sophisticated homeostatic mechanism in man (calcium homeostasis being a close rival). When such a system breaks down, as it may often do in patients with neoplasia, it implies a fairly serious disruption of one or more of the controlling factors. The neoplastic cell may show a number of abnormalities in the way it handles glucose. Intriguingly, several of these abnormalities may be common to tumours associated with hyperglycaemia and those associated with hypoglycaemia.

In the normal peripheral cell, glucose enters under the influence of insulin, and is rapidly phosphorylated by the action of hexokinase, before being metabolised in one of several ways. Much will be converted to pyruvate by glycolysis, involving the production of six high energy ATP molecules from ADP and inorganic phosphate, for every molecule of glucose. In the healthy cell a great deal of this pyruvate will now be fully oxidised via the Krebs cycle, producing 30 ATP molecules per molecule of glucose.

The evidence suggests that neoplastic cells may differ in several ways:

The Cell Wall

Venuta and Rubin (1973) demonstrated that glucose influx increased markedly following the transformation of chick embryo fibroblasts by Rous sarcoma virus. Similar findings were reported by Hatanaka (1974), and it was suggested that glucose entry to the neoplastic cell was down a concentration gradient, rather than specifically in response to insulin. Since glucose is rapidly 'removed' on the intracellular side by phosphorylation, this change would result in very high rates of glucose influx.

Glycolysis

Warburg (1930) demonstrated a markedly increased rate of glycolysis in tumour cells despite adequate oxygen availability—an observation later to be known as the 'Warburg effect'. Enhanced glycolysis is normally only seen in anaerobic conditions in which the Krebs cycle cannot function adequately. The mechanism by which the 'Warburg effect' is initiated is not clear. It has been suggested that an increased growth rate, or increased cell density, is responsible. This latter explanation now seems to be the most probable (Bissell *et al.*, 1972). The functional significance of accelerated glycolysis is seen by some as an adaptation of the neoplastic cell for later life, when anaerobic conditions may prevail (Levin and Gevers, 1981).

Lactate Accumulation

As a result of excessive glycolysis, NADH accumulates, upsetting the normal balance of NADH/NAD. This occurrence in any cell, neoplastic or not, will favour the reduction of pyruvate to lactate, with the accompanying oxidation of NADH back to NAD. Unless an early reversal of this situation occurs, lactate accumulates and re-enters the circulation, often with some increase in plasma levels.

These then are abnormalities of the neoplastic cell. An intact mechanism for glucose homeostasis should rarely, if ever, be troubled by these events. This implies that disturbances of glucose homeostasis involve other tissues and their regulating mechanisms, which will now be discussed under the general headings of hyperglycaemia and hypoglycaemia.

HYPERGLYCAEMIA

Prevalence

Glucose intolerance in association with malignant disease was first described in 1885 (Freund, 1885). The occurrence of an abnormal glucose tolerance test in cancer was subsequently found to be so commonplace that it was even suggested that it might be a suitable screening test for malignant disease. Treatment of the malignant lesion was shown to result in improvement in glucose tolerance (Slosse and Reding, 1927), implying that the abnormality was the result of the malignant lesion. Others suggested that the finding of abnormal glucose tolerance imparts a worse prognosis for treatment of the tumour (Jackson, 1929). Needless to say, many of these early studies are open to criticism. In a large and carefully controlled study, Glicksman and Rawson (1956) confirmed the high frequency of abnormal glucose tolerance in 950 patients with both benign and malignant lesions. Their findings, shown in summary form in Table 5.1, suggest a prevalence of glucose intolerance of 36·7% in patients with malignant lesions, and 9·3% in those with benign tumours. Other groups studying smaller numbers reached similar conclusions.

TABLE 5.1

Frequency of the Finding of Glucose Intolerance with Various Tumours

	Malignant tumours		Benign tumours	
	Abnormal GTT (%)	*Number studied*	*Abnormal GTT (%)*	*Number studied*
All	36.7	628	9.3	322
Respiratory system	35.7	84	10.0	30
Skin/soft tissues/bone	35.5	74	5.1	39
Gastrointestinal tract	36.1	178	17.5	40
Genito-urinary/ gynaecological	35.0	120	7.7	104
Lymphoma/leukaemia	44.0	50	—	—
Breast	35.0	100	—	—

The table shows the prevalence of glucose intolerance during an oral glucose tolerance test in 950 patients with various benign and malignant tumours (based on Glicksman and Rawson, 1956). The glucose load given was 1·75 g/kg body weight, and the criteria for definition of abnormal glucose tolerance were *all three* of: (1) one value greater than 11 mmol/litre, (2) a 2-hour value greater than 5·6 mmol/litre, and (3) a 3-hour value greater than the fasting glucose level.

Aetiology

Most cases of hyperglycaemia in association with malignant disease are not the result of specific endocrine syndromes, and are not associated with pancreatic tumours. They are however characterised by certain features; these are described below.

The Cori cycle

Excessive lactate produced by cancer cells (as already described) cannot be further metabolised at that site. Gluconeogenesis takes place in the liver, and to a lesser extent in the kidney, the rate of flux being determined mainly by substrate supply (e.g. lactate, alanine, glycerol) and the prevailing insulin level; low levels promoting gluconeogenesis. Lactate, produced in excess by neoplastic cells, therefore supports increased gluconeogenesis and thus increases hepatic glucose output. This situation is represented diagrammatically in Fig. 5.1. This glucose/lactate/glucose cycle is known as the Cori cycle.

Holroyde *et al.* (1975) and Waterhouse (1974) have demonstrated, in sophisticated studies, that the rate of gluconeogenesis is markedly increased in patients with malignant neoplasia *and* weight loss. For every molecule of glucose cycled once around the Cori cycle, four ATP molecules are lost (since six are used in gluconeogenesis), and it has been suggested that this

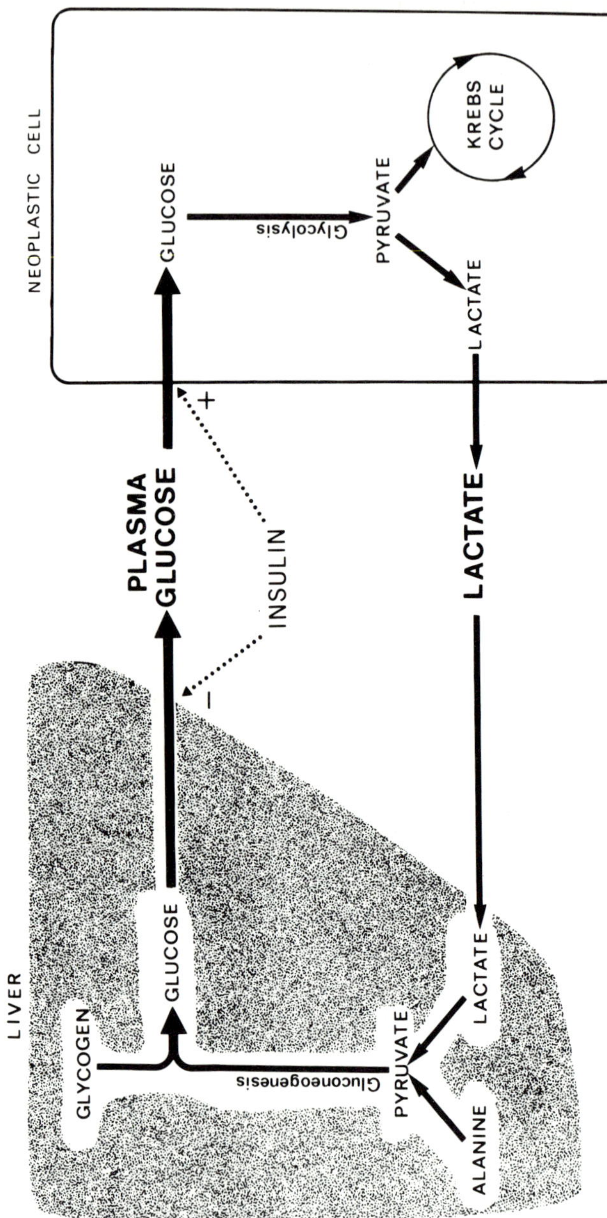

Fig. 5.1. *The Cori cycle. Insulin will both inhibit hepatic glucose output, and stimulate uptake of glucose into most types of peripheral cell. Glucose entry to neoplastic cells is less dependent on insulin than normal cells.*

energy wasting situation contributes to the cachexia of cancer. Stein (1978) has argued that amino acids may also play a part in enhanced gluconeogenesis. Neoplastic cells may selectively trap certain amino acids, in order to meet specific metabolic needs. This process could result in an incomplete complement of amino acids being available for normal functions (e.g. protein synthesis in muscle), causing weight loss and an increased supply of gluconeogenic amino acids (e.g. alanine) to the liver. Nevertheless, it remains difficult to see how enhanced Cori cycling can lead to hyperglycaemia. An imperfect analogy is that of the bathtub, with taps running and plug out. In normal circumstances the taps run slowly, and no water accumulates. If the taps are now turned on more forcefully, *and* the plughole is enlarged (as happens with excessive Cori cycling) still no water accumulates. In these circumstances an event which now turns the taps full on *and* partially blocks the plughole causes the bath to fill up and overflow. This critical event (as can be seen from Fig. 5.1) must be either deficient insulin secretion, or inadequate action (insulin resistance). Can such defects be identified?

Impairment of insulin secretion

Jasani *et al.* (1978) examined the plasma insulin response to glucagon in patients with cancer (with and without cachexia), and in control subjects; a clearly insufficient insulin response was demonstrated only in those patients with weight loss. They also noted that this group were hypoalbuminaemic, and proposed that protein deficiency was a cause of the inadequate insulin response. It has been shown both in animals (Weinkove *et al.*, 1976) and man (Smith *et al.*, 1975) that malnutrition is accompanied by decreased insulin responsiveness to various stimuli. Schein *et al.* (1979) also report a slightly impaired insulin response during an oral glucose tolerance test in patients with malignant disease and weight loss.

Multiple factors regulate insulin release. Of particular note in the present context are somatostatin, the α-adrenergic effects of adrenaline and noradrenaline, serotonin and prostaglandin E, all of which inhibit insulin release. Whilst several groups have searched for and failed to find abnormal somatostatin concentrations in patients with malignant disease, the possible role of these other β-cell inhibitors is not clear.

Insulin resistance

Bishop and Marks (1959) reported that the fall in blood glucose in response to an intravenous injection of insulin was significantly smaller in a group of patients with carcinoma, lymphoma or leukaemia than in age-matched controls. Schein *et al.* (1979) produced similar results during a continuous intravenous insulin infusion, although *in vitro* measurement of insulin receptors on mononuclear cells from these same patients were normal. Free fatty acid uptake is a sensitive indicator of peripheral insulin effect, but no abnormality of fatty acid uptake was found in this group. These rather perplexing results suggest a selective resistance to glucose uptake in response to insulin. However, in the presence of excessive gluconeogenesis, caution should be exercised in their interpretation. It should be possible using modern glucose 'clamp' techniques with radio-labelled substrate infusions to determine if insulin resistance does exist.

In summary, it seems clear that excessive Cori cycle activity exists in patients with malignant disease. This would allow amplification of defects in insulin secretion or action, which otherwise might appear insignificant. Whether these defects are the result of neoplasia itself, of weight loss, or coexist by chance, is not yet clear. The techniques now exist for determining the answers to these questions.

Hyperglycaemia following Neoplastic Involvement of the Pancreas

A close association between carcinoma of the pancreas and diabetes has long been recognised. Although difficult to demonstrate conclusively, it seems unlikely that diabetes is an aetiological factor in the genesis of carcinoma of the pancreas. Animal studies in which pancreatic cancer is induced by nitrosamine administration suggest that diabetes is secondary to the tumour.

Schwartz *et al.* (1978) undertook a prospective controlled study of hyperglycaemia following pancreatic cancer, and found an incidence of 81% in 32 patients. This is well above the frequency that would be expected from the hyperglycaemia associated with malignancy described above. In this study, insulin, C-peptide and glucagon levels during a glucose tolerance test were measured. It was found that this syndrome was characterised by impaired insulin release. This might have resulted from B-cell destruction, although it is probable that 80–90% of the B-cell mass would have to be lost before diabetes resulted, signifying a very extensive tumour. Glucagon did not differ between the pancreatic cancer and control group; this would appear to argue against simple pancreatic destruction, and in favour of disturbance in the subtle processes governing insulin release from the B-cell. Elevated levels of somatostatin—a peptide that is known to inhibit insulin secretion—have not been demonstrated in this condition.

Miscellaneous

Several tumours of endocrine tissue produce clinical syndromes which may include hyperglycaemia, e.g. Cushing's syndrome, acromegaly, the glucagonoma syndrome; but these will not be discussed further here.

Treatment of malignant disease may by itself produce hyperglycaemia as a result of the use of drugs such as steroids (glucocorticoids and anabolic steroids) which induce resistance to the action of insulin, L-asparaginase (which may also be associated with a haemorrhagic pancreatitis), and cyclophosphamide in diabetic patients, which has been reported to interfere with sulphonylurea metabolism.

Pancreatic resection (e.g. for carcinoma of the pancreas) may produce an insulin-dependent diabetes, depending on the extent of the resection.

Investigation

For practical purposes the investigation of hyperglycaemia is of importance mainly in the choice of hypoglycaemic treatment, and thus may be confined to a fasting blood glucose, and perhaps a glucose tolerance test. Although hyperglycaemia may improve with treatment of the neoplasm, it provides a poor marker of disease progress because of its dependence on several variables. Factors such as the lactate production rate might provide a more useful disease marker, but this would require systematic evaluation.

Management

The aims of treatment of diabetes when *not* associated with malignant disease can be stated as follows:

a) To maintain the patient free of symptoms, e.g. polyuria, polydipsia, malaise and infection.
b) To maintain as near normal metabolic control as possible in order to limit the risk of later development of the renal, retinal and vascular complications of diabetes.

In hyperglycaemia associated with malignant disease, only the first of these treatments aims usually need apply, since complications of diabetes take 10–20 years to develop. To this end, diet, sulphonylurea drugs and occasionally insulin may be used.

Dietary therapy should probably not be pursued with great zeal in view of the possible co-existence of weight loss and anorexia. High fibre diets may improve glucose tolerance to the extent that hyperglycaemic symptoms disappear, but may be inappropriate when diarrhoea or frequency of bowel movements are the result of neoplasia, or its surgical treatment. Sulphonyl-urea therapy (e.g. chlorpropamide, glibenclamide) are usually well tolerated in the presence of malignant disease. Excessive dosage that might result in hypoglycaemia, particularly if meals are sometimes missed as a result of ill health, should be avoided. If maintaining regular food intake is a problem, it may be valuable to use one of the shorter acting sulphonylureas (e.g. gliquidone) which can be taken with each meal.

Biguanides (e.g. metformin) are probably best avoided. As has been discussed, hyperlactataemia already exists in many patients with this syndrome. Biguanide therapy will interfere with hepatic utilisation of lactate (contributing to an improvement in hyperglycaemia), with the result that lactate will accumulate in the circulation, and may lead to lactic acidosis. This effect is well recognised with phenformin, but may also occur with metformin.

Insulin therapy is only infrequently required in treating diabetes associated with malignant disease, but may be needed in subjects with pre-existing diabetes, following pancreatic infiltration by tumour, or after surgical pancreatectomy. In the first situation, control of symptoms can usually be obtained with a once daily injection of a medium–long acting insulin (e.g. Lente or Monotard insulin). As with once daily sulphonylurea therapy, care should be taken to ensure that adequate meals are taken. If this is not possible it is probable that the patient will still need some insulin, although perhaps in reduced dosage. In order to judge this, some form of diabetes monitoring will be required, and for most purposes in this situation, urine testing for glucose will suffice. For the hospital patient, measurement of the venous or capillary blood glucose gives information that is easier to interpret, and some patients may prefer to use capillary blood glucose measurements at home.

Similar insulin regimens to those described above may be effective in patients with a non-functioning pancreas—either due to tumour invasion or surgical removal. It is sometimes argued that these patients have an inadequate glucagon response to hypoglycaemia, and hence that long acting insulin regimens are undesirable because of the risk of serious nocturnal hypoglycaemia. Twice daily insulin regimens may therefore be more suitable, e.g. using an injection of soluble and isophane insulin in the morning, with soluble alone, or soluble and a small dose of isophane insulin in the evening. With all patients treated in this way, the physician should be ready to adapt the insulin regimen, perhaps at frequent intervals, as the disease progresses or regresses with treatment.

HYPOGLYCAEMIA

Hypoglycaemia is a much less frequent association with malignant disease than hyperglycaemia, but is inevitably more dangerous. All of the causes of hypoglycaemia shown in Table 5.2 may occur coincidentally in patients with malignant disease, and these are reviewed in detail elsewhere (Marks and Rose, 1981). The investigation of hypoglycaemia is discussed later in this chapter; the demonstration of hypoglycaemia with inappropriate hyper-

TABLE 5.2

Causes of Hypoglycaemia other than that Associated with Tumours (For a detailed discussion see Marks and Rose (1981))

Congenital:
  Glycogen storage disease
  Fructose intolerance
  Galactosaemia
Acquired:

Endocrine causes	*Drugs/poisons:*
Insulinoma	Insulin
Carcinoid syndrome	Sulphonylureas
Hypopituitarism	Biguanides
Adrenal insufficiency	Alcohol
Neonatal nesidioblastosis	Salicylates
Secondary to other disease	Barbiturates
Liver disease	Tryptophan
Pancreatitis	Monoamine oxidase inhibitors
Others	Propanalol
Exercise	
Starvation	
Reactive hypoglycaemia	

insulinaemia is indicative of sulphonylurea or insulin use or abuse, or of an insulinoma (or very rarely a carcinoid tumour).

Tumour-Associated Hypoglycaemia (TAH)

Hypoglycaemia associated with malignant disease is a condition that has been recognised for over 50 years, and has been associated with virtually

TABLE 5.3

Tumour Types Associated with Hypoglycaemia

Fibrosarcoma	26%
Hepatoma	16%
Carcinoma (all types)	16%
Mesothelioma	10%
Lymphoma (including Hodgkin's disease)	6%
Haemangiopericytoma	4%
Leiomyosarcoma	3%
Others	19%

The table shows the frequency of the association of various tumour types with the hypoglycaemic syndrome, and is based on a survey of 292 reports in the literature.

every type of tumour histology. Nevertheless, the cause remains unclear in most cases. A survey of 292 published cases suggests mesenchymal tumours, hepatoma and carcinoma are the most commonly associated tumours (*see* Table 5.3). Inevitably, this type of survey cannot give a true indication of the frequency of the association with any tumour type. Of interest, however, is the high position in this 'league table', occupied by the relatively rare haemangiopericytoma.

Aetiology

In any situation, hypoglycaemia will only occur if glucose disposal exceeds hepatic glucose output. It might, therefore, seen remarkably simple to identify the causes of TAH, but this has not been the case. It is still frequently taught that TAH results from excessive consumption of glucose by tumour tissue. This is almost certainly a misleading oversimplification, and therefore will be discussed first.

Excessive consumption of glucose by tumour

This subject was well reviewed by Unger (1966), and there has been little evidence since then to cause revision of his view that this abnormality *alone* would be an exceedingly rare cause of TAH. This is based on the knowledge that, the calculated glucose consumption rate for a number of very large tumours associated with the hypoglycaemia syndrome is not adequate or, at best, is barely adequate, to exceed a normal maximal hepatic glucose output. It is not disputed that many tumours do consume glucose excessively for reasons discussed at the beginning of this chapter (deficient cell wall barrier and accelerated glycolysis), but if hypoglycaemia is to occur one must postulate a co-existent hepatic defect. In the next four sections we shall examine the possibilities—that the liver has been damaged by metastases, that the inhibition of hepatic glucose output by insulin, or insulin-like growth factors is involved, and finally that some other abnormality of hepatic metabolism is responsible.

Hepatic destruction by metastases

This cannot clearly be a universal explanation for TAH since many cases of the syndrome without hepatic metastases have been described. Moreover, hepatic destruction would have to be extensive—major surgical resection of the liver (e.g. for trauma) is not usually associated with hypoglycaemia. The finding that many patients with TAH and extensive liver metastases do respond (if only partially) to glucagon injection as a therapeutic measure also argues against this. Impaired liver function and diminished glycogen storage may however contribute to other factors in this syndrome.

Ectopic insulin secretion

A number of ectopic hormone syndromes are distinct clinical and pathological entities. A very reasonable explanation for TAH might be the ectopic secretion of insulin by a tumour. With the exception of carcinoid tumours however it is very doubtful that this ever occurs. In nearly all cases of TAH, plasma insulin levels are appropriately low—a diagnostically useful point. Skrabanek and Powell (1978) reviewed 120 cases of TAH and considered especially the seven with inappropriately elevated insulin levels. Three of these cases were probably carcinoid tumours, one had a coincidental islet-cell adenoma, and one had metastases in the pancreas. Neither of the two remaining cases with fibrosarcoma came to autopsy, and there may possibly have been a separate islet-cell adenoma in these cases. Ectopic insulin secretion does not therefore appear to be a real entity—which is perhaps surprising in itself. Rees *et al.* (1974) described a bronchial tumour releasing multiple hormones including insulin, but which was not associated with hypoglycaemia.

Insulin-like growth factors

Long before the advent of the radioimmunoassay for insulin, it was realised that the bio-assayable insulin-like activity of normal plasma could not be entirely explained by insulin itself. The addition of antibodies raised against insulin to a serum sample only suppressed the insulin-like activity to a small extent. The remaining activity was named the non-suppressible insulin-like activity (NSILA). Non-suppressible insulin-like activity could be shown to consist of several substances covering a range of molecular weights. Very little is known about most of the NSILA, but two peptides have now been well characterised and sequenced (Rinderknecht and Humbel, 1978). These are known as the insulin-like growth factors (IGF I and II), having molecular weights of about 7500, and showing considerable structural homogeneity with pro-insulin (*see* Fig. 5.2).

Insulin-like growth factors are potent growth stimulating peptides, but have only a fraction of the metabolic potency of insulin (*see* Fig. 5.3). It has been suggested that secretion of IGFs from tumour tissue might account for some cases of the TAH syndrome. In several of the published reports of this condition, raised insulin-like activity of the plasma has been reported (*see* Skrabanek and Powell, 1978) in the presence of low insulin levels as detected by radioimmunoassay. One laboratory, using a radioreceptor assay believed to measure IGF II, has consistently been able to identify elevations of this substance in about 40% of patients with TAH (Megyesi, 1974; Kahn, 1980; Gorden *et al.*, 1981). Others dispute this (Widmer *et al.*, 1982) and show that neither IGF I or II are elevated when measured by a radioimmuno-assay. It may be that an as yet undiscovered peptide is responsible for these

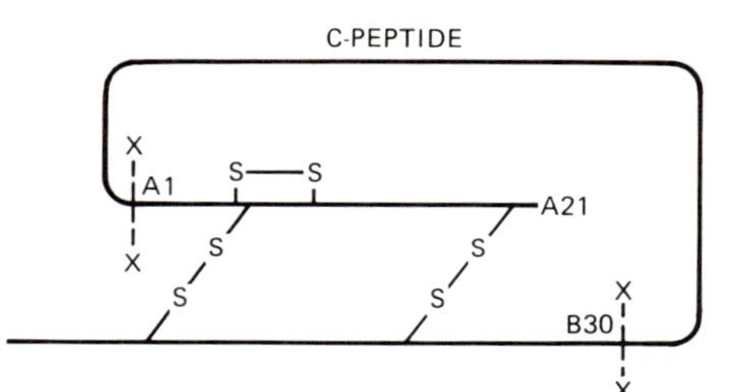

Fig. 5.2.   *Primary and secondary structures of human pro-insulin and insulin-like growth factors I and II(IGF I and II) . The primary structure of all three peptides is shown in the upper half of the figure, with shaded areas representing regions of sequence homology. Whilst there is extensive similarity in the A and B chain regions, the C chain differs markedly. The pro-insulin C-peptide(lower part of figure) is excised enzymatically at the points marked X–X in the B-cell, before secretion in equimolar quantities with insulin. C-peptide has a longer half-life in the circulation than insulin, and no known physiological function.*

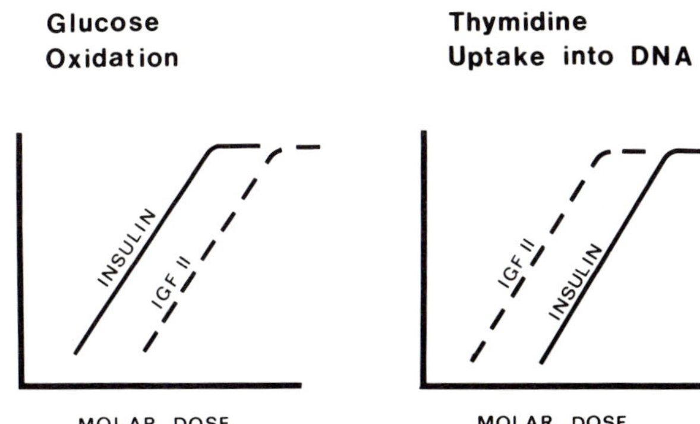

Fig. 5.3. *Dose–response curves of insulin and IGF II with respect to metabolic functions (e.g. glucose oxidation) and growth-promoting functions (e.g. ^3H thymidine uptake into DNA).*

findings, having the receptor stimulating properties of IGF II, but no immunological cross-reactivity. Synthesis and secretion of IGFs by tumour tissue has not yet been demonstrated.

It seems that we shall have to await further dissection of the NSILA fraction of serum before further conclusions on the role of these substances in TAH can be drawn.

Abnormalities of hepatic regulation

In healthy subjects the exogenous administration of glucagon or adrenaline stimulates glycogenolysis and gluconeogenesis in the liver, resulting in a rise in plasma glucose. Frequently, when this response has been examined in patients with TAH, it has been found to be inadequate. Further evidence for deficient gluconeogenesis comes from the occasional finding of elevated lactate levels—which should normally be taken up from the circulation by the liver. It might, therefore, seem reasonable to postulate that the excess or deficiency of some regulating metabolite, co-factor, or hormone, could account for the failure of hepatic glucose output. Tryptophan in excess will inhibit phosphoenolpyruvate carboxykinase (an important step in gluconeogenesis); excess has been demonstrated in some cases of TAH (Silverstein *et al.*, 1966). Deficient glucagon release in response to hypoglycaemia has also been demonstrated in some cases (Silbert *et al.*, 1976), and would account for impaired gluconeogenesis. The search for any factor inhibiting glucagon release (e.g. excess somatostatin) has not been fruitful.

Although the causes of TAH are less well defined at present than tumour hyperglycaemia, it seems probable that most cases must involve some degree of glucose overconsumption by the tumour, *and* some failure of hepatic glucose output. The next few years should see an answer to the difficult question of the role of IGFs.

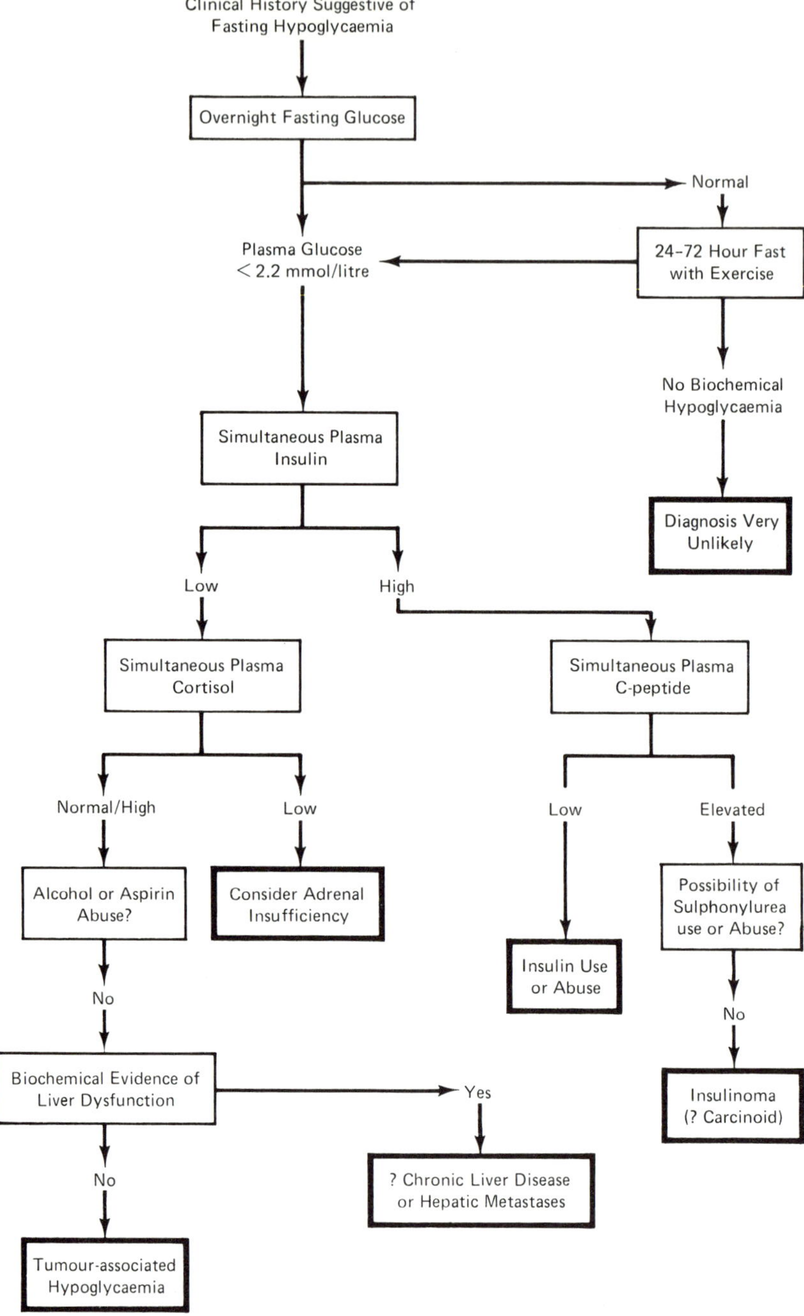

Fig. 5.4. *A scheme of investigation of hypoglycaemia in adult patients with neoplastic disease. See text and references for discussion.*

Investigation

Hypoglycaemia associated with malignant disease produces symptoms that closely resemble those of any other type of hypoglycaemia. The time from the first symptoms of hypoglycaemia to diagnosis of this complication is often shorter than for other causes of the condition. The possibility of hypoglycaemia should always be considered in any patient with malignant disease who exhibits episodes of strange behaviour, or lapses in consciousness. Such events may often be mistakenly attributed to cerebral metastases or general ill-health.

Once hypoglycaemia is suspected, a more precise diagnosis is dependent on taking a blood sample during an episode of hypoglycaemia (i.e. a venous blood glucose of less than 2.2 mmol/litre). To this end, it may be necessary to fast the patient for up to 72 hours with occasional periods of exercise. If hypoglycaemia does not develop during this time, the diagnosis is very unlikely. In the event of hypoglycaemia occurring, additional blood samples should be taken for insulin, C-peptide, sulphonylurea levels (if available) and cortisol. The flow diagram (Fig. 5.4) demonstrates the way these results can be used to make a precise diagnosis in adult patients with neoplastic disease. The further investigation of insulinoma is discussed in the section on this condition.

Management

Clinical symptoms and signs of hypoglycaemia associated with malignant disease are essentially the same as those of hypoglycaemia resulting from any other cause. Treatment of the individual attack with oral carbohydrate, intravenous glucose or glucagon injection is effective. The long-term prevention of hypoglycaemia is more difficult. Complete surgical removal of the tumour is the preferred treatment, but this is often not possible. Nevertheless, removal of the bulk of the tumour and its metastases (including those in the liver) often prevents hypoglycaemia recurring. Both chemotherapy and radiotherapy to the tumour will reduce the risk of hypoglycaemia.

If treatment of the tumour in this way fails, or is not warranted, patients can often be maintained in normoglycaemia with a combination of frequent meals and glucose-containing drinks together with glucagon injections. Glucagon (1 mg i.m.) at bedtime is often useful in preventing nocturnal hypoglycaemia, and works in most cases, supporting the suggestion that gluconeogenesis is inadequate. Glucagon may have unpleasant cardiovascular effects, and is sometimes accompanied by late reactive hypoglycaemia, resulting from its effect in stimulating insulin secretion. Other drugs have been used with less success; glucocorticoids are probably the most effective of this group. Growth hormone and diazoxide are occasionally helpful.

Streptozotocin, which may be useful in treating insulinoma, usually has no beneficial effect in hypoglycaemia resulting from malignant disease.

OTHER CAUSES OF HYPOGLYCAEMIA

Insulinoma

Insulinoma tissue has the histological appearance of a mass of B-cells, and can be shown to store and secrete insulin and C-peptide (*see* Fig. 5.2). Ten to twenty per cent of cases are malignant, in which case metastases are usually found in the liver. Patients with benign insulinomas often present with a long history (sometimes several years) of psychiatric or neurological symptoms. Symptoms of hypoglycaemia, either on exercise or whilst fasting are characteristic. Weight gain may also be a feature.

Treatment is ideally by surgical resection of the tumour. There is debate about the value of pre-operative localisation (e.g. with arteriography, trans-hepatic portal venography, CT scanning or ultrasound), and must depend to a great extent on the local expertise. Intra-operative localisation of insulinomas is also dependent on the skill of the surgeon and is facilitated to some extent by the knowledge that many tumours appear darker than surrounding tissues as a result of their greater vascularity. It is useful to try to confirm the histology of any putative insulinoma on frozen section. If a tumour cannot be identified pre- or intra-operatively, either a distal (partial) pancreatectomy may be undertaken, or one can opt for medical treatment with diazoxide and a thiazide diuretic. In the case of an inoperable malignant insulinoma, streptozoticin treatment is often very effective.

Carcinoid Tumours

Carcinoid tumours secreting insulin may also present with hypoglycaemia, although often the carcinoid syndrome is also present. Such tumours are probably the only true cases of ectopic insulin secretion.

Post-Gastrectomy Reactive Hypoglycaemia

This strange condition is more commonly recognised as a complication of gastric surgery for peptic ulcer disease, although it can occur after gastrectomy or gastro-jejunostomy for treatment or palliation of carcinoma of the stomach. Symptoms are of reactive hypoglycaemia, 2–3 hours after meals, and diagnosis may be made following a 4–6 hour oral glucose tolerance test.

Attempts at surgical correction of the condition are often inappropriate. High fibre diets are probably the treatment of choice.

SUMMARY

Abnormalities of glucose homeostasis give several fascinating insights into metabolism in general, and the metabolism of neoplastic tissue in particular. It may yet be possible that a useful marker of progress of malignant disease could be identified.

Several areas of knowledge are incomplete however, and a number of recently devised metabolic investigative techniques could be usefully applied in this area of cancer research.

REFERENCES

Bishop J.S., Marks P.A. (1959). Studies on carbohydrate metabolism in patients with neoplastic disease II. Response to insulin administration. *J. Clin. Invest*; **38**: 668–72.

Bissell M.J., Hatie C., Rubin H. (1972). Patterns of glucose metabolism in normal and virus-transformed chick cells in tissue culture. *J. Natl. Cancer Institute*; **49**: 555–65.

Freund E. (1885). Zur diagnose des Carcinoms. *Wien Med. Bull*; **8**: 268–9.

Glicksman A. S., Rawson R. W. (1956). Diabetes and altered carbohydrate metabolism in patients with cancer. *Cancer*; **9**: 1127–34.

Gorden P., Hendricks C. M., Kahn C. R., Megyesi K., Roth J. (1981). Hypoglycaemia associated with non-islet cell tumour and insulin-like growth factors. A study of the tumour types. *N. Engl. J. Med*; **305**: 1452–5.

Hatanaka M. (1974). Transport of sugars in tumour cell membranes. *Biochim. biophys. acta*; **355**: 77–104.

Holyroyde C.P., Gabuzda T.G., Putnam R. C., Paul P., Reichard G.A. (1975). Altered glucose metabolism in metastatic carcinoma. *Cancer Res*; **35**: 3710–14.

Jackson D. (1929). Carbohydrate metabolism in cancer. *Texas State J. Med*; **24**: 622–9.

Jasani B., Donaldson L.J., Ratcliffe J.G., Sakhi G.S. (1978). Mechanism of impaired glucose tolerance in patients with neoplasia. *Brit. J. Cancer*; **38**: 287–91.

Kahn C.R. (1980). The riddle of tumour hypoglycaemia revisited. *Clinics Endocrinol. Metabol*; **9**: 335–60.

Levin L., Gevers W. (1981). Metabolic alterations in cancer: Carbohydrate metabolism. *S. Afr. med. J.*; **59**: 518–21.

Marks V., Rose F.C. (1981). *Hypoglycaemia*, 2nd edn. London: Blackwell Scientific Publications.

Megyesi K., Kahn C.R., Roth J., Gorden P. (1974). Hypoglycaemia in association with extrapancreatic tumours: Demonstration of elevated plasma NSILA-s by a new radioreceptor assay. *J. Clin. Endocrinol. Metab*; **38**: 931–4.

Rees L.H., Bloomfield G.A., Rees G. M., Corrin B., Franks L.M., Ratcliffe J.G. (1974). Multiple hormones in a bronchial tumour. *J. Clin. Endocrinol. Metab*; **38**: 1090–97.

Rinderknecht E., Humbel R. E. (1978). Primary structure of human insulin-like growth factor II. *FEBS Letters*; **89**: 283–6.

Schein P.S., Kisner D., Haller D., Blecher M., Hamash M. (1979). Cachexia of malignancy. Potential role of insulin in nutritional management. *Cancer*; **43**: 2070–76.

Schwartz S.S., Zeidler A., Moossa A.R., Kuku S.F., Rubenstein A.H. (1978). A prospective study of glucose tolerance, insulin, C-peptide, and glucagon responses in patients with pancreatic carcinoma. *Digestive Diseases*; **23**: 1107–14.

Skrabanek P., Powell D. (1978). Ectopic insulin and Occam's razor: Reappraisal of the riddle of tumour hypoglycaemia. *Clin. Endocrinol*; **9**: 141–54.

Silbert S. K., Rossini A., Guazvinian S., Widrick W.C., Marks L.J., Sawin C.T. (1976). Tumour hypoglycaemia. Deficient splanchnic output and deficient glucagon secretion. *Diabetes*; **25**: 202–6.

Silverstein M.N., Wakin K.G., Bahn R.C. (1966). Tryptophan metabolites in hypoglycaemia associated with neoplasia. *Cancer*; **19**: 2024–8.

Slosse A., Reding R. (1927). Etudes des alterations humorales dans le cancer et le precancer. *Bull. Acad. Roy. de med de Belgique*; **7**: 405–38.

Smith S. R., Edgar P.J., Pozefsky T., Chhetri M.K., Prout T.E. (1975). Insulin secretion and glucose tolerance in adults with protein-calorie malnutrition. *Metabolism*; **24**: 1073–84.

Stein T. P. (1978). Cachexia, gluconeogenesis, and progressive weight loss in cancer patients. *J. Theor. Biol*; **73**: 51–9.

Unger R.H. (1966). The riddle of tumour hypoglycaemia. *Amer. J. Med*; **40**: 325–30.

Venuta S., Rubin H. (1973). Sugar transport in normal and Rous sarcoma virus-transformed chick-embryo fibroblasts. *Proc. Natl. Acad. Sci*; **70**: 653–7.

Warburg O. (1930). *Metabolism of Tumours*. London: Constable.

Waterhouse C. (1974). Lactate metabolism in patients with cancer. *Cancer*; **33**: 66–71.

Weinkove C., Weinkove E.A., Pimstone B.L. (1976). Glucose tolerance and insulin release in malnourished rats. *Clin. Sci. Mol. Med*; **50**: 153–63.

Widmer U., Zapf J., Froesch E.R. (1982). Is extrapancreatic tumour hypoglycaemia associated with elevated levels of insulin-like growth factor II? *J. Clin. Endocrinol. Metab*; **55**: 833–9.

Chapter 6

Michael W.J. Davie

Disorders of Mineral Metabolism

INTRODUCTION

Tissue undergoing neoplastic change may affect calcium and magnesium metabolism in several ways. Malignancy may occur in glands that normally synthesise hormones, such as the parathyroid or thyroid glands, thus leading to the consequences expected from supraphysiological dosage of the respective hormones. Over 40 years ago, however, Albright suggested that neoplastic involvement of non-endocrine organs might also lead to production of substances capable of influencing calcium metabolism (Albright, 1941), whereas normal tissue was not able to synthesise these substances. Since then this prophecy has been more than fulfilled. Several mediators of neoplastic hypercalcaemia have been recognised and there are undoubtedly others that await characterisation. More has become known about the process involved in the resorption of calcium from bone and of the relationship of tumour deposits to bone destruction. Malignant disease may also give rise to forms of bone disease other than simple osteolysis, whilst treatment of cancer can also lead to disturbance of calcium and magnesium homeostasis. It is with the effect of tumours on bone, the mechanisms of osteolysis, the humoral agents produced by tumours, the consequences of treatment and the management of hypercalcaemia that this chapter is concerned.

HYPERCALCAEMIA

Incidence

In the general population, hypercalcaemia is relatively uncommon, 178 cases being found from 15 903 otherwise normal subjects undergoing a screening procedure (Christensson *et al.*, 1976). Of those patients with malignant disease, up to 20% may experience hypercalcaemia at some stage of their illness (Myers, 1973).

Although primary hyperparathyroidism appears to occur with unexpected frequency amongst subjects with neoplasia (Farr *et al.*, 1973), the most frequent cause of malignancy associated with hypercalcaemia is the neoplasm itself. Secondary deposits in bone are found in 75% of cases with malignant disease and hypercalcaemia (Fisken *et al.*, 1980), although the secondary tumour is not necessarily the cause of hypercalcaemia. The incidence of hypercalcaemia depends upon the primary tumour. Carcinoma of the breast, which accounted for over half of the cases, was the tumour most frequently associated with hypercalcaemia in one series (Myers, 1973), whilst bronchial carcinoma headed the list of a series collected in Birmingham (UK) (Fisken *et al.*, 1980). In most series the primary sites most often associated with hypercalcaemia are breast, bronchus, renal and urinary tract. However, myeloma is the tumour most likely to give rise to a high serum calcium, followed by thyroid, bronchus and breast (Fisken *et al.*, 1980). Conversely, it is unusual for hypercalcaemia to complicate tumours of the large bowel or stomach (Fisken *et al.*, 1980). Obvious neoplastic deposits in bone are found almost universally in myeloma and in carcinoma of the breast. They occur less frequently with tumours of the oesophagus, bronchus and renal tract, primary tumours in these sites being often associated with a biochemical state akin to hyperparathyroidism. It is also unusual for hypercalcaemia to be discovered before the tumour becomes clinically obvious. Out of 153 cases of hypercalcaemia in the Birmingham survey, only 14 were the result of malignancy and presented before the diagnosis was made. In only one subject was the neoplasm not discovered at once (Fisken *et al.*, 1981). Neither are serum calcium measurements likely to be a valuable means of screening for cancer; out of the series of almost 16 000 subjects screened for hypercalcaemia only two had malignancy-associated hypercalcaemia (Christensson *et al.*, 1976).

Furthermore, such endeavours might also lead to false conclusions, since hypercalcaemia has been reported in association with benign breast lesions, removal of which was followed by a fall of the serum calcium level (Marx *et al.*, 1977).

Pathophysiology

Elevated serum calcium levels can arise from enhanced bone resorption, reduced bone accretion, increased intestinal calcium absorption, diminished endogenous intestinal calcium secretion or impaired renal excretion of calcium. The results of investigations into all these possibilities are broadly consistent. Intestinal calcium absorption is usually normal or may indeed be low (Coombes *et al.*, 1976), a finding that is consistent with the low serum 1,25-dihydroxy vitamin D (1,25-$(OH)_2$D) levels found in hypercalcaemia of humoral origin (Stewart *et al.*, 1980). Endogenous faecal calcium is not affected (Table 6.1).

Removal of calcium by the kidney is likely to be the most serious limitation to the maintenance of normocalcaemia. Urinary calcium ex-

TABLE 6.1
Hypercalcaemia and Neoplasia

Investigators	Calcium turnover	Calcium pool	Intestinal calcium absorption	Endogenous faecal calcium secretion
1. Lafferty and Pearson (1963) Hypercalcaemia M −	↑	↑	N	
2. Myers (1973, Review) Normocalcaemia	↓	slight ↓	N	
Hypercalcaemia M +	↑			
Pseudohyper-parathyroid		↓	N	N
3. Coombes *et al.* (1976)		(^{47}Ca space)		↓
Normocalcaemia M −			N	N
Normocalcaemia M +		↑	↓	N
Hypercalcaemia M −			↓	
Hypercalcaemia M +		↑	↓	N or ↑
4. Szymendera (1970) Hypercalcaemia	↑	↑		N

Notes 1)
↑   Increased;
↓   Decreased;
N   Normal;
M − No metastases;
M + Metastases present.

2)   Techniques used by different investigators differ and the results have been pooled into the general categories, as above. The ^{47}Ca space measured by Coombes *et al.* (1976) correlates well with bone accretion rate, and a high ^{47}Ca space was correlated with high serum calcitonin levels. In general, metastases increase calcium turnover and the calcium pool, and may increase endogenous faecal calcium. Endogenous faecal calcium is normal and intestinal calcium absorption normal or low in hypercalcaemia of malignancy.

cretion corresponds to filtered calcium, less any calcium reabsorbed by the renal tubules. Parathyroid hormone (PTH) promotes tubular reabsorption of calcium, whereas PTH deficiency leads to higher urinary calcium excretion for any serum calcium level compared with normal subjects. The role of renal handling of calcium has been investigated in a number of malignant diseases, notably myeloma. Renal tubular reabsorption of calcium is within the normal range in myeloma, but the urinary (calcium/creatinine) ratio falls for any given serum calcium level as the serum creatinine rises (Nordin, 1976). Nordin has suggested that the term (urinary calcium/urinary creatinine)/serum creatinine is useful in delineating cases of hypercalcaemia that are primarily renal in origin and those in whom resorption is the dominant component. The upper limit compatible with normocalcaemia is 0·3 mg/100 ml glomerular filtrate. Analysis of cases with hypercalcaemia associated with myeloma showed that reduced GFR was the major factor in hypercalcaemia in 30% of cases, and increased entry of calcium into the blood was primarily responsible in another 30% (Nordin, 1976). In 40% of cases both factors were operating, and it has been shown that mithramycin is capable of exerting an additional hypocalcaemic effect in myeloma after initial lowering of serum calcium levels using a saline diuresis (Heyburn *et al.*, 1981). Under certain circumstances high serum calcium levels in myeloma may not cause complications. Abnormal binding of calcium by high concentrations of myeloma protein can raise total serum calcium concentration whilst ionised calcium levels remain within the normal range, thus giving no systemic manifestations (Lindgärde and Zettervall, 1973).

HYPOPHOSPHATAEMIA

Hypophosphataemia not uncommonly occurs in neoplastic disease, often associated with hypercalcaemia or in a form associated with hypophosphataemic osteomalacia. The association with hypercalcaemia (Fisken *et al.*, 1981) lends support to the proposition that ectopic PTH might be produced by tumours. In association with carcinoma of the breast, it has been suggested that hypercalcaemia might lead to hypophosphataemia through a phosphaturic action of calcium upon the renal tubules, even in the presence of an increased phosphate load. Infusion of saline led to a fall of serum calcium and to increased tubular absorption of phosphate (Schussler *et al.*, 1972). Hypophosphataemia may complicate leukaemia. It is associated with a pronounced leukocytosis, and its presence may warn of the tumour lysis syndrome (q.v.) occurring on starting chemotherapy (Zamkoff and Kirschner, 1980; Colman *et al.*, 1983).

BONE AND MALIGNANT DISEASE

Although the capacity of the renal tubule to excrete calcium is important in maintaining the high serum calcium level, hypercalcaemia arises largely from increased mobilisation of calcium from bone.

The extent of bone resorption with secondary tumour and the subsequent hypercalcaemia depends upon the tumour type. Similarly, tumours vary in their ability to destroy bone and cause hypercalcaemia in the absence of secondary spread. Thus, epidermoid carcinoma of the lung is more frequently associated with hypercalcaemia than any other lung tumour, even though bone metastases occur with greater frequency in other types (Bender and Hansen, 1974). Tumours of the large bowel have a high incidence of secondary involvement of bone but a low incidence of associated hypercalcaemia (Fisken *et al.*, 1980). It is also unlikely that the mass of secondary tumour is important (Ralston *et al.*, 1982), but in those tumours that are associated with hypercalcaemia, a large tumour load generally exists by the time elevation of the serum calcium is detected (Stewart *et al.*, 1982*b*). Hypercalcaemia of malignancy can occur in the absence of metastases, and although these may be difficult to detect (Lafferty, 1966), use of ^{99m}Tc diphosphonate scanning is valuable in locating bone involvement, and false negatives are becoming increasingly less common (Ralston *et al.*, 1982).

Such circumstantial evidence for the existence of mediators of bone resorption led to efforts to isolate substances capable of resorbing bone, either locally (being synthesised by tumour deposits), or of exerting a general effect upon bone after being produced at some remote site. Possible hormone mediators of bone resorption are discussed later, but an account is given here of local effects of tumours leading to bone resorption.

Bone is a tissue that is undergoing constant remodelling, and tumours may affect both the formation and the resorption of bone. The importance of the ratio of bone synthesis to bone breakdown on the level of serum calcium is emphasised by the finding of hypocalcaemia in association with tumours.

Neoplasia of both breast and bronchus has been associated with hypocalcaemia (Sackner *et al.*, 1960; Hall *et al.*, 1966). Whilst enhanced synthesis of bone could give rise to hypocalcaemia, a decline in the rate of bone resorption is also a possibility. A more frequent finding is the uncoupling of the synthesis: resorption process, leading to a situation favouring bone resorption. Histological examination of bone in a subject with squamous carcinoma and hypercalcaemia revealed that osteoclast numbers were increased whilst osteoblasts were absent (Stewart *et al.*, 1982*a*), an appearance strikingly in contrast with hyperparathyroidism in which both osteoclast and osteoblast numbers are increased.

Metastatic tumour invading bone does not destroy tissue only by direct invasion. Direct breakdown of bone by metastatic lesions of bronchial neoplasms is rare compared with more complex processes involving release of bone cell activators or initiation of a host response leading to bone destruction. Interpretation of tumour–bone relationships is influenced by histological concepts of the appearances of ischaemia, metabolic activation and osteolysis. Nevertheless, attempts have been made to explain bone breakdown in terms of the histological findings (Cramer *et al.*, 1981). Loss of bone trabeculae and enhanced bone cell activity in remaining trabeculae typified the appearance of secondary tumour from epidermoid or adeno-carcinoma of the lung, whilst empty osteocytic lacunae and an absence of viable bone cells were features of malignancy derived from small cell tumours of the lung. Each tumour appears capable of inducing an individual response. Bone resorption experiments '*in vitro*' have shown that many stimuli associated with bone resorption including PTH, 1,25-$(OH)_2$D, and prostaglandin E2 are capable of attracting human monocytes (Mundy *et al.*, 1978*a*), cells which may be the precursors of osteoclasts. In the study of Cramer *et al.* (1981) there was no accumulation of monocytes indicating that other resorptive factors are involved.

CLINICAL FEATURES OF HYPERCALCAEMIA OF MALIGNANCY

A case of hypercalcaemia will occur in a general hospital up to three times per week (Fisken *et al.*, 1981), and over 90% of these will be caused by malignant tumours or by hyperparathyroidism. The differential diagnosis of causes other than these two will not be further considered. Distinguishing malignant disease from hyperparathyroidism is not easy and in one series 20% of cases of malignant disease had undergone neck exploration for primary hyperparathyroidism (Lafferty, 1966). It is unusual for hypercalcaemia to be the presenting feature of malignancy, and probably because it is a late finding, is associated with a poor prognosis (Fisken *et al.*, 1980).

TABLE 6.2

Humoral Hypercalcaemia (HH) and Primary
Hyperparathyroidism (Primary HPT)

	1° HPT	*HH*	
Serum:			
Calcium	↑	↑ ↑	
Phosphate	↓ ↓	↓	
Chloride	↑	N	
Chloride/phosphate	↑	slight ↑	
PTH	↑	↓ or N	
1,25-$(OH)_2D_3$	↑	↓	
Calcitonin	N	↑	
Urine:			
Cyclic AMP	↑	↑	(Group 1)
		↓	(Group 2)
Fasting calcium	slight ↑ or N	↑	

Note
  ↑ Increased;
  ↓ Decreased;
  N Normal.

Anorexia, a substantial degree of weight loss, and symptoms occurring over a short period, favour a neoplastic cause. Fatigue occurs with equal incidence in both groups, whereas a history of renal stones or a long duration of symptoms are more usually associated with primary hyperparathyroidism (Fisken *et al.*, 1980). The diagnosis of malignancy is favoured by finding lymphadenopathy, hepatomegaly or a tumour mass.

Biochemical means of distinction have included serum phosphate, serum chloride, the serum chloride/phosphate ratio and multivariate analysis. Primary hyperparathyroidism tends to give a lower serum phosphate, higher chloride and a higher chloride/phosphate ratio. This ratio has been found valuable in some centres (Palmer *et al.*, 1974), but not in others (Fisken *et al.*, 1981). Although PTH levels have not been as valuable as initially hoped, levels in primary hyperparathyroidism are often higher than those encountered in malignancy-associated hypercalcaemia, irrespective of the antibody used, although levels are not low in malignancy-associated hypercalcaemia (Stewart *et al.*, 1980; Fisken *et al.*, 1981). Other measurements (Table 6.2) may also be helpful. Levels of plasma 1,25-$(OH)_2D$ are high in primary hyperparathyroidism and low in malignancy-associated hypercalcaemia (Stewart *et al.*, 1982), a finding that will be more useful when assays for the hormone are less time consuming. Serum calcitonin levels may also have valuable discriminatory powers. In primary hyperparathyroidism, levels remain low or within the normal range, whereas levels are raised in malignancy-associated hypercalcaemia (Morita *et al.*, 1978).

The steroid suppression test, originally introduced to distinguish hyperparathyroidism from sarcoidosis (Anderson *et al.*, 1954), has enjoyed some popularity in differentiating the cause of hypercalcaemia. The high incidence of failed suppression in non-parathyroid disease makes this test useful but not diagnostic. If serum calcium falls to a normal range after administration of hydrocortisone 150 mg/day for 10 days, hyperparathyroidism is very unlikely, although there are occasional reports of suppression in primary hyperparathyroidism (Gwinup and Sayle, 1961).

MEDIATORS OF HYPERCALCAEMIA IN MALIGNANCY

Pseudohyperparathyroidism (Humoral Hypercalcaemia)

The term pseudohyperparathyroidism has been widely used to describe a syndrome of hypercalcaemia, hypophosphataemia and malignant disease without secondary spread. It is best avoided, as the number of cases with true ectopic production of PTH is probably very small indeed. Since the biochemical characteristics suggest the presence of hyperparathyroidism, evidence for production of the hormone has been sought by immunological reactivity or by examination of the tumour for PTH activity. The parathyroid glands themselves are normal (Sherwood *et al.*, 1967). Levels of immunoassayable PTH in plasma are often less than might be expected for the prevailing level of hypercalcaemia.

Comparison with known forms of hyperparathyroidism showed that the highest levels of PTH occurred in chronic renal failure followed by parathyroid adenoma. Cases of bronchogenic carcinoma displayed levels that were less impressively elevated (Berson and Yalow, 1966), and other workers reached similar conclusions (Benson *et al.*, 1974), leading to the suggestion that the calcium/PTH ratio might be of diagnostic value. Tumours themselves have, however, been found to have immunoassayable PTH, and resection of tumours has led to a fall of both serum calcium and of PTH (Sherwood *et al.*, 1967; Knill-Jones *et al.*, 1970). It is, however, noteworthy that there is little experience of the syndrome of 'hungry bones' that occurs occasionally following removal of benign parathyroid tumours. For the same degree of hypercalcaemia, removal of a malignant neoplasm would be expected to require measures to maintain the serum calcium level.

The possibility that tumour may stimulate the parathyroid glands, thereby increasing the level of PTH, has not been extensively studied. In one reported case however, hypercalcaemia consequent upon an epidermoid carcinoma of the cervix was found to be independent of the presence of the parathyroids. All four parathyroid glands had been removed in an effort to control hypercalcaemia, which nevertheless persisted until death supervened 18 days later (Myers, 1973).

Much early work relied upon anti-bovine PTH serology. More recently, attempts have been made to correlate the known physiologic actions of PTH with immunoassayable levels. Hypercalcaemia in malignant disease may be associated with either high or low nephrogenous cyclic AMP levels in urine; PTH levels, measured by a variety of antisera directed against different parts of the PTH molecule, are normal or even low in the presence of raised nephrogenous cyclic AMP levels. Moreover, the low level of serum 1,25-$(OH)_2D$ occurring in this condition is telling evidence against excess secretion of PTH (Stewart *et al.*, 1980). Synthesis of this hormone is stimulated by PTH, hypophosphataemia and hypocalcaemia (Holick and DeLuca, 1978), and in primary hyperparathyroidism levels are high. Thus, although there may be a slight increase of immunoassayable PTH in malignancy-associated hypercalcaemia, it is not capable of stimulating 1-α-hydroxylation, indicating a relative degree of hypoparathyroidism. An indirect method of assessing nephrogenous cyclic AMP production is by measuring glucose-6-phosphate dehydrogenase activity in renal tubular cells. Tumour extracts increased the activity of the enzyme but this was only partially inhibited by (32–47%) adding anti-PTH antiserum (Goltzman *et al.*, 1981), whereas activity induced by PTH was completely counteracted by the same antiserum. Using gel chromatography the molecular weight of the activity in fractions from tumour extracts was measured and then compared with the molecular weight of the activity of serum of a patient with primary hyperparathyroidism and with the molecular weight of radiolabelled intact PTH (1–84) and with the 1–34 PTH fragment. In primary hyperparathyroidism most of the activity eluted with the intact molecule. In humoral hypercalcaemia the activity was more widely distributed, with the greater part of it eluting at molecular weights greater that the 1–84 PTH moiety, although in one case some activity was coincidental with the native hormone.

Further evidence against the secretion of PTH by tumours comes from the application of hybridisation technology. P^{32} labelled complementary DNA probes coded for human and bovine PTH have been used to detect mRNA for PTH. The process, capable of detecting as little as 1 μm of parathyroid hormone mRNA, did not reveal any mRNA in either human or animal tumours. Hypercalcaemia was recorded in five instances of human tumours and was associated with normal levels of PTH ('inappropriate secretion') in four subjects. The DNA probe contained 300 base pairs and is thought capable of detecting as few as 15 successive identical pairs. Since no base pairing was detected, the mRNA sequence of any altered form of PTH that might be synthesised by the tumour is unlikely to resemble that of native PTH (Simpson *et al.*, 1983). The failure to detect PTH by this technique contrasts with the success claimed in detecting calcitonin mRNA in small cell tumours of the bronchus (Ferry *et al.*, 1983).

Other evidence against PTH secretion in humoral hypercalcaemia has come from studies on bone. Parathyroid hormone is able to increase osteoblast number, if not the activity of each individual cell, whilst osteoclasts are also stimulated (Rasmussen and Bordier, 1974). Although the osteoblast and osteoclast are no longer believed to derive from the same cell, the osteoblast originating from a connective tissue line and the osteoclast from marrow cells (Owen, 1980), the activity of the two cells is evenly balanced under most circumstances, although the rate of bone turnover may alter. Tumour-free iliac crest bone biopsies from subjects with humoral hypercalcaemia showed that osteoclast surface and number were increased, whereas osteoblast surface and osteoid volume were diminished. Such an appearance has been termed uncoupling (Stewart *et al.*, 1982*a*), and the relative inactivity of the osteoblast may play a part in hypercalcaemia by preventing the uptake of calcium into bone, and account for the absence of the 'hungry bone syndrome' after removal of a tumour.

Tumours, therefore, are capable of secreting substances that increase urinary cyclic AMP, stimulate phosphaturia, increase osteoclastic activity and possibly inhibit osteoblasts. In a minority of cases PTH activity is present, but in the majority there is another mediator. The nature of the mediator(s) and the relationship to those that may exist in tumour associated hypophosphataemic osteomalacia remain to be established.

Prostaglandins and Bone Resorption

Prostaglandins are a family of substances derived from arachidonic acid. All contain a 20 carbon fatty-acid chain and incorporate a cyclopentane ring. The metabolic pathways are summarised in Fig. 6.1. The most important prostaglandins connected with bone resorption are those of the PGF and PGE series. A keto group at position nine distinguishes PGF from PGE in which position nine is filled by an hydroxyl group. The numerical designation (PGE$_1$, PGE$_2$, PGE$_3$, etc.) refers to the number of double bonds in the fatty-acid chain. The most frequently occurring group, the PGE$_2$ series, has an additional double bond between carbons five and six. Prostaglandin E and F are rapidly metabolised in a first pass through the lung, the ensuing oxidation and degradation of the fatty-acid chain increasing their water solubility.

The major urinary metabolite, 7α-hydroxy-5-11-diketotetranor-prostane-1-16 dioic acid (PGEM) has been used as an index of prostaglandin secretion. The extensive degradation of PGE by the lung makes venous plasma samples an unreliable means of assessing prostaglandin output from a tumour.

Although both PGE$_1$ and PGE$_2$ are capable of inducing bone resorption *in vitro* (Tashjian *et al.*, 1972), most work has been done on the compound most frequently encountered, i.e. PGE$_2$. Tumour cells are themselves able to produce PGE$_2$ (Tashjian *et al.*, 1972), although, as with much of the data

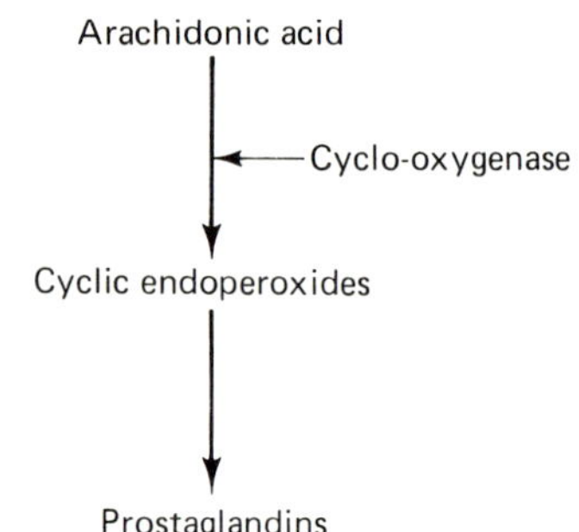

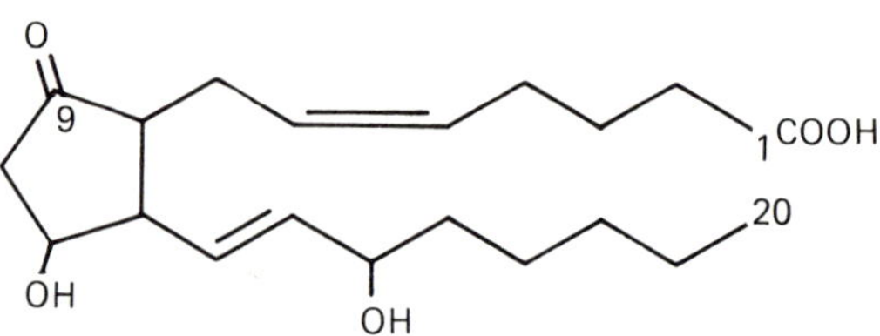

Fig. 6.1. *Prostaglandin synthesis from arachidonic acid, showing site of action of cyclo-oxygenase. The prostaglandin illustrated is PGE$_2$; the numbers indicate the sequence of the carbon atoms.*

relating hypercalcaemia to prostaglandin synthesis, animal evidence is more convincing than that obtained from human studies. Under certain circumstances monocytes may be induced to secrete prostaglandins (Bockman, 1980) and, as these cells are attracted by resorbing bone (Mundy *et al.*, 1978*b*), additional production may be derived from this source.

Animal tumour models that provide compelling evidence for a PGE role in bone resorption are the VX_2 carcinoma in the rabbit, the mouse fibrosarcoma, and the Walker carcino-sarcoma tumour (Tashjian *et al.*, 1972; Powles *et al.*, 1973; Voelkel *et al.*, 1975). All these tumours produce PGE_2, levels of which may be lowered by indomethacin, an inhibitor of cyclo-oxygenase. Marked hypercalcaemia accompanies the VX_2 tumour, together with bone resorption, both effects being inhibited by indomethacin (Voelkel *et al.*, 1975). Although indomethacin lowers PGE_2 levels in animals, a related effect of PGE_2 and hypercalcaemia must not be considered proven. In human subjects with hypercalcaemia, indomethacin may lower plasma PGE_2 levels without affecting the hypercalcaemia (Brenner *et al.*, 1982), and the level of plasma prostaglandin is a poor predictor of success of the treatment of hypercalcaemia with indomethacin.

Animal tumours have been of value in understanding the process of bone resorption due to prostaglandins. Tumour cell deposits in bone following injection of Walker tumour cells into rats were not detectable radiologically if animals were pretreated with indomethacin and treatment continued after the injection of the malignant cells. However, there was no reduction in the weight of the tumour that appeared in the indomethacin treated animals (Powles *et al.*, 1973). The poor detection rate of secondary tumour using x-rays has been mentioned previously, but it appears that indomethacin prevented local osteolysis in bone without inhibiting tumour growth. Such a conclusion reinforces the concept that bone destruction is mediated by chemicals secreted locally.

The frequency of prostaglandin-associated hypercalcaemia arising from tumours is difficult to establish, and many reports exist to bolster the hypothesis that prostaglandins play an important role in hypercalcaemia without providing control data. Plasma prostaglandin levels were, however, significantly elevated in 14 subjects with hypercalcaemia and neoplasia, whereas no normocalcaemic subject had high values in one series (Demers *et al.*, 1977). Urinary PGEM levels, evaluated in 29 male subjects with malignant tumours, 14 of whom were hypercalcaemic, were increased in 12 subjects. Six subjects treated with indomethacin experienced a fall of both serum calcium and of PGEM (Seyberth *et al.*, 1975). Nevertheless, lowering an elevated PGE_2 level with indomethacin does not necessarily reduce serum calcium levels, and only 20% of subjects may have prostaglandin-mediated hypercalcaemia (Brenner *et al.*, 1982).

Solid tumours are those most likely to lead to high levels of PGE, hypercalcaemia occurring in haematological tumours (myeloma, lymphoma) being associated with normal levels of PGEM. Extracts of a hypernephroma obtained from a patient who was pre-operatively hyper-calcaemic, revealed that this tumour was able to release calcium from bone previously labelled with ^{45}Ca. Indomethacin inhibited this calcium release but not that induced by PGE_2. Because indomethacin does not inhibit the action of PGE_2 on bone resorption, it has been concluded that tumour extracts do not contain PGE_2 but synthesise a factor that promotes prostaglandin production from arachidonic acid (Minkin *et al.*, 1981). Culture fluid from the mononuclear cells of peripheral blood, derived from a T-cell tumour, resorbed bone *in vitro*, and this resorption was partially inhibited by indomethacin. However, PGE_2 levels were lower than those found to induce bone resorption in this assay (Grossman *et al.*, 1981). The pitfalls that are possible in the interpretation of PGE-induced hyper-calcaemia are illustrated by the VX_2 carcinoma in the rabbit. Animals with this tumour remain normocalcaemic unless a high calcium diet is fed. Hypercalcaemia occurring under these circumstances disappears when indomethacin is given, but it was also found that indomethacin reduced daily food intake substantially. The high calcium diet was no longer being eaten, thereby introducing a further variable into the hypocalcaemic response (Doppelt *et al.*, 1982).

Prostaglandins may also stimulate bone resorption by other agents. Since PGE is so readily destroyed by the lung, very little will reach the systemic circulation. One site in which PGE might function is in the kidney tubule where 1-α-hydroxylation of 25-hydroxycholecalciferol takes place. This reaction may be stimulated by many factors including prostaglandin (Trechsel *et al.*, 1980). $1,25$-$(OH)_2D$ is a potent resorber of bone. The previously mentioned data relating $1,25$-$(OH)_2D$ levels to hypercalcaemia do not suggest however that this process is important.

Prostaglandin-mediated hypercalcaemia is probably a real entity and may arise from a number of cell species. Prostaglandin is the most likely compound responsible for hypercalcaemia, but the biochemical changes leading to enhanced synthesis are ill understood. Inhibitors of cyclo-oxygenase reduce release of ^{45}Ca from bone *in vitro* and may be of limited value in lowering serum calcium levels, but there are at present no reliable means of predicting the response to these agents.

Osteoclast Activating Factor

Tumours of lymphoid tissue, particularly multiple myeloma—a β-cell tumour—are among the tumours most frequently associated with hyper-calcaemia. Investigation of leucocyte-dependent bone resorption revealed that supernatants of normal leucocyte cultures were able to release ^{45}Ca from fetal rat long bones (Raisz *et al.*, 1975). Stimulation of an osteoclast activating factor (OAF) has been achieved by treatment with phytohaemag-glutinin, a T-cell activator. Osteoclast activating factor production by mononuclear cells was impaired by irradiation, thereby implicating lymphocytes as a major source. Purified lymphocytes do not by themselves produce OAF but require the presence of macrophages to facilitate OAF release (Horton *et al.*, 1974). Osteoclast activating factor production by peripheral blood leucocytes *in vitro* falls when cyclo-oxygenase inhibitors are exhibited, suggesting a role for prostaglandin in its release (Yoneda and Mundy, 1979), but additional PGE_2 does not necessarily increase production (Raisz *et al.*, 1975).

Osteoclast activating factor production by tumours has been investigated in cell lines from myeloma, Burkitt lymphoma, and T-cell lymphoma. The curves relating OAF concentration to ^{45}Ca release from fetal long bones, showed that OAF from normal lymphocytes was similar to that obtained from tumours and had the dose–response characteristics associated with PTH rather than PGE_2 or 1,25-$(OH)_2D$ (Mundy *et al.*, 1974*a*). Heating to 30°C causes variable loss of activity, but this effect may be reduced if the heating is done in the presence of plasma. Osteoclast activating factor has been partially purified and found to exist in two forms. Determination of molecular weight by gel chromatography indicates that the factor from normal leucocytes is excluded between 13 700 and 25 000 daltons. It is retained by a 10 000 dalton filter. Under conditions of high ionic strength this material dissociates to a smaller fraction having a molecular weight between 1330 and 3500 daltons. This moiety retains calcium mobilising activity and reverts back to the higher molecular weight from when the ionic strength is lowered. Analysis of the fractions eluting from the chromatographic column failed to reveal the presence of either prostaglandins, and the molecular weight excluded any vitamin D metabolite. Both big and little OAF may be inhibited by proteolytic enzymes, suggesting that proteins makes up at least part of the material (Mundy and Raisz, 1977). Osteoclast activating factor from myeloma cells is excluded from gel filtration columns at a molecular weight similar to that from normal leucocytes (Mundy *et al.*, 1974*b*).

The release of calcium by OAF from normal leucocytes is not increased by PTH but may be inhibited by calcitonin (Raisz *et al.*, 1975). The inhibition of OAF-mediated calcium release was not permanent and declined after four days of culture. Cortisone also inhibits OAF-induced bone resorption at a concentration of 10^{-7} M compared with 10^{-5} M required to inhibit PTH-induced bone resorption. Indomethacin, at a concentration of 10^{-4} M, does not inhibit OAF activity. The value of corticosteroids in treating hypercalcaemia of non-solid tumours is underlined by studies on a lymphosarcoma cell line in which ^{45}Ca release was markedly reduced in the presence of 10^{-8} M cortisol (Mundy *et al.*, 1978*a*). Inhibition of collagen synthesis is a feature of both OAF and of PTH. Incorporation of [3H]-proline into collagenase-digestible protein fell by over 50% in the presence of either PTH or of OAF; 1,25-$(OH)_2D$ is less effective. Prostaglandins also inhibit collagen synthesis, but only at concentrations considerably in excess of those effective at mediating bone resorption (Raisz *et al.*, 1975).

The importance of OAF in clinical practice is not clear. Injected OAF has no effect on serum calcium, suggesting that rapid degradation takes place or that a substantial number of OAF-producing cells in close proximity to bone are required before hypercalcaemia is brought about. Histological studies in myeloma show large multinucleate osteoclasts in bone, with extensive osteoclast resorption only taking place adjacent to myeloma cell infiltrates; osteocytic lacunae were not prominent (Mundy *et al.*, 1974*b*). Myeloma cell mass also correlates with OAF activity. However, it is not possible to show that there is a difference between OAF activity in patients with a normal serum calcium and those with high serum calcium levels. No particular immunoglobulin cell type is associated with high OAF levels, although those with IgA myeloma have an unexpectedly high cell mass and OAF levels (Durie *et al.*, 1981), and slightly higher incidence of hypercalcaemia (Heyburn *et al.*, 1981). Treatment directed towards hypercalcaemia does not affect OAF activity (Grossman *et al.*, 1981).

Calcitriol Production by Tumours

Under normal circumstances the synthesis of the hormone calcitriol (1,25 dihydroxyvitamin D) from 25 hydroxyvitamin D takes place only in the kidney and the placenta. Production from ectopic sites was originally encountered in patients with hypercalcaemia caused by sarcoidosis, a major feature of which is the proliferation of activated T-lymphocytes (Crystal *et al.*, 1984). Since abnormal calcitriol synthesis continues in anephric subjects it is inferred that the source of the hormone is sarcoid tissue itself (Barbour *et al.*, 1981), and direct evidence for this exists (Mason *et al.*, 1984).

Elevated serum calcitriol levels associated with hypercalcaemia have been described in three patients with lymphatic neoplasia, including one subject whose tumour was determined to be a T-cell lymphoma (Breslau *et al.*, 1984). Treatment with corticosteroids rapidly lowers both the elevated serum calcium and calcitriol levels.

Growth Factors

Growth-inducing factors have been discovered in a variety of cells, both normal and neoplastic. These substances, including epidermal growth factor and platelet-derived growth factor may stimulate bone resorption as well as increase fibroblast replication, but their role in overall bone turnover has yet to be defined. Growth factors isolated from tumours associated with hypercalcaemia have been postulated as causes of humoral hypercalcaemia (Ibbotson *et al.*, 1982).

TUMOUR-ASSOCIATED OSTEOMALACIA

A case of osteomalacia, apparently associated with a tumour, was first reported in 1947 (McCance, 1947). Subsequently there have been reports of this rare syndrome being associated with many different tumours, the majority of which have a mesenchymal origin.

The diagnosis should be borne in mind in patients presenting with osteomalacia, in whom hypophosphataemia is the predominant biochemical feature. That is not to say, however, that all such cases will turn out to have an underlying malignancy; Dent and Stamp (1971) describe nine cases of primary hypophosphataemic osteomalacia. Long follow-up is required, since there may be a long prodromal period of symptoms before the tumour becomes apparent. Instances of 4 years, 5 years, 9 years and, in the case of the patient of McCance (1947) probably even longer, have been recorded (Salassa *et al.*, 1970; Linovitz *et al.*, 1976; Wyman *et al.*, 1977).

Symptoms include generalised bone pain, especially affecting the spine, together with muscle weakness so profound that lifting of the head or sitting without support becomes impossible. A similar clinical picture can complicate the epidermal naevus syndrome (Aschinberg *et al.*, 1977). Many reports emphasise the sudden nature of the onset of pain, and there are instances of several centimetres of height being lost. Examination confirms the muscle weakness, largely proximal, the bone tenderness, kyphosis and other skeletal deformities.

The biochemical results relative to normal values appear in Table 6.3. Outstanding features are the low serum phosphate, high urinary phosphate

TABLE 6.3

Biochemical Features of Tumour-associated
Osteomalacia

Serum	
Calcium	Normal
Phosphorus	Low
Alkaline phosphatase	Raised
Parathormone	Normal
$1,25\text{-}(OH)_2D_3$	Low
$24,25\text{-}(OH)_2D_3$	Normal
Urine	
pH	Acid
Amino acids	Usually increased
Calcium	Normal
Tubular reabsorption } Phosphate	Reduced
Creatinine clearance	Normal

excretion, normal PTH, and low serum 1,25-(OH)$_2$D levels. Conversely, serum 24,25-(OH)$_2$D levels are normal (Sweet *et al.*, 1980). Bone biopsy shows a large proportion of osteoid with defective mineralisation, and Looser's zones may be found on skeletal surveys.

The spectrum of tumours associated with this syndrome extends yearly. There is an undoubted preponderance of mesenchymal tumours with haemangioma, haemangiopericytoma, and malignant bone tumours figuring prominently in a recent series (Linovitz *et al.*, 1976), whilst prostatic carcinoma (Lyles *et al.*, 1980) and neurofibroma have also to be considered. The rarity of the syndrome and the lack of a suitable animal model have combined to make experimental observations rare. Sufficient fibroangiomatous tissue was, however, obtained from a subject with the epidermal naevus syndrome, to allow homogenisation and injection of an extract into a dog. A marked phosphaturia occurred and was maintained for at least 2 hours (Aschinberg *et al.*, 1977). It was thus postulated that the tumour was secreting a phosphaturic substance and, as PTH levels were normal, involvement of this hormone is unlikely. Removal of a tumour frequently restores phosphate excretion to normal, heals Looser's zones and the abnormal bone histology, and relieves both pain and weakness. The chemical response precedes the clinical response, the latter occurring within one to two months, although improvement within two days of tumour removal is known.

Low levels of 1,25-(OH)$_2$D in serum have been found in this disease (Drezner and Feinglos, 1977; Haussler *et al.*, 1979; Sweet *et al.*, 1980). Treatment of a case of giant cell tumour of bone with 3 μg 1,25-(OH)$_2$D daily, a dose within the physiological range, led to a marked biochemical improvement, resolution of the histological bone defects and positive calcium and phosphate balances (Drezner and Feinglos, 1977). Resistance to cholecalciferol exists and the specific inhibition of 1-α-hydroxylation is emphasised by the normal values for other serum metabolites of vitamin D, including 24,25-(OH)$_2$D. It is difficult however, to account for all the pathological findings by implicating low levels of plasma 1,25-(OH)$_2$D alone. Whereas other syndromes with low levels of this hormone (autosomal recessive vitamin D resistant rickets type 1 and possibly some cases of simple rickets) are associated with weakness and back pain, low serum calcium levels and elevated PTH are also present. Conversely, the presence of normal serum calcium and PTH levels is more in keeping with the inherited forms of hypophosphataemic rickets. Although rachitic and osteomalacic changes are found in these subjects, muscle weakness is never as profound as is found with tumour-associated osteomalacia. If low levels of serum 1,25-(OH)$_2$D are confirmed, these exist in the presence of two powerful stimuli for the synthesis of this hormone, namely hypophosphataemia and PTH (Holick and DeLuca, 1978). The phosphaturia is independent of PTH activity, since additional phosphaturia may be induced by PTH even in the presence of tumour phosphaturic substance. The two compounds probably exert their effects at different sites in the renal tubule (Nortman *et al.*, 1979).

Surgical resection of the tumour is usually attended by considerable clinical and biochemical improvement. Treatment with 1,25-(OH)$_2$D has been successful in some patients, but not invariably. Symptoms arising from an osteosarcoma of the jaw were not improved, nor much impact made upon the biochemical changes during treatment with 1,25-(OH)$_2$D, whereas surgical resection led to marked clinical and biochemical improvement (Nomura *et al.*, 1982). Thus, reduction of tumour size remains the most valuable therapeutic option.

ECTOPIC CALCITONIN PRODUCTION

Calcitonin is normally secreted by the medullary C-cells of the thyroid gland, and considerable increases in concentration may accompany medullary carcinoma of thyroid. Serum calcitonin levels may also be increased in malignancy associated with hypercalcaemia (*see* above), and, although part may originate from the thyroid C-cells, it is also probable that calcitonin may be secreted by non-thyroid tumours. Originally described in oat cell carcinoma of the bronchus, hypercalcitonaemia has been found in all forms of bronchial neoplasms as well as breast, larynx, pancreas and prostate (Roos *et al.*, 1980; Becker *et al.*, 1982). Venous catheterisation studies have indicated a tumour origin in some cases, but high concentrations have also been found in the thyroidal veins of subjects with bronchial neoplasms (Silva *et al.*, 1979). Thus, a thyroidal source may be implicated in some instances.

Continuous cultures of human epidermoid bronchial carcinoma provide a readily accessible means of studying tumour calcitonin. Following speculation that ACTH and calcitonin might be derived from one precursor molecule in the rat pars intermedia, it was suggested that the two moieties might also derive from a single molecule in ectopic hormone-producing situations. In the course of showing that this was not so, two forms of immunoreactive calcitonin of tumour origin were discovered (Bertagna *et al.*, 1978). With molecular weights of between 7000 and 14 000 daltons and of about 75 000 daltons, both forms were considerably larger than native calcitonin (3500 daltons). Other studies have confirmed that the molecular weights lie between 10 000 and 14 000 daltons and around 40 000 daltons compared with 25 000, 10 000 and 3500 daltons obtained from extracts of medullary thyroid carcinoma (Ham *et al.*, 1980). There may also be a separate immunoreactive calcitonin of 13 000 daltons, but hydrolysis of all forms of ectopic calcitonin results in the appearance of the 10 000 dalton form; no 3500 dalton material is produced (Lumsden *et al.*, 1980). Whilst these forms of calcitonin were active in binding to calcitonin antibodies, binding was markedly inferior in a calcitonin receptor binding system using bronchial epidermoid carcinoma compared with native 3500 dalton calcitonin (Ham *et al.*, 1980). Immunoreactivity displayed by big calcitonin from bronchial neoplasms may be abolished by heating. Heat labile immunoreactivity is a non-specific effect and is largely confined to epidermoid and anaplastic bronchial neoplasms, a property that may be helpful in establishing cell type (Roos *et al.*, 1980).

Messenger RNA for calcitonin with either 1050 or 1500 base pairs, both of which combine with a complimentary DNA probe, has been found in small cell carcinoma of the bronchus (Ferry *et al.*, 1983), and more widespread application of recombinant DNA technology will probably clarify the origins of the different calcitonin molecules.

Measurement of ectopic calcitonin production may also have a role to play in assessing the response of a tumour to treatment. High levels of calcitonin in bronchial neoplasia may be lowered by a variety of therapeutic measures directed against the tumour, a decline being found most frequently in subjects showing the greatest clinical improvement (Silva *et al.*, 1979). Since calcitonin levels may be increased by a number of non-malignant pulmonary diseases, further work characterising the nature and origin of this hormone is necessary before it can be considered a reliable marker of a neoplasia.

OTHER FACTORS INFLUENCING CALCIUM HOMEOSTASIS IN MALIGNANCY

An osteolytic factor obtained from human breast neoplasms and which was soluble in organic solvents was reported in 1966. Injection of this factor into parathyroidectomised rats led to hypercalciuria, but it was not possible to purify the material sufficiently for characterisation. It was termed an osteolytic sterol (Gordon *et al.*, 1966), but there have been no subsequent observations to confirm such a compound. Hypercalcaemia has also been reported in the watery diarrhoea syndrome, and a direct action of vasoactive intestinal polypeptide upon intestinal calcium absorption was proposed (Holdaway *et al.*, 1977). In any case of hypercalcaemia there arises the possibility that immobilisation is partially responsible. This entity is most frequently found in young subjects or in Paget's disease of bone and may be related to a high bone turnover rate. Unexpectedly, PTH levels are increased and fall to normal when mobilisation takes place (Lerman *et al.*, 1977).

Treatment of tumours is becoming an increasingly common cause of perturbation of calcium homeostasis. Tamoxifen, an anti-oestrogen drug used in carcinoma of the breast, leads to hypercalcaemia in up to 20% of subjects. This usually occurs early in treatment and may be associated with worsening of bone pain (Veldhuis, 1978). A similar phenomenon has accompanied oestrogen treatment (Swaroop and Krant, 1973). The tumour lysis syndrome, consisting of hypocalcaemia, hyperphosphataemia, hyperuricaemia, azotaemia, and sometimes hyperkalaemia, may be initiated by chemotherapy, lymphatic tumours, or granulocytic leukaemia (Zusman *et al.*, 1973; Cervantes *et al.*, 1982). Clinical manifestations include weakness and lethargy. The sudden fall of serum calcium is ascribed to the considerable hyperphosphataemia caused by the destruction of immature cells, which, relative to their mature counterparts, contain a high proportion of phosphate. Infusion of calcium gluconate is a life saving measure under these circumstances.

Hypocalcaemia has also arisen as a result of treatment with cytotoxic drugs or antibiotics administered concurrently with tumour chemotherapy. Some cases may be associated with hypomagnesaemia, which unless corrected may lead to a syndrome akin to hypoparathyroidism. However, therapy with cytotoxic drugs may lead to hypocalcaemia and low PTH levels in the presence of a normal serum magnesium concentration (Grieve *et al.*, 1982). Parathyroid hormone production is evidently not stimulated even by the low serum calcium level, and direct inhibition by drugs has been considered. Cisplatin and the aminoglycoside group of antibiotics are the drugs most commonly associated with hypocalcaemia, although in many of the reported cases a number of drugs have been administered simultaneously (Gonzales and Villasanta, 1982; Keating *et al.*, 1977).

Specific bone disturbance following antitumour therapy is less common. Increased urinary and faecal calcium excretion has accompanied methotrexate therapy and has been suggested as a possible cause of osteoporosis (Nevinny *et al.*, 1965). Revival of osteoblastic cellular activity can follow therapy of acute granulocytic leukaemia and lead to enhanced osteoid production, calcification of which is delayed. This has been termed osteomalacia, but closer delineation of the defect of the calcification front is necessary before this diagnosis can be accepted (Okita and Block, 1979).

Maintenance of nutrition by parenteral feeding is receiving increasing attention in cancer (Brennan, 1981). Hypercalcaemia occurred in 8% of subjects receiving parenteral nutrition and two cases of neoplasia were amongst those with hypercalcaemia (Gilligan *et al.*, 1982). In the few cases in which both serum PTH levels and intestinal calcium absorption were measured, they were low. Bone in subjects undergoing long-term total parenteral nutrition (TPN) shows many features of osteomalacia and serum levels of $1,25\text{-}(OH)_2D$ are depressed. The level returns to normal if TPN is discontinued with improvement in clinical symptoms. The syndrome does not appear to result from simple vitamin D deficiency, and possible factors include high concentrations of calcium or phosphate in the infusing solution (Klein *et al.*, 1980; Klein *et al.*, 1981; Shike *et al.*, 1980). The possible role of toxic quantities of trace elements has also to be considered; infusion of these in even small quantities may lead to higher inputs than normal, since many are effectively excluded by the intestinal mucosa when taken by mouth. Recent experience with aluminium toxicity in the osteomalacia of chronic renal failure has highlighted possible roles for inorganic elements in the aetiology of osteomalacia (Ott *et al.*, 1982).

MAGNESIUM AND CANCER

Reabsorption of magnesium by the kidney occurs largely in the ascending limb of the loop of Henle and is linked with calcium and sodium. An increase in the excretion of the latter two ions enhances magnesium excretion, leading to hypomagnesaemia (Rude and Singer, 1981). Hypomagnesaemia from a variety of causes may lead to hypocalcaemia, resolution of which occurs when the magnesium status is restored. This probably reflects increased PTH secretion and improved end organ sensitivity (Wiegmann and Kaye, 1977; Rude and Singer, 1981). Hypomagnesaemia may follow treatment of leukaemia, but appropriate supplements of magnesium and calcium together with 1-α-hydroxy vitamin D will prevent any tendency to hypomagnesaemia or associated hypocalcaemia (Freedman *et al.*, 1982).

Aminoglycoside therapy may lead to low levels of magnesium as well as calcium in the presence of low PTH levels and normal calcitonin concentrations (Keating *et al.*, 1977). These drugs inhibit renal tubular magnesium reabsorption, causing a markedly negative magnesium balance. Restoration of magnesium levels does not necessarily improve serum calcium levels if these are also low. Cisplatin is also associated with renal tubular magnesium loss and hypomagnesaemia (Gonzales and Villasanta, 1982).

Dietary-induced experimental hypomagnesaemia in the rat predisposes to the development of blast-like lymphocytes in the thymic cortex, leading to malignant lymphoma (Averdunk *et al.*, 1982). The mechanism whereby magnesium deficiency induces this change is unclear, but such changes are not unique to hypomagnesaemia since similar changes, but not lymphoma, have been associated with zinc deficiency.

MANAGEMENT OF HYPERCALCAEMIA

The severity of the hypercalcaemia and the stage in the progress of the tumour dictate the treatment regimen. In the presence of dehydration, vomiting or confusion, urgent measures to lower the serum calcium level are essential. A severe degree of hypercalcaemia (> 3.5 mmol/litre) without symptoms also warrants close attention. During the initial stages of treatment, rehydration and establishing a diuresis are important; later, inhibition of osteoclastic activity is valuable.

Up to 10 litres of normal (0·9%) saline may be necessary over the first 24 hours, though it is usually sufficient to aim for 6 litres over this period. Administration of sodium sulphate or sodium phosphate has been used with success, but there is a theoretical risk of precipitation of insoluble calcium salts in the tissues and their use has waned. In addition to saline, frusemide may be given for its calciuretic effect. Up to 100 mg/h intravenously has been given (Suki *et al.*, 1970), but conventional dosages of 40–80 mg intravenously are usually sufficient. Intravenous saline is attended by the risk of heart failure, hypokalaemia and hypomagnesaemia. Clinical examination is necessary to monitor heart failure and a venous pressure gauge may be needed. Use of frusemide will reduce the risk of heart failure but will tend to exacerbate the electrolyte abnormalities. Frequent monitoring of electrolytes is mandatory, with appropriate replacement being given as necessary.

Other regimens may also be valuable. Because of the danger of electrolyte abnormalities, associated with the use of saline or frusemide, a combination of calcitonin and corticosteroids has been evaluated and found to be successful (Binstock and Mundy, 1980). Salmon calcitonin (100–200 units 12-hourly) and prednisone (30–60 mg/day) led to a significant fall of serum calcium after 2–3 days in all patients with lymphoproliferative malignancies and most patients with solid tumours. Calcitonin alone is successful initially but its effect is short lived. Successful reduction of serum calcium has also been achieved using intravenous dichloromethylene diphosphonate (Cl_2MDP). Infusion of 2·5 mg/kg body weight on day 1, followed by 5 mg/kg on each of six ensuing days caused serum calcium levels to fall to the normal range. Urinary calcium and urinary hydroxproline also declined (Jacobs *et al.*, 1981). The onset of the hypocalcaemic action of Cl_2MDP is delayed for 1–2 days when used intravenously, but is more rapid than the action of the original diphosphonate drug, EHDP, whose action is delayed for up to one week (Jung *et al.*, 1981*a*).

Whilst resolution of acute hypercalcaemia may be difficult in some cases, necessitating even dialysis, long-term maintenance of a normal serum calcium level may be an even more difficult undertaking. Mithramycin, corticosteroids and the diphosphonate group of drugs are the most valuable adjuncts to therapy at this stage; occasionally indomethacin has been successful, and resort is sometimes made to oral phosphate therapy.

Mithramycin is an inhibitor of osteoclastic activity, although this is not its only effect *in vivo*. The hypocalcaemic effect is usually delayed for 48 hours, and it is therefore started at the same time as the intravenous saline regimen. The dosage is 25 µg/kg body weight per day over 4 hours in 1 litre of normal saline. Urinary calcium usually falls and normocalcaemia can be maintained by intermittent intravenous dosage as required.

Oral corticosteroids are the drugs to which resort is most frequently made. High dosage prednisolone (60 mg/day) may be necessary, but the dose is lowered to the minimum compatible with control of the hypercalcaemia. The side effects of corticosteroids must be weighed against the natural history of the tumour. These drugs inhibit intestinal calcium absorption and the ensuing hypocalcaemia in normal subjects has been held responsible for the high PTH levels found in corticosteroid treated subjects (Hahn, 1978). The high PTH levels in turn have been implicated in the osteopenia of hypercortisolism. Corticosteroids also inhibit osteoblast function (Meunier and Bressôt, 1982), a property that might oppose any hypocalcaemic action. Corticosteroids also inhibit arachidonic acid release (Hong and Levine, 1976), an action that may be of importance in prostaglandin-mediated bone resorption.

Possibly the most promising form of treatment lies in the diphosphonate drugs. The prototype drug, EHDP, has been used successfully in Paget's disease of bone, but skeletal mineralisation and osteoblastic activity are inhibited as well as osteoclastic activity. The newer drugs, APD and Cl_2MDP, are more specific in their effect upon the osteoclast. All diphosphonates are badly absorbed from the intestine. Nevertheless, oral treatment with 3200 mg Cl_2MDP daily has been continued for periods of up to eight weeks and serum calcium levels remain lower than before treatment was started. Some subjects, however, required other forms of therapy intermittently (intravenous diphosphonates or mithramycin) to help keep serum calcium levels in an acceptable range (Chapuy *et al.*, 1980; Jung *et al.*, 1981*a*; Jacobs *et al.*, 1981). High dosage oral diphosphonate therapy, like oral phosphate treatment, frequently causes diarrhoea which may be treated with codeine. EHDP taken by mouth is of no value in hypercalcaemia. Intermittent treatment with diphosphonates intravenously can control hypercalcaemia and has been found to reduce the considerable negative calcium balance that accompanies metastatic bone disease (Jung *et al.*, 1981*b*).

After the initial suppression of acute hypercalcaemia, the management of the tumour frequently supersedes that of the serum calcium. In this phase of management, tumour removal, or reduction of the tumour load, may benefit treatment of hypercalcaemia. Malignancy-associated hypercalcaemia in gynaecological tumours is accompanied by a large tumour burden (Stewart *et al.*, 1982*b*). Removal of tumour surgically can cause not only serum calcium to fall, but also abnormalities of nephrogenous cyclic AMP and tubular maximum reabsorption of phosphate to return to values in the normal range (Stewart *et al.*, 1982*b*; Gottlieb *et al.*, 1982).

Management of the patient with recurring tendency to hypercalcaemia demands a flexible approach that allows for relief of hypercalcaemia in the context of tumour spread. Hypercalcaemia does not necessarily indicate metastatic spread to bone, and removal of a tumour may be countenanced even in the presence of hypercalcaemia. Surgery may also be considered to control hypercalcaemia if it is believed that the benefits will outweigh the trauma of surgery.

REFERENCES

Albright F. (1941). Case records of the Massachusetts General Hospital. *N. Engl. J. Med*; **225**: 789–91.

Anderson J., Dent C.E., Harper C., Philpott G.R. (1954). Effect of cortisone on calcium metabolism in sarcoidosis with hypercalcaemia. *Lancet*; **2**: 720–4.

Aschinberg L.C., Solomon L.M., Zeis P.M., Justice P., Rosenthal I.M. (1977). Vitamin D-resistant rickets associated with the epidermal naevus syndrome: Demonstration of a phosphaturic substance in the dermal lesions. *J. Ped*; **91**: 56–60.

Averdunk R., Bippus P.H., Gunther T., Merker H.J. (1982). Development and properties of malignant lymphoma induced by magnesium deficiency in rats. *J. Cancer. Res. Clin. Oncology*; **104**: 63–73.

Barbour G.L., Coburn J.W., Slatopolsky E., Norman A.W., Horst R.L. (1981). Hypercalcaemia in an anephric patient with sarcoidosis: Evidence for extrarenal generation of 1,25 dihydroxyvitamin D. *N. Engl. J. Med*; **305**: 440–3.

Becker K.L., Silva O.L., Snider R.H., Moore C.F., Geelhoed G.W. (1982). The surgical implications of hypercalcitonaemia. *Surg. Gyn. Obst*; **154**: 897–908.

Bender R.A., Hansen H. (1974). Hypercalcaemia in bronchogenic carcinoma. *Ann. Int. Med*; **80**: 205–208.

Benson R.C., Riggs B.L., Pickard B.M., Arnaud C.D. (1974). Radioimmunoassay of parathyroid hormone in hypercalcaemic patients with malignant disease. *Am. J. Med*; **56**: 821–6.

Berson S.A., Yalo R.S. (1966). Parathyroid hormone in plasma in adenomatous hyperparathyroidism uremia and bronchogenic carcinoma. *Science*; **154**: 907–909.

Bertagna X.Y., Nicholson W.E., Pettergill O.S., Sorensen G.D., Mount C.D., Orth D.N. (1978). Ectopic production of high molecular weight calcitonin and corticotrophins by human small cell carcinoma cells in tissue culture: Evidence for separate precursors. *J. Clin. End. Metab*; **47**: 1390–3.

Binstock M.L., Mundy G.R., (1980). Effect of calcitonin and corticosteroids in combination on the hypercalcaemia of malignancy. *Ann. Int. Med*; **93**: 269–72.

Bockman R.S., (1980). Hypercalcaemia in malignancy. *Clin. End. Metab*; **9**: 317–33.

Brennan M.F. (1981). Total parenteral nutrition in the management of the cancer patient. *Ann. Rev. Med*; **32**: 233–43.

Brenner D.E., Harvey H.A., Lipton A., Demers L. (1982). A study of prostaglandin E2, parathormone and response to indomethacin in patients with hypercalcaemia of malignancy. *Cancer*; **49**: 556–61.

Breslau N.A., McGuire J.L., Zerwekh J.E., Frenkel E.P., Pak C.Y.C. (1984). Hypercalcaemia associated with increased serum calcitriol levels in three patients with lymphoma. *Ann. Int. Med*; **100**: 1–7.

Cervantes F., Ribera J.M., Granena A., Montserrat E., Rozman C. (1982). Tumour lysis syndrome with hypocalcaemia in accelerated chronic granulocytic leukaemia. *Acta. Haematol*; **68**: 157–9.

Chapuy M.C., Meunier P.J., Alexandre C.M., Vignon E.P. (1980). Effects of disodium dichloromethylene diphosphonate on hypercalcaemia produced by bone metastases. *J. Clin. Invest*; **65**: 1243–7.

Christensson T., Hellstrom K., Wengle B., Alveryd A., Wikland B. (1976). Prevalence of hypercalcaemia in a health screening in Stockholm. *Acta Med. Scand*; **200**: 131–7.

Colman P., Firkin B.G., van der Weyden M.B. (1983). Severe hypophosphataemia in T-cell lymphoblastic lymphoma. *Brit. Med. J*; **286**: 105–106.

Coombes R.C., Ward M.K., Greenberg P.B. *et al.* (1976). Calcium metabolism in cancer. *Cancer*; **38**: 2111–120.

Cramer S.F., Fried L., Carter K.J. (1981). The cellular basis of metastatic bone disease in patients with lung cancer. *Cancer*; **48**: 2649–60.

Crystal R.G., Bitterman P.B., Rennard S.I., Hance A.J., Keogh B.A. (1984). Interstitial lung diseases of unknown cause. *N. Engl. J. Med*; **310**: 235–44.

Demers L.M., Allegra J.C., Harvey H.A. *et al.* (1977). Plasma prostaglandins in hypercalcaemic patients with neoplastic disease. *Cancer*; **39**: 1559–62.

Dent C.E., Stamp T.C.B. (1971). Hypophosphataemic osteomalacia presenting in adults. *Q. J. Med*; **40** (NS): 303–29.

Doppelt S.H., Slovik D.M., Neer R.M., Nolan J., Zusman R.M., Potts J.T. (1982). Gut mediated hypercalcaemia in rabbits bearing VX_2 carcinoma: New mechanism for tumour induced hypercalcaemia. *Proc. Natl. Acad. Sci. USA*; **79**: 640–4.

Drezner M.K., Feinglos M.N. (1977). Osteomalacia due to 1α25 dihydroxy-cholecalciferol deficiency. Association with a giant cell tumour of bone. *J. Clin. Invest*; **60**: 1046–53.

Durie B.G.M., Salmon S.E., Mundy G.R. (1981). Relation of osteoclast activating factor production to extent of bone disease in multiple myeloma. *Brit. J. Haematol*; **47**: 21–30.

Farr H.W., Fahey T.J., Nash A.G. *et al.* (1973). Primary hyperparathyroidism and cancer. *Am. J. Surg*; **126**: 539–43.

Ferry S., Kumar A., Schworer M.E., Orth D.N., Jacobs J.W. (1983). *Calc. Tiss. Intl*; **35**: 654 (Abstract).

Fisken R.A., Heath D.A., Bold A.M. (1980). Hypercalcaemia—A hospital survey. *Q. J. Med*; **44** (NS): 405–18.

Fisken R.A., Heath D.A., Somers S., Bold A.M. (1981). Hypercalcaemia in hospital subjects. *Lancet*; **1**: 202–207.

Freedman D.B., Shannon M., Dandena P., Prentice H.G., Hoffbrand A.V. (1982). Hypoparathyroidism and hypocalcaemia during treatment for acute leukaemia. *Brit. Med. J*; **284**: 700–702.

Gilligan J.E., Hagley S., Worthley L.I.G. *et al.* (1982). Hypercalcaemia associated with parenteral amino acid and dextrose infusion. *Amer. J. Clin. Nutr*; **35**: 993–6.

Goltzman D., Stewart A.F., Broadus A.E. (1981). Malignancy-associated hypercalcaemia: Evaluation with a cytochemical assay for parathyroid hormone. *J. Clin. End. Metab*; **53**: 899–904.

Gonzales C., Villasanta U. (1982). Life threatening hypocalcaemia and hypomagnesaemia associated with cisplatin chemotherapy. *Obstet. Gynaecol*; **59**: 732–4.

Gordon G.S., Cantino T.J., Erhardt L., Hansen J., Lubich W. (1966). Osteolytic sterol in human breast cancer. *Science*; **151**: 1226–8.

Gottlieb S., Rude R.K., Sharp C.F., Singer F.R. (1982). Humoral hypercalcaemia of malignancy: A syndrome in search of a hormone. *Am. J. Med*; **73**: 751–5.

Grieve R.J., Roberts H., Dixon P.F., Hunter R.D. (1982). Hypoparathyroidism and hypocalcaemia occurring during cancer chemotherapy. *Brit. Med. J*; **284**: 1877.

Grossman B., Schecter G.P., Horton J.E., Pierce L., Jaffe E., Wahl L. (1981). Hypercalcaemia associated with T-cell lymphoma-leukaemia. *Amer. J. Clin. Path*; **75**: 149–55.

Gwinup G., Sayle B. (1961). Cortisone responsive hypercalcaemia in proved hyperparathyroidism. *Ann. Int. Med*; **55**: 1001–1004.

Hahn T.J. (1978). Corticosteroid induced osteopenia. *Arch. Intern. Med*; **138**: 882–5.

Hall T.C., Griffiths C.T., Petranek J.R. (1966). Hypocalcaemia—An unusual complication of breast cancer. *N. Eng. J. Med*; **275**: 1474–7.

Ham J., Ellison M.L., Lumsden J. (1980). Tumour calcitonin. *Biochem. J*; **199**: 545–50.

Haussler M.R., Drezner M.K., Pike J.W., Chandler J.S., Hagan L.A. (1979). Assay of 1,25 dihydroxyvitamin D and other active vitamin D metabolites in serum: Application to animals and humans. In *Vitamin D Basic Research and its Clinical Application* (Norman A.W. *et al.* eds.) pp. 189–96. Berlin: Walter de Gruyter & Co.

Heyburn P.J., Child J.A., Peacock M. (1981). Relative importance of renal failure and increased bone resorption in the hypercalcaemia of myelomatosis. *J. Clin. Pathol*; **34**: 54–7.

Holdaway I.M., Evans M.C., Clarke E.D. (1977). Watery-diarrhoea syndrome with episodic hypercalcaemia. *Aust. New Zealand J. Med*; **7**: 63–5.

Holick M.F., DeLuca H.F. (1978). Metabolism of vitamin D. In *Vitamin D* (Lawson D.E.M., ed.) pp. 75–7. London: Academic Press.

Hong S.L., Levine L. (1976). Inhibition of arachidonic acid release from cells as the biochemical action of anti-inflammatory corticosteroids. *Proc. Natl. Acad. Sci. USA*; **73**: 1730–4.

Horton J.E., Oppenheim J.J., Mergenhagen S.E., Raisz L.G. (1974). Macrophage lymphocyte synergy in the production of osteoclast activating factor. *J. Immunol*; **113**: 1278–87.

Ibbotson K., D'Souza S.M., Osborne C.K., Niall M., Wah K., Martin T.J., Mundy G.R. (1982). Evidence that a tumour derived growth factor is responsible for the humoral hypercalcaemia of malignancy. *Calc. Tiss. Intl*; **34** Suppl. 1, S31.

Jacobs T.P., Siris E.S., Bilezikian J.P., Baquiran D.C., Shane E., Canfield R.E. (1981). Hypercalcaemia of malignancy: Treatment with intravenous dichloromethylene diphosphonate. *Ann. Int. Med*; **94**: 312–16.

Jung A., van Ouwenaller C., Chantraine A., Courvoisier B. (1981*a*). Parenteral diphosphonates for treating malignant hypercalcaemia. *Cancer*; **48**: 1922–5.

Jung A., van Ouwenaller C., Chantraine A., Donath A., Rosini S. (1981*b*). Use of dichloromethylene diphosphonate in metastatic bone disease. *N. Engl. J. Med*; **305**: 343–4.

Keating M.J., Sethi M.R., Bodey G.P., Samaan N.A. (1977). Hypocalcaemia with hypoparathyroidism and renal tubular dysfunction associated with aminoglycoside therapy. *Cancer*; **39**: 1410–14.

Klein G.L., Ament M.E., Bluestone R., *et al.* (1980). Bone disease associated with total parenteral nutrition. *Lancet*; **2**: 1041–4.

Klein G.L., Herst R.L., Norman A.W., Ament M.E., Slatopolsky E., Coburn J.W. (1981). Reduced serum levels of 1α25 hydroxyvitamin D during long term total parenteral nutrition. *Ann. Int. Med*; **94**: 638–43.

Knill-Jones R.P., Buckle R.M., Parsons V., Calne R.Y., Williams R. (1970). Hypercalcaemia and increased parathyroid hormone like activity in a primary hepatoma. *N. Engl. J. Med*; **282**: 704–708.

Lafferty F.W. (1966). Pseudohyperparathyroidism. *Medicine (Baltimore)*; **45**: 247–60.

Lafferty F.W., Pearson O.H. (1963). Skeletal, intestinal and renal calcium dynamics in hyperparathyroidism. *J. Clin. End. Metab*; **23**: 891–902.

Lerman S., Canterbury J.M., Reiss E. (1977). Parathyroid hormone and the hypercalcaemia of immobilization. *J. Clin. End. Metab*; **45**: 425–8.

Lindgärde F., Zettervall O. (1973). Hypercalcaemia and normal serum calcium in a case of myelomatosis. *Ann. Int. Med*; **78**: 396–9.

Linovitz R.J., Resnick D., Keissling P., *et al.* (1976). Tumour induced osteomalacia and rickets: A surgically curable syndrome. *J. Bone and Joint Surg*; **58A**: 419–23.

Lumsden J., Ham J., Ellison M.L. (1980). Purification and partial characterization of high molecular weight forms of ectopic calcitonin from a human bronchial carcinoma cell line. *Biochem. J*; **191**: 239–46.

Lyles K.W., Berry W.R., Haussler M., Harrelson J.M., Drezner M.K. (1980). Hypophosphataemic osteomalacia: Association with prostatic carcinoma. *Ann. Int. Med*; **93**: 275–8.

Marx S.J., Zusman R.M., Umiker W.O. (1977). Benign breast dysplasia causing hypercalcaemia. *J. Clin. End. Metab*; **45**: 1049–52.

Mason R.S., Frankel T., Chan Y.L., Lissner D., Posen S. (1984). Vitamin D conversion by sarcoid lymph node homogenate. *Ann. Int. Med*; **100**: 59–61.

McCance R.A. (1947). Osteomalacia with Looser's nodes (Milkman's syndrome) due to raised resistance to vitamin D acquired about the age of 15 years. *Q. J. Med*; **16** (NS): 33–46.

Meunier P.J., Bressôt C. (1982). Endocrine influences on bone cells and bone remodelling evaluated by clinical histomorphometry. In *Endocrinology of Calcium Metabolism*. (Parsons J.A. ed.) pp. 456–7. New York: Raven Press.

Minkin C., Fredericks R.S., Pokness S. *et al.* (1981). Bone resorption and humoral hypercalcaemia of malignancy: Stimulation of bone resorption *in vitro* by tumour extracts is inhibited by prostaglandin synthesis inhibitors. *J. Clin. End. Metab*; **53**: 941–7.

Morita R., Fukunaga M., Dokop S., Yamamoto I., Torizaka K. (1978). Differential diagnosis of hypercalcaemia by measurement of parathyroid hormone, calcitonin and 25 hydroxyvitamin D. *J. Nucl. Med*; **19**: 1225–30.

Mundy G.R., Raisz L.G. (1977). Big and little forms of osteoclast activating factor. *J. Clin. Invest*; **60**: 122–8.

Mundy G.R., Luben R.A., Raisz L.G., Oppenheim J.J., Buell D.N. (1974a). Bone resorbing activity in supernatants from lymphoid cell lines. *N. Engl. J. Med*; **290**: 867–71.

Mundy G.R., Raisz L.G., Cooper R.A., Schechter G.P., Salmon S.E. (1974b).

Evidence for the secretion of an osteoclast stimulating factor in myeloma. *N. Engl. J. Med*; **291**: 1041–6.

Mundy G.R., Rick M.E., Turcotte R., Kowalski M.A. (1978*a*). Pathogenesis of hypercalcaemia in lymphosarcoma cell leukaemia. *Am. J. Med*; **65**: 600–606.

Mundy G.R., Varani J., Orr W., Gendek M.D., Ward P.A. (1978*b*). Resorbing bone is chemotactic for monocytes. *Nature*; **275**: 132–5.

Myers W.P.L. (1973). Hypercalcaemia associated with malignant disease. In *Endocrine and Non Endocrine Hormone-producing Tumours*. pp. 147–71. Chicago: Year Book Medical Publishers.

Nevinny H.B., Krant M.J., Moore E.W. (1965). Metabolic studies of the effects of methotrexate. *Metabolism*; **14**: 135–40.

Nomura G., Koshino Y., Morimoto H., Kida H., Nomura S., Tamai K. (1982). Vitamin D resistant hypophosphataemic osteomalacia associated with osteosarcoma of mandible: Report of a case. *Jap. J. Med*; **21**: 35–9.

Nordin B.E.C. (1976). Plasma calcium and plasma magnesium homeostasis. In *Calcium, Phosphate and Magnesium Metabolism*. (Nordin B.E.C., ed.) pp. 186–216. Edinburgh: Churchill Livingstone.

Nortman D.F., Coburn J.W., Brautbar N. *et al.* (1979). Treatment of mesenchymal tumour associated osteomalacia (MTAO) with $1,25(OH)_2D_3$. Report of a case. In *Vitamin D Basic Research and its Clinical Application*. (Norman A.W. *et al.* eds.) pp. 1167–8. Berlin: Walter de Gruyter & Co.

Okita H., Block M. (1979). Osteomalacic new bone formation during chemotherapy of acute granulocytic leukaemia. *Am. J. Clin. Pathol*; **71**: 645–50.

Ott S.M., Maloney N.A., Coburn J.W., Alfrey A.C., Sherrard D.J. (1982). The prevalence of bone aluminium deposition in renal osteodystrophy and its relation to the response to calcitriol therapy. *N. Engl. J. Med*; **307**: 709–13.

Owen M. (1980). The origin of bone cells in the postnatal organism. *Arth. Rheum*; **23**: 1073–80.

Palmer F.J., Nelson J.C., Bacchus H. (1974). The chloride phosphate ratio in hypercalcaemia. *Ann. Int. Med*; **80**: 200–204.

Powles T.J., Clark S.A., East D.M., Easty G.C., Neville A.M. (1973). The inhibition by aspirin and indomethacin of osteolytic tumour deposits and hypercalcaemia in rats with Walker tumour, and its possible application to human breast cancer. *Brit. J. Cancer*; **28**: 316–21.

Raisz L.G., Luben R.A., Mundy G.R., Dietrich J.W., Horton J.E., Trummel C.L. (1975). Effect of osteoclast activating factor from human leukocytes on bone metabolism. *J. Clin. Invest*; **56**: 408–13.

Ralston S., Gardner M.D., Fogelman I., Boyle I.T. (1982). Hypercalcaemia and metastatic bone disease: Is there a causal link? *Lancet*; **2**: 903–905.

Rasmussen H., Bordier P. (1974). *The Physiological and Cellular Basis of Metabolic Bone Disease*. pp. 153–60. Baltimore: Williams & Wilkins.

Roos B.A., Lindall A.W., Baylin S.B. *et al.* (1980). Plasma immunoreactive calcitonin in lung cancer. *J. Clin. End. Metab*; **50**: 245–59.

Rude R.K., Singer F.R. (1981). Magnesium deficiency and excess. *Ann. Rev. Med*; **32**: 245–59.

Sackner M.A., Spivack A.P., Balian L.J. (1960). Hypocalcaemia in the presence of osteoblastic metastases. *N. Eng. J. Med*; **262**: 173–6.

Salassa R.M., Jowsey J., Arnaud C.D. (1970). Hypophosphataemic osteomalacia associated with non endocrine tumours. *N. Engl. J. Med*; **283**: 65–70.

Schussler G.C., Verso M.A., Nemoto T. (1972). Phosphaturia in hypercalcaemic breast cancer patients. *J. Clin. End. Metab*; **35**: 497–504.

Seyberth H.W., Segre G.V., Morgan J.L., Sweetman B.J., Potts J.Y., Oates J.A. (1975). Prostaglandin as mediators of hypercalcaemia associated with certain types of cancer. *N. Engl. J. Med*; **293**: 1278–83.

Sherwood L.M., O'Riordan J.L.H., Aurbach G.D., Potts J.T. (1967). Production of parathyroid hormone by nonparathyroid tumours. *J. Clin. End. Metab*; **27**: 140–6.

Shike M., Harrison J.E., Sturtridge W.C. *et al.* (1980). Metabolic bone disease in patients receiving long term total parenteral nutrition. *Ann. Int. Med*; **92**: 343–50.

Silva O.L., Broder L.E., Doppman J.L. *et al.* (1979). Calcitonin as a marker for bronchogenic cancer. *Cancer*; **44**: 680–4.

Simpson E., Mundy G.R., D'Souza S.M., Ibbotson K.J., Bockman R., Jacobs J.W. (1983). Absence of parathyroid hormone messenger RNA in nonparathyroid tumours associated with hypercalcaemia. *N. Engl. J. Med*; **309**: 325–30.

Stewart A.F., Horst R., Deftos L.J., Cadman E.C., Lang R., Broadus A.E. (1980). Biochemical evaluation of patients with cancer associated hypercalcaemia. *N. Engl. J. Med*; **303**: 1377–83.

Stewart A.F., Vignery A., Silverglate A. *et al.* (1982*a*). Quantitative bone histomorphometry in humoral hypercalcaemia of malignancy: Uncoupling of bone cell activity. *J. Clin. End. Metab*; **55**: 219–27.

Stewart A.F., Romero R., Schwartz P.E., Kohorn E.I., Broadus A.E. (1982*b*). Hypercalcaemia associated with gynaecologic malignancies. *Cancer*; **49**: 2389–94.

Swaroop S., Krant M.J. (1973). Rapid oestrogen induced hypercalcaemia. *JAMA*; **223**: 913–14.

Sweet R.A., Males J.L., Hamstra A.J., DeLuca H.F. (1980). Vitamin D metabolite levels in oncogenic osteomalacia. *Ann. Int. Med*; **93**: 279–80.

Suki W.N., Yuim J.J., Von Hinden M., Saller-Herbert L., Eknoyan G., Martinez-Maldonado M. (1970). Acute treatment of hypercalcaemia with furosemide. *N. Engl. J. Med*; **283**: 836–40.

Szymendera J. (1970). Bone mineral metabolism in cancer. *Recent Results Cancer Res*; **27**: 84.

Tashjian A.H., Voelkel E.F., Levine L., Goldharber D. (1972). Evidence that the bone resorption stimulation factor produced by mouse fibrosarcoma cells is prostaglandin E_2. *J. Exp. Med*; **136**: 1329–43.

Trechsel U., Taylor C.M., Bonjour J.P., Fleisch H. (1980). Influence of prostaglandins and of cyclic nucleotides on the metabolism of 25-hydroxyvitamin D_3 in primary chick kidney cell culture. *BBRC*; **93**: 1210–16.

Veldhuis J.D. (1978). Tamoxifen and hypercalcaemia. *Ann. Int. Med*; **88**: 574–5.

Voelkel E.F., Tashjian A.M., Franklin R., Wasserman E., Levine L. (1975). Hypercalcaemia and tumour prostaglandins. The VX_2 carcinoma model in the rabbit. *Metabolism*; **24**: 973–86.

Wiegmann T., Kaye M. (1977). Hypomagnesaemic hypocalcaemia. *Arch. Int. Med*; **137**: 953–5.

Wyman A.L., Paradinas F.J., Daly J.R. (1977). Hypophosphataemic osteomalacia associated with a malignant lymphoma of the tibia: Report of a case. *J. Clin. Path*; **30**: 328–35.

Yoneda T., Mundy G.R. (1979). Prostaglandins are necessary for osteoclast activating factor production by activated peripheral blood leucocytes. *J. Exp. Med*; **149**: 279–83.

Zamkoff K.W., Kirschner J.J. (1980). Marked hypophosphataemia associated with acute myelomonocytic leukaemia. *Arch. Int. Med*; **140**: 1523–4.

Zusman J., Brown D.M., Nesbit M.E. (1973). Hyperphosphataemia, hyperphosphaturia and hypocalcaemia in acute lymphoblastic leukaemia. *N. Engl. J. Med*; **289**: 1335–40.

Chapter 7

Martin O. Savage

Growth and Development

INTRODUCTION

Normal growth in childhood is dependent on the integrity of the central nervous system control of hypothalamic–pituitary endocrine function. Growth at adolescence and normal pubertal development depend, in addition, on the integrity of the pituitary–gonadal axis. Any neoplastic process which interferes with anterior pituitary function, and specifically with growth hormone secretion, will thus disturb the pattern of normal growth. Similarly, puberty may be either delayed or advanced by factors acting locally in the region of the hypothalamus or pituitary to alter the normal pattern of gonadotrophin secretion.

Inappropriate secretion of sex steroids by gonadal tumours may also disturb normal growth and puberty. Androgens stimulate linear growth but the end result may be short stature due to early epiphyseal closure. Androgen and oestrogen secretion during the prepubertal period may produce precocious virilisation and feminisation, respectively, giving rise to so-called pseudoprecocious puberty. Excess cortisol and sex steroid production by tumours of the adrenal cortex may also suppress growth and lead to inappropriate virilisation or feminisation.

The aim of this chapter is to review the major disturbances of growth and pubertal development caused by malignant disease in childhood. The chapter is divided into three main sections. The first discusses central nervous system malignancies, the second malignancies of other endocrine glands which may disturb growth and puberty, and the third, the investigation and management of endocrine disturbance.

MALIGNANT TUMOURS OF THE CENTRAL NERVOUS SYSTEM

Primary tumours arising in the region of the pituitary and hypothalamus constitute an important cause of abnormal growth and development. The most frequent of these, the craniopharyngioma, is a benign neoplasm and will not be considered here. Endocrine disturbance may result from direct interference with pituitary function by the tumour, causing deficiency of anterior pituitary trophic hormones. Alternatively, there may be disturbance of the normal hypothalamic–pituitary relationship, which can produce either pituitary insufficiency or hypersecretion of anterior pituitary hormones, principally gonadotrophins. Secretion of human chorionic gonadotrophin (HCG) by a midline cerebral tumour is also a recognised cause of precocious sexual development. The cerebral tumours most frequently associated with abnormal growth and pubertal development are the following: optic glioma, gliomas of the hypothalamus, suprasellar germinoma, and pineal tumours (Table 7.1).

TABLE 7.1
Malignant Childhood CNS Tumours
Affecting Growth and Development

Tumours which may cause impaired growth
    Optic glioma
    Glioma of the hypothalamus
    Suprasellar germinoma
    Histiocytosis X
Tumours which may cause delayed puberty
    Optic glioma
    Suprasellar germinoma
    Parenchymal pinealoma
Tumours which may cause precocious puberty
    Optic glioma
    Gliomas of the hypothalamus
    Suprasellar germinoma
    Midline β-HCG-secreting tumours

TUMOURS WHICH MAY CAUSE IMPAIRED GROWTH

Optic Glioma

Glial tumours of the optic nerve and chiasm are rare, however about 70% present during the first decade of life (Reese, 1963). This neoplasm may occur either as a solitary entity or may be a component of neurofibromatosis. The incidence of neurofibromatosis in the majority of large series of patients with optic glioma is in the region of 30% (Oxenhandler and Sayers, 1978; Danoff *et al.*, 1980). Visual disturbance is the principal presenting feature of optic glioma. However, if the disease spreads to or above the chiasm, compression of the third ventricle and injury to the pituitary stalk may

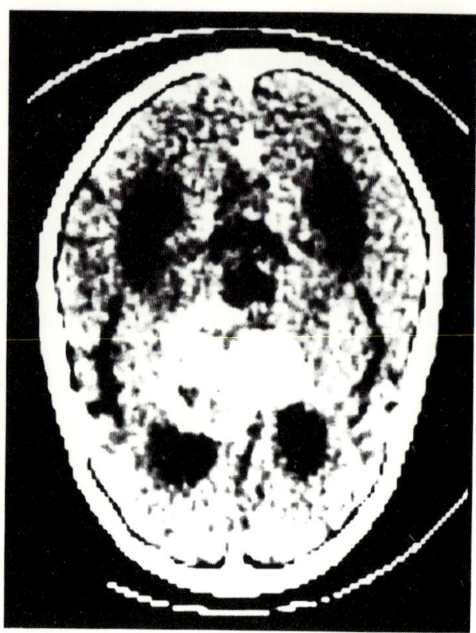

Fig. 7.1. *Cranial CT scan showing large hypothalamic tumour (not biopsied).
The patient (Fig. 7.2) presented with the diencephalic syndrome and developed
precocious puberty (Fig. 7.3) following radiotherapy to the tumour.*

disturb hypothalamic–pituitary function. There is little data on endocrine
function in children with optic gliomas, however impaired growth and
deficient growth hormone secretion have been described as part of the
diencephalic syndrome (*see* below, Danoff *et al.*, 1980).

Gliomas of the Hypothalamus

Gliomas of the hypothalamus (Fig. 7.1) may cause two distinct clinical
pictures, depending on the age of onset. These are the diencephalic
syndrome (Fig. 7.2), and precocious puberty (Fig. 7.3). Occurring usually
before the age of four years, the diencephalic syndrome is most often
associated with gliomas of the anterior hypothalamus and third ventricle.
The most frequent tumours are astrocytomas followed by spongioblastoma,
astroblastoma, ependymoma, ganglioglioma, oligodendroglioma and dysgerminoma (Burr *et al.*, 1976).

The Diencephalic Syndrome

The recognition of this syndrome is generally attributed to Russell (1951).
The essential features comprise a tumour of the diencephalon associated

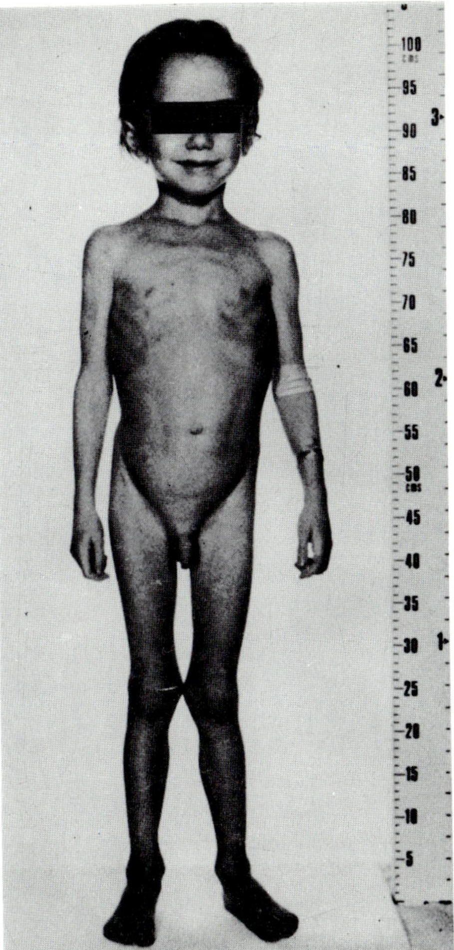

Fig. 7.2. *Diencephalic syndrome in a four-year-old boy caused by a hypothalamic tumour (Fig. 7.1).*

with emaciation and minimal neurological signs in infants and children. The child's weight is always grossly reduced whereas the height may be initially normal or even increased with advanced bone age (Drop *et al.*, 1980), but growth may ultimately fail as the syndrome progresses (Costin, 1979). The peak incidence is at six months of age (Burr *et al.*, 1976), and the presence of a tumour may not be confirmed until the clinical features are well established. Other recognised features are hyperkinesis, alert appearance, inappropriate euphoria, vomiting, pallor, nystagmus and reduced visual acuity. Tumour cells may or may not be present in the cerebrospinal fluid and elevation of cerebrospinal fluid protein concentration may be seen. The

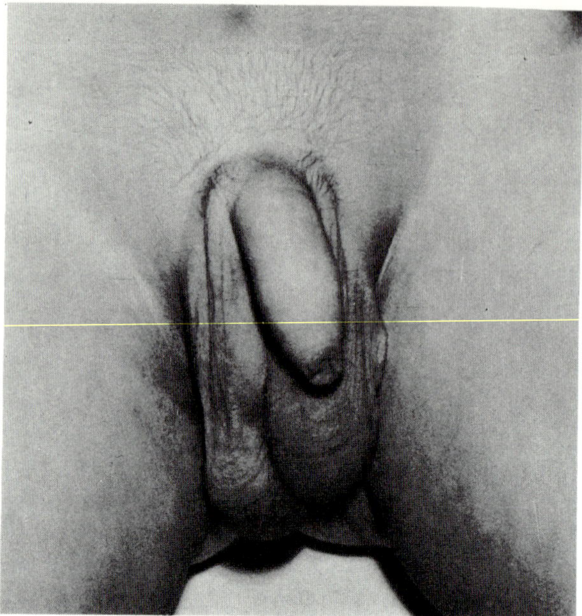

Fig. 7.3. *Precocious puberty in the same patient (Fig. 7.2) following radiotherapy to his hypothalamic tumour.*

endocrine abnormalities are variable, but elevated basal growth hormone
concentration (Drop *et al.*, 1980) and paradoxical growth hormone responses to hyper- and hypoglycaemia (Häger and Thorell, 1973) have been
described.

Suprasellar Germinoma

Growth delay is perhaps less recognised as a complication of suprasellar
germinoma than other endocrine presentations such as diabetes insipidus or
precocious puberty. Growth hormone deficiency, however, appears to be a
common complication of this neoplasm in childhood and may be associated
with other anterior pituitary hormone deficiencies. Pomerade *et al.* (1982)
reported that 11 out of 13 children with histologically proven germinoma,
conforming to the criteria of Russell and Rubinstein (1977), had growth
hormone deficiency and five had short stature at the time of presentation.
Similar findings were described by Newman *et al.* (1981), and by Sklar *et al.*
(1981) who reported some degree of anterior pituitary dysfunction in all ten
patients with germinoma in their series. Growth was retarded in five and
growth hormone deficiency present in all seven tested. The combination of
diabetes insipidus and growth hormone deficiency may be an ominous

prelude to the subsequent presentation of a suprasellar germinoma in childhood (Pomerade *et al.*, 1980).

Histiocytosis X

Histiocytosis X is still a potentially fatal condition. However, there is debate as to whether it qualifies as a true malignancy (Pritchard, 1979). The presence of growth failure secondary to growth hormone deficiency in histiocytosis is now an established entity (Latorre *et al.*, 1974). Diabetes insipidus is a common finding and may be associated with growth hormone deficiency; both possibly being due to a single hypothalamic lesion (Braunstein and Kohler, 1972). It has also been suggested that impaired growth velocity might be related to abnormal fluid balance, improving after treatment of diabetes insipidus (Calzada *et al.*, 1979). Replacement of growth hormone is usually required, contrasting with other anterior pituitary hormones which appear to be characteristically normal (Calzada *et al.*, 1979).

TUMOURS WHICH MAY CAUSE DELAYED PUBERTY
(Table 7.2)

Delayed puberty can be defined as complete lack of secondary sexual development at an age two standard deviations beyond the mean (Tanner, 1962). In practical terms this means 15 years in boys and 14 years in girls. Intracranial tumours causing gonadotrophin deficiency accounted for 9·5% of males and 19% of females in a series of 200 patients with delayed puberty

TABLE 7.2
Tumours of Endocrine Glands
Affecting Growth and Puberty

Adrenocortical tumours[a]
Testicular tumours
    Leydig cell tumour[a]
    Gonadal stromal tumour[a,b]
    Gonadoblastoma[b]
Ovarian tumours
    Granulosa cell[b]
    Granulosa theca cell[b]
    Androblastoma[a]
    Gonadoblastoma[a,b]

Tumours causing principally virilisation[a] and feminisation[b].

(Chaussain, 1981). As with growth delay, craniopharyngioma is the most frequent neoplasm. As gonadotrophin and growth hormone secretion are closely related structurally in the anterior pituitary, most of the neoplasms described above may also disturb gonadotrophin production. Delayed puberty has specifically been documented in optic glioma, suprasellar germinoma (Sung Duk *et al.*, 1978; Sklar *et al.*, 1981), and in pineal tumours of parenchymal origin (Kitay, 1954).

TUMOURS WHICH MAY CAUSE PRECOCIOUS PUBERTY

Intracranial tumours in the region of the diencephalic structures constitute an important cause of precocious puberty, particularly in males (Balagura *et al.*, 1979). In this situation the neurogenic inhibitory control of hypothalamic–pituitary–gonadal function is apparently removed, showing increased secretion of LH-RH from the hypothalamus and in turn gonadotrophins and sex steroids. The affected children, most commonly boys, in a ratio of 5:1, are tall with advanced skeletal age, and have the signs of puberty associated with gonadal maturation (Costin, 1979). The tumours most frequently associated with precocious puberty are optic glioma, hypothalamic astrocytoma and teratoma, suprasellar germinoma and pi-nealoma. A further cause is the ectopic secretion of HCG by a midline tumour.

Optic Glioma and Hypothalamic Gliomas

Precocious puberty is a well recognised complication of optic gliomas which spread to the chiasm or infiltrate adjacent structures in the region of the hypothalamus (Danoff *et al.*, 1980). Neurofibromatosis is often the primary disorder (Riccardi, 1981). The progression of puberty may not, however, be arrested by radiotherapy to the primary tumour, precocious puberty being demonstrated in seven out of 54 children with optic glioma extending beyond the optic nerve (Kalifa *et al.*, 1981). It has also been reported to develop after radiotherapy in another child with optic glioma (Iraci *et al.*, 1980). In a review of 82 cases of true precocious puberty, Balagura *et al.* (1979) reported that astrocytoma was the most frequently occurring primary hypothalamic tumour, with a peak incidence between the ages of three and seven years. Neurofibromatosis and tuberous sclerosis were frequent associated disorders.

Tumours in the Pineal Region (Suprasellar Germinoma)

Precocious puberty is the endocrine abnormality that is most widely associated with pineal tumours (Axelrod, 1977; Giovanelli, 1982). The mechanism of this association is unclear. It is possible either that tumours cause loss of pineal anti-gonadotrophin effect, that other areas normally inhibiting sexual development are destroyed by the tumour or that an ectopic gonadotrophin is produced. Most cases of precocious puberty develop in young males with non-parenchymatous tumours (Kitay, 1954), the most frequent being a germinoma. Suprasellar germinoma or ectopic pinealoma (Russell and Rubinstein, 1977) is typical of most midline cerebral tumours in that it may disseminate into the ventricular system and metastasise to the cerebral or spinal subarachnoid space. The tumour, however, is highly sensitive to radiotherapy (Sung Duk *et al.*, 1978). Precocious puberty occurred in two out of 16 patients reported by Sung Duk *et al.* (1978), and in 22 histologically verified cases reported by Balagura *et al.* (1979). Numerically, however, precocious puberty may be less common in childhood germinoma than diabetes insipidus and growth hormone deficiency (Pomerade *et al.*, 1982).

Primary HCG-producing Intracranial Tumours

Human chorionic gonadotrophin can be produced by midline cerebral tumours (Vaitukaitis, 1973) and this may be associated with premature sexual development (Romshe and Sotos, 1975). Most HCG-producing tumours appear to be of germ cell origin and in only a few cases has the nature of the ectopic hormone been documented by the use of a specific HCG assay (Kubo *et al.*, 1977). Tumours producing human chorionic gonadotrophin in the region of the pineal gland are extremely rare, however there have been three recent fully documented reports; two of germinomas (Sklar *et al.*, 1981; Ahmed *et al.*, 1983), and the other a pineal choriocarcinoma (Wass *et al.*, 1982). The presence of the HCG-producing brain tumours provides an alternative mechanism for precocious puberty of cerebral origin. In this situation the hypothalamic–pituitary system would remain immature, with prepubertal LH and FSH levels. The low secretion of FSH, normally necessary for female pubertal development, might explain why precocious puberty, due to HCG production, is much commoner in boys (Sklar *et al.*, 1981).

TUMOURS OF OTHER ENDOCRINE GLANDS AFFECTING GROWTH AND DEVELOPMENT

Tumours of the Adrenal Cortex

Tumours of the adrenal cortex are rare in childhood, accounting for only two in 100 000 of all childhood malignancies (Levine, 1978). An exception is the relative frequency of adrenal carcinoma in certain high risk groups, notably children with Beckwith–Weidemann syndrome and with hemi-hypertrophy (Tank and Kay, 1979). The histological distinction between benign and malignant adrenocortical tumours is often not clear-cut, and may only be made with certainty when the adrenal capsule is invaded by the tumour or when metastases develop (Forest, 1981). Endocrine disturbances are, however, a common feature of childhood adrenal malignancy, the most frequent being abnormal virilisation (Hughes, 1982) which may be associated with hypercortisolism. Virilising adrenal tumours are more likely to occur in young children under the age of two years with a female to male ratio of two to one (Hayles *et al.*, 1966); most are carcinomas. In a review of 44 previously reported cases of functioning childhood adrenal tumours by Drago *et al.* (1979), 25 presented with virilism, ten with Cushing's syndrome, seven with combined virilism and Cushing's syndrome, and two with virilism and gynaecomastia. This contrasts with the predominance of Cushing's syndrome in adults with adrenal carcinoma (Didolkar *et al.*, 1981).

In children, the virilisation constitutes a form of pseudoprecocious puberty and usually presents as penile or clitoral enlargement with pubic hair growth. Linear growth is accelerated due to androgen stimulation of skeletal maturation. True pubertal development will be delayed or arrested because of suppression of gonadotrophins by the high circulating sex steroids, and in boys the testes remain infantile. The characteristic hormonal feature of adrenal tumours is the excessive production of $\Delta 5$ pregnene steroids (Forest, 1981; Honour *et al.*, 1984). Over production of dehydroepiandrosterone and its sulphate, and of their normal or abnormal metabolites, is a constant finding (Cahen *et al.*, 1978; Gregory *et al.*, 1979).

Patients presenting with Cushing's syndrome usually have growth retardation (Lee *et al.*, 1975) often associated with obesity and hypertension. The mechanism of the growth-suppressing effect of cortisol is unclear and is likely to be multifactorial. Growth hormone production during sleep may be impaired as may its peripheral metabolism by suppression of somatomedin secretion (Elders *et al.*, 1975).

Feminising adrenal tumours are considerably less common than their virilising counterparts. In boys, gynaecomastia is present (Sultan *et al.*, 1979), either alone or with signs of virilisation (Itami *et al.*, 1982). In girls there is usually sexual precocity with premature breast development, pubic or axillary hair growth and possibly premature menarche (Wohltmann *et al.*, 1980). Growth and skeletal maturation is advanced in both sexes and hormonal studies have shown a combination of increased oestrogen and androgen excretion, with androgen production being approximately half that found in predominantly virilising adrenal tumours (Forest, 1981; Benaily *et al.*, 1975).

Testicular Tumours

Testicular tumours are the seventh most common neoplasm in the paediatric age group and represent 1% of all cases of malignant disease in childhood (Sabio *et al.*, 1974). The majority of these tumours are not endocrinologically functional. An exception is the Leydig cell tumour which constitutes a well established cause of pseudoprecocious puberty (Root *et al.*, 1972; Colodny and Hopkins, 1977; Röttger *et al.*, 1981). Detailed hormonal studies have been performed in several children with Leydig cell tumours which have been shown to produce androstenedione and testosterone (Wegienka and Kolb, 1967), as well as oestrogens and dehydroepiandrosterone (Ilondo *et al.*, 1981). These tumours are, however, relatively benign in childhood.

Steroid metabolism was studied in a gonadal stroma tumour by De Niepowniszcze *et al.* (1982) who demonstrated deficient activity of the enzymes 17–20 desmolase and 3β-hydroxysteroid dehydrogenase within the tumour. Fligiel *et al.* (1976) reported a child with bilateral Sertoli cell tumours, which produced both virilising and feminising effects. A further rare type of childhood testicular tumour is the gonadoblastoma, which may develop in a dysgenetic testis. This is a well known occurrence in patients with male pseudohermaphroditism due to deficient gonadal differentiation, but has also been described in the newborn period (Hung *et al.*, 1981).

Ovarian Tumours

Ovarian tumours are rare in childhood and adolescence, accounting for approximately 1% of all childhood malignancy (Breen and Maxson, 1977). The majority occur between the ages of 10 and 14 years and the overall incidence of malignancy varies from 22–55%. The most common ovarian neoplasms are of germ cell origin, and these are usually endocrinologically inactive. It is the group of sex cord stromal tumours which are often functional, and they account for most cases of both isosexual and heterosexual precocious puberty of ovarian origin.

In 43 cases of isosexual precocious puberty, the relative frequency of associated histological diagnosis was as follows: granulosa cell 27–29%, granulosa theca cell 14%, immature teratoma 14%, Sertoli cell 4·7%, choriocarcinoma 7%, embryonal carcinoma of the vagina with follicle cysts of the ovaries 2·3%. In 11 cases (25·6%), the only identifiable lesions were non-neoplastic follicle cysts (Breen and Maxson, 1977). Granulosa cell (Eberlein *et al.*, 1960) and granulosa theca cell tumours (Lack *et al.*, 1981) are the most important oestrogen-producing neoplasms. They are also capable of causing virilisation and one patient developed hyperprolactinaemia and galactorrhoea (Lack *et al.*, 1981). Isosexual precocity is manifested by breast development, maturation of external genitalia and accelerated growth. There is often associated anovulatory vaginal bleeding.

Virilising ovarian tumours are less frequent (Groeber, 1963), and the most important is the androblastoma, known also as Sertoli–Leydig cell tumour or arrhenoblastoma (Roth *et al.*, 1981). Virilisation will present as pubic hair growth, clitoromegaly, and advanced growth, and the cause must be distinguished from late-presenting congenital adrenal hyperplasia. Granulosa theca cell tumours may also secrete androgens (Lack *et al.*, 1981), as may a lipid-cell tumour (Ammann *et al.*, 1967; Scully *et al.*, 1982). A further ovarian tumour which is occasionally functional is the gonadoblastoma. This typically develops in dysgenetic gonads (Frasier *et al.*, 1964), and may cause either feminisation or virilisation (Griffiths *et al.*, 1966).

DIAGNOSIS AND MANAGEMENT OF ENDOCRINE DISTURBANCE

Investigation of Suspected Intracranial Lesion

Hypothalamic–pituitary deficiency (Tables 7.3 and 7.4)

The clinical signs of anterior pituitary deficiency may be subtle and often develop over a considerable length of time. A history of visual disturbance or symptoms suggestive of raised intracranial pressure associated with thirst

TABLE 7.3
Assessment of Hypothalamic–Pituitary Function

Clinical assessment
History: Disturbance of growth, pubertal development
 Symptoms of raised intracranial pressure
 Intellectual changes
 Symptoms of diencephalic syndrome
 Visual disturbances
 Signs of neurofibromatosis
Fundoscopy, visual fields

Auxological assessment
Height, height velocity
Puberty ratings
Testicular volume
Skin-fold thicknesses

Radiological assessment
Skull x-ray (pituitary fossa)
Bone age
Cranial CT scan

TABLE 7.4

Laboratory Assessment of Hypothalamic–Pituitary Function

Anterior pituitary
Basal hormone concentrations: T_3, T_4
                                   Cortisol (12 pm and 9 am)
                                   Testosterone, oestradiol
                                   Prolactin

Stimulation tests:
  Growth hormone, ACTH
     1) Insulin tolerance test (0·1 units/kg i.v.)
     2) Glucagon stimulation test (100 μg/mg i.m.)
  TSH, prolactin
    TRH test (200 μg i.v.)
  LH, FSH
    LHRH test (100 μg i.v.)

Posterior pituitary
  24-hour fluid balance
  Early morning simultaneous plasma and urine osmolalities
  Water deprivation test
  DDAVP test

---

and polyuria may indicate a lesion in the hypothalamic–pituitary region. Growth failure or delayed puberty suggest anterior pituitary deficiency. Clinical examination should include fundoscopy and visual field assessment, with detailed anthropometric assessment of height, height velocity (Cameron ,1978) and pubertal development (Tanner, 1962; Zachmann *et al.*, 1974). Skull x-ray and cranial CT are also essential, and measurement of visual evoked responses may be helpful.

The laboratory investigation of anterior pituitary function consists of examination of basal plasma concentrations of thyroxine, cortisol, sex steroids and prolactin. Dynamic tests examine anterior pituitary hormone reserve and are usually combined as a single stimulation test (Table 7.4), i.e. insulin tolerance test, TRH test, and LH-RH test (Milner and Burns, 1982). In children with suspected ACTH deficiency, half the normal dose of insulin should be used (i.e. 0·05 units/kg).

Hypothyroidism, if present, should be corrected before assessment of growth hormone secretion. In children under 4 years of age an insulin tolerance test is dangerous, and an intramuscular glucagon stimulation test (Vanderschueren–Lodeweyckx *et al.*, 1974), which provides effective stimulation of growth hormone and ACTH secretion, is preferable.

Posterior pituitary function is assessed by measurement of 24-hour fluid balance, simultaneous early morning plasma and urine osmolalities and, if necessary, a water deprivation test, followed by administration of DDAVP.

Investigation of true and pseudoprecocious puberty (Tables 7.5 and 7.6)

Precocious pubertal development requires urgent investigation. True hypothalamic–pituitary precocity must be distinguished from pseudoprecocity due to abnormal secretions of sex steroids from the gonads or the adrenal cortex. In either situation a malignant neoplasm may be the cause. Clinical examination should include detailed assessment of height, height

TABLE 7.5

Clinical Assessment of Precocious Puberty

History:
    Timing of onset of puberty
    Symptoms of raised intracranial pressure
    Visual disturbances

General examination:
    Fundoscopy, visual fields
    Signs of neurofibromatosis or McCune-Albright syndrome
    Rectal examination (for ovarian mass)
    Blood pressure

Auxological assessment:
    Height, height velocity
    Puberty ratings
    Testicular volume
    Possible clitoromegaly

Radiological assessment:
    Skull x-ray (pituitary fossa)
    Bone age
    Cranial CT scan
    Abdominal ultrasound
    Abdominal CT scan

TABLE 7.6

Laboratory Assessment of Precocious Puberty

Plasma androgens:	testosterone
	dehydroepiandrosterone
Urinary androgens:	17-oxosteroids
Plasma oestrogen:	oestradiol
Plasma cortisol:	17-OH progesterone
Gonadotrophins:	basal LH, FSH
	LHRH stimulation test (100 µg i.v.)

velocity and pubertal status, looking particularly for signs of heterosexual development such as clitoromegaly or gynaecomastia. In boys, symmetrical testicular enlargement is suggestive of premature hypothalamic–pituitary activity whereas virilisation in the presence of prepubertal testes suggests adrenal androgen secretion. Signs of hypercortisolism such as obesity, acne, virilism and hypertension are particularly suggestive of an adrenocortical tumour. In true precocious puberty, radiological studies should include a skull x-ray and cranial CT scan. In pseudoprecocity, abdominal ultrasound or CT scan should be performed to exclude an adrenocortical or ovarian neoplasm.

Laboratory assessment consists of determination of basal plasma concentrations of sex steroids, adrenal androgens, 17-hydroxyprogesterone, β-HCG, cortisol, ACTH and urinary 17-oxosteroids. An LH-RH stimulation test (Chaussain *et al.*, 1978) will show a pubertal response of LH and FSH in true precocious puberty compared with a suppressed response in pseudo-precocity. In Cushingoid patients, a dexamethasone suppression test should be performed to distinguish between adrenal hyperplasia and an adrenal neoplasm.

MANAGEMENT OF ENDOCRINE DISTURBANCE

Hypopituitarism is managed by replacement of the deficient hormones. For example, growth hormone deficiency is treated by injections of human growth hormone throughout the remaining period of the child's growth (Preece, 1982). Adrenocorticotrophic hormone deficiency is treated by hydrocortisone replacement ($20\,mg/m^2$ surface area), and TSH deficiency by thyroxine replacement. In gonadotrophin deficiency, male puberty is usually induced by sex steroid replacement using either depot testosterone given by monthly injection (100–500 mg monthly) or by oral testosterone undecanoate (40 mg t.d.s.). Human chorionic gonadotrophin may also be given by injection (1000–2000 units weekly) to stimulate endogenous testosterone secretion. In girls, oestrogen and progesterone replacement may be given as ethinyloestradiol (10–30 μg daily) and progesterone as medoxyprogesterone acetate (5 mg daily for seven days in each month).

Diabetes insipidus is managed on the principal that as much water is available to the child as is necessary to avoid a hyperosmolar state. Antidiuretic hormone replacement is given in the form of an analogue, DDAVP, which is available in a solution of 0·1 mg/ml. DDAVP is administered intra-nasally, usually twice daily, in a dose of 0.5–1.0 μg in infants and 2·5 μg in older children.

The management of precocious puberty is aimed at removal of the primary tumour, whether this be of cerebral, gonadal or adrenal origin. Some intracranial neoplasms are inoperable, due either to their inaccessibility or involvement of vital structures. In these cases, radiotherapy or chemotherapy may be indicated. In the presence of progressive sexual precocity the most effective agent is probably cyproterone acetate ($70-150\,\text{mg}/\text{m}^2$ surface area) (Kauli *et al.*, 1976). Cyproterone acetate has been shown to effectively arrest secondary sexual development, however its growth-suppressing properties have yet to be confirmed (Bierich *et al.*, 1980). Recently, research on long acting analogues of LHRH suggest that these are effective in arresting precocious pubertal development (Mansfield *et al.*, 1983).

REFERENCES

Ahmed S.R., Shalet S.M., Price D.A., Pearson D. (1983). Human chorionic gonadotrophin secreting pineal germinoma and precocious puberty. *Arch. Dis. Child*; **58**: 743–5.

Ammann A.J., Kaufman S., Gilbert A. (1967). Virilising ovarian tumour in a $2\frac{1}{2}$ year old girl. *J. Pediatr*; **70**: 782–7.

Axelrod L. (1977). Endocrine dysfunction in patients with tumours of the pineal region. In *Pineal Tumours* (Schmidek H.H., ed.) pp. 61–77. USA: Masson Publishing.

Balagura S., Shulman K., Sobel E.H. (1979). Precocious puberty of cerebral origin. *Surg. Neurol*; **11**: 315–26.

Benaily M., Schweisguth O., Job J.C. (1975). Adrenocortical tumours in children. Retrospective study of 34 cases observed between 1954 and 1973. *Arch. Fr. Pediatr*; **32**: 441–54.

Bierich J.R., Heinrich J.G., Esteves P.E. (1980). Experiences in the treatment of idiopathic precocious puberty with cyproterone acetate. In *Pathophysiology of Puberty* (Cacciani E., Prader A., eds.) pp. 245–55. London: Academic Press.

Braunstein G.D., Kohler P.O. (1972). Pituitary function in Hand–Schuller–Christian disease: Evidence for deficient growth-hormone release in patients with short stature. *N. Engl. J. Med*; **286**: 1225–9.

Breen J.L., Maxson W.S. (1977). Ovarian tumours in children and adolescents. *Clinical Obstet. Gynaecol*; **20**: 607–23.

Burr I.M., Slonim A.E., Danish R.K., Gadoth N., Butler I.J. (1976). Diencephalic syndrome revisited. *J. Pediatr*; **88**: 439–44.

Cahen L.A., Villee D.B., Powers M.L., Crigler J.F. (1978). A virilising adrenocortical tumour in a female infant: *In vivo* and *in vitro* biochemical characteristics. *J. Clin. Endocrinol. Metab*; **47**: 300–6.

Calzada L.D., Chaussain J.L., Job J.C. (1979). Le retard de Croissance an Cours de l'histiocytose X. *SEM Hop Paris*; **54** (41–42): 1251–6.

Cameron N. (1978). The methods of auxological anthropometry. In *Human Growth* (Falkner F., Tanner J.M., eds.) pp. 35–87. New York: Plenum.

Chaussain J.L. (1981). Late puberty. In *Clinical Paediatric Endocrinology* (Brook C.G.D., ed.). pp. 240–7. Oxford: Blackwell Scientific Publications.

Chaussain J.L., Savage M.O., Nahoul K., Brijana A., Canlorbe P., Job J.C. (1978). Hypothalamo-pituitary-gonadal function in male central precocious puberty. *Clin. Endocrinol*; **8**: 437–44.

Colodny A., Hopkins T.B. (1977). Testicular tumours in infants and children. In *The Urologic Clinics of North America Symposium on Testicular Tumours*; 4 October: pp. 347–58. Philadelphia: W.B. Saunders Company.

Costin G. (1979). Endocrine disorders associated with tumours of the pituitary and hypothalamus. Symposium on Paediatric Endocrinology. In *The Pediatric Clinics of North America*; **26**: 15–31. (Kaplan S.A., ed.). Philadelphia: W.B. Saunders Company.

Danoff B.F., Kramer S., Thompson N. (1980). The radiotherapeutic management of optic nerve gliomas in children. *Int. J. Radiot. Oncol. Biol. Phys*; **6**: 45–50.

De Niepowniszcze A.B., Rivarola M.A., Chemes H.E., Bergada C. (1982). Steroid metabolism by a tumour of the specific gonadal stroma in a child. *Acta Endocrinol*; **99**: 624–9.

Didolkar M.S., Bescher R.A., Elias E.G., Moore R.H. (1981). Natural history of adrenal cortical carcinoma. *Cancer*; **47**: 2153–61.

Drago J.R., Olstein J.S., Tesluk H., Sheikholislam B., Palmer J.M., Link D. (1979). Virilising adrenal cortical carcinoma with hypertrophy of spermatic tubules in childhood. *Urology*; **14**: 70–5.

Drop S.L.S., Guyda H.J., Colle E. (1980). Inappropriate growth hormone release in the diencephalic syndrome of childhood: Case report and 4-year endocrinological follow up. *Clin. Endocrinol*; **13**: 181–7.

Eberlein W.R., Bongiovanni A.M., Jones I.T., Yakovac N.C. (1960). Ovarian tumour and cysts associated with sexual precocity. *J. Pediatr*; **57**: 484–97.

Elders M.J., Winfield B.S., McNatt M.L. (1975). Glucocorticoid therapy in children. Effect on somatomedin secretion. *Am. J. Dis. Child*; **129**: 1393–6.

Fligiel Z., Kaneko M., Leiter E. (1976). Bilateral Sertoli cell tumour of testes with feminising and masculinising activity occurring in a child. *Cancer*; **38**: 1853–8.

Forest M.G. (1981). Adrenal steroid excess. In *Clinical Paediatric Endocrinology* (Brook C.G.D., ed.) pp. 429–452. Oxford: Blackwell Scientific Publications.

Frasier S.D., Bashore R.A., Mosier H.D. (1964). Gonadoblastoma associated with pure gonadal dysgenesis in monozygous twins. *J. Pediatr*; **64**: 740–5.

Giovanelli G. (1982). Pineal region tumours: Endocrinological aspects. *Child's Brain*; **9**: 267–73.

Gregory T., Gardner L.I., Gower D.B., Bicknell D.C., Barlow M.J. (1979). Studies of 16-androstenes in an infant with virilising adrenal carcinoma. *Am. J. Dis. Child*; **133**: 294–7.

Griffiths K., Grant J.K., Browning M.C.K., Whyte W.G., Sharp J.L. (1966). Steroid synthesis *in vitro* by tumour tissue from a dysgenetic gonad. *J. Endocrinol*; **34**: 155–62.

Groeber W. (1963). Ovarian tumours during infancy and childhood. *Am. J. Obstet. Gynecol*; **86**: 1027–35.

Häger A., Thorell J.I. (1973). Studies on growth hormone secretion in a patient with the diencephalic syndrome of emaciation. *Acta Paed. Scand*; **62**: 231–40.

Hayles A.B., Hahn H.B., Sprague R.G., Bahn R.C., Priestley J.T. (1966). Hormone-secreting tumours of the adrenal cortex in children. *Pediatrics*; **37**: 19–25.

Honour J.W., Price D.A., Taylor N.F., Marsden H.B., Grant D.B. (1984). Steroid biochemistry of virilizing adrenal tumours in childhood. *Eur. J. Pediat* (in press).

Hughes I.A. (1982). Congenital and acquired disorders of the adrenal cortex. In *Clinics in Endocrinology and Metabolism. Paediatric Endocrinology.* (Bailey J.D., ed.) pp. 89–125. London: W.B. Saunders Company Ltd.

Hung W., Randolph J.G., Chandra R., Belman A.B. (1981). Gonadoblastoma in dysgenetic testis causing male pseudohermaphroditism in newborn. *Urology*; **17**: 584–7.

Ilondo M.M., Van den Mooter F., Marchal G. *et al.* (1981). A boy with Leydig cell tumour and precocious puberty. Ultrasonography as a diagnostic aid. *Eur. J. Pediatr*; **137**: 221–7.

Iraci G., Geroso M., Scanarini M. *et al.* (1980). Anterior optic gliomas with precocious or pseudoprecocious puberty. *Child's Brain*; **7**: 314–24.

Itami R.M., Amundson G.M., Kaplan S.A., Lippe B.M. (1982). Prepubertal gynaecomastia caused by an adrenal tumour. *Am. J. Dis. Child*; **136**: 584–6.

Kalifa C., Ernest C., Rodary C., Sarrizin D., Bloch-Michel E., Lemerle J. (1981). Les gliomes du chiasma optique chez l'enfant. Etude retrospective de 57 traites par irradiation. *Arch. Fr. Pediat*; **38**: 309–13.

Kauli R., Pertzelan A., Prager-Lewin R., Grunebaum M., Laron Z. (1976). Cyproterone acetate in treatment of precocious puberty. *Arch. Dis. Child*; **51**: 202–208.

Kitay J.I. (1954). Pineal lesions and precocious puberty. A review. *J. Clin. Endocrinol. Metab*; **14**: 622–30.

Kubo O., Yamasaki N., Kamijo Y., Amano K., Kitamura K., Demura R. (1977). Human chorionic gonadotrophin produced by ectopic pinealoma in a girl with precocious puberty. *J. Neurosurg*; **47**: 101–105.

Lack E., Perez-Atayde A.R., Murthy A.S.K., Goldstein D.P., Crigler J.F., Vawter G.F. (1981). Granulosa theca cell tumours in premenarchal girls. *Cancer*; **48**: 1846–54.

Latorre H., Kenney F.M., Lahey M.E., Drash A. (1974). Short stature and growth hormone deficiency in histiocytosis X. *J. Pediatr*; **85**: 813–6.

Lee P.A., Veldon V.V., Migeon C.J. (1975). Short stature as the only clinical sign of Cushing's syndrome. *J. Pediatr*; **86**: 89.

Levine G.W. (1978). Adrenocortical carcinoma in two children with subsequent primary tumours. *Am. J. Dis. Child*; **132**: 238–40.

Mansfield M.J., Beardsworth D.E., Loughlin J.S., Crawford J.D., Bode H.H., Rivier J., Vale W., Kushner D.C., Crigler J.F., Crowley W.F. (1983). Long term treatment of central precocious puberty with a long-acting analogue of luteinising hormone-releasing hormone: Effects on somatic growth and skeletal maturation. *New Engl. J. Med*; **309**: 1286–90.

Milner R.D.G., Burns E.C. (1982). Investigation of suspected growth hormone deficiency. *Arch. Dis. Child*; **57**: 944–7.

Newman C.B., Levine L.S., New M.I. (1981). Endocrine function in children with intrasellar and suprasellar neoplasms. *Am. J. Dis. Child*; **135**: 259–62.

Oxenhandler D.C., Sayers M.P. (1978). The dilemma of childhood optic gliomas. *J. Neurosurg*; **48**: 34–41.

Pomerade R., Czernichow P., Rappaport R., Royer P. (1980). Le diabete insipide pipresso sensible, chez l'enfant II Etude de 93 Cas observes entre 1955 et 1978. *Arch. Fr. Pediatr*; **37**: 37–46.

Pomerade R., Czernichow P., Finidori J., *et al.* (1982). Endocrine aspects and tumoral markers in intra-cranial germinoma. An attempt to delineate the diagnostic procedure in 14 patients. *J. Pediatr*; **101**: 374–8.

Preece M.A. (1982). Diagnosis and treatment of growth hormone deficiency. In *Clinics in Endocrinology and Metabolism. Paediatric Endocrinology.* (Bailey J.D., ed.) pp. 1–24. London: W.B. Saunders Company Ltd.

Pritchard J. (1979). Histiocytosis X: Natural history and management in childhood. *Clin. Exp. Dermat*; **4**: 421–33.

Reese A.B. (1963). *Tumours of the Eye.* pp. 162–71. New York: Harper and Row, Hoeber Medical Division.

Riccardi V.M. (1981). Von Recklinghausen neurofibromatosis. *New Engl. J. Med*; **305**: 1617–27.

Romshe C.A., Sotos J.F. (1975). Intracranial human chorionic gonadotrophin-secreting tumour with precocious puberty. *J. Pediatr*; **86**: 250–2.

Root A., Steinberger E., Smith K., Steinberger A., Russ D., Somers L., Rosenfield R. (1972). Isosexual pseudoprecocity in a 6-year-old boy with interstitial cell adenoma. *J. Pediatr*; **80**: 264–8.

Roth L.M., Anderson M.C., Govan A.D.T., Langley F.A., Gowing N.F.C., Woodcock A.S. (1981). Sertoli-Leydig cell tumours: A clinico-pathologic study of 34 cases. *Cancer*; **48**: 187–97.

Röttger J., Hadden D.R., Morrison E., McKeown F. (1981). Isosexual precocious puberty in a 9-year-old boy: Nodular interstitial cell hyperplasia. *J. Royal Soc. Med*; **76**: 66–8.

Russell A. (1951). A diencephalic syndrome of emaciation in infancy and childhood. *Arch. Dis. Child*; **26**: 274–84.

Russell D.S., Rubinstein L.J. (1979). *Pathology of the Nervous System.* pp. 283–98. Baltimore: Williams and Wilkins.

Sabio H., Burgert E.O., Farron G.M., Kelalis P.P. (1974). Embryonal carcinoma of the testis in childhood. *Cancer*; **34**: 2118–21.

Scully R., Mark E.J., McNeely B.U. (1982). Case records of the Massachusetts General Hospital. *New Engl. J. Med*; **306**: 1348–55.

Sklar C.A., Conte F.A., Kaplan S.L., Grumbach M.M. (1981). Human chorionic gonadotrophin-secreting pineal tumour: Relation to pathogenesis and sex limitation of sexual precocity. *J. Clin. Endocrinol. Metab*; **53**: 656–60.

Sklar C.A., Grumbach M.M., Kaplan S.L., Conte F.A. (1981). Hormonal and metabolic abnormalities associated with central nervous system germinoma in children and adolescents and the effect of therapy. Report of 10 patients. *J. Clin. Endocrinol. Metab*; **52**: 9–16.

Sultan C., Descomps B., Garandeau P., Bressot N., Jean R. (1979). Pubertal gynaecomastia due to an oestrogen-producing adrenal adenoma. *J. Pediatr*; **95**: 744–6.

Sung Duk I.L., Harisiadis L., Chang Chuh (1978). Midline pineal tumour and suprasellar germinomas: Highly curable by irradiation. *Radiology*; **128**: 745–51.

Tank E.S., Kay R. (1979). Neoplasms associated with hemihypertrophy, Beckwith-Wiedemann syndrome and Aniridia. *J. Urol*; **124**: 266–8.

Tanner J.M. (1962). The development of the reproductive system. In *Growth and Adolescence*, 2nd edn. pp. 28–39. Oxford: Blackwell Scientific Publications.

Vaitukaitis J.L. (1973). Immunologic and physical characterisation of human chorionic gonadotrophin (HCG) secreted by tumours. *J. Clin. Endocrinol. Metab*; **37**: 505–14.

Vanderschueren–Lodeweyckx M., Wolter R., Malvaux P. (1974). The glucagon stimulation test: Effect on plasma growth hormone and on immunoreactive insulin, cortisol and glucose in children. *J. Pediatr*; **85**: 182–7.

Wass J.A.H., Jones A.E., Rees L.H., Besser G.M. (1982). HCG β-producing pineal choriocarcinoma. *Clin. Endocrinol*; **17**: 423–31.

Wegienka L.C., Kolb F.O. (1967). Hormonal studies of a benign interstitial cell tumour of the testes producing androstenedione and testosterone. *Acta Endocrinol*; **56**: 481–9.

Wohltmann H., Mathur R.S., Williamson H.O., Wesby E., Moody L., Landgrebe S. (1980). Sexual precocity in a female infant due to feminising adrenal carcinoma. *J. Clin. Endocrinol. Metab*; **50**: 186–9.

Zachmann M., Prader A., Kind H.P., Hafliger H., Budliger H. (1974). Testicular volume during adolescence. Cross-sectional and longitudinal studies. *Helv. Paediatr. Acta*; **29**: 61–72.

Chapter 8

Harvey S. Besterman

Hypopituitarism

Non-specific symptoms such as tiredness, weakness, anorexia, nausea and weight loss are common in cancer patients. These may be secondary to the malignant disease itself (perhaps due to secretion of as yet unrecognised peptides) or to the side effects of chemotherapy or radiotherapy. In a small number of patients, however, these general complaints may be due to hypopituitarism. If this diagnosis is considered and a failure of pituitary secretion of one or more trophic hormones detected, then these symptoms are extremely amenable to treatment with the appropriate hormone replacement.

Hypopituitarism may result from metastatic spread either to the pituitary itself or, it may be secondary to failure of release of hypothalamic factors. The hormonal abnormality will reflect the exact anatomical site of tumour spread. Thus, metastases in the region of the supra-optic, paraventricular and supra-chiasmatic nuclei in the hypothalamus, as well as in the posterior lobe of the pituitary, may cause diabetes insipidus (these aspects will be covered in Chapter 9).

Metastatic spread from carcinomas of breast and bronchus is the commonest cause of anterior pituitary dysfunction, and this will be discussed subsequently. Other causes of neoplastic hypopituitarism include pituitary tumours and tumours arising in the parasellar region. In addition, cancer patients are also susceptible to the full spectrum of causes of hypopituitarism as listed in Table 8.1. This differential diagnosis should be borne in mind when considering the possibility of hypopituitarism in a patient known to have cancer and, although likely, it should not be immediately assumed to be secondary to metastatic disease.

HYPOTHALAMIC LESIONS PRODUCING HYPOPITUITARISM

Neoplastic invasion of the hypothalamus may occur as a result of primary neoplasms developing in this region. The commonest type is the pilocytic astrocytoma (Daniel and Treip, 1977). Hypothalamic gliomas may present insiduously, either with pituitary failure or with progressive visual failure

TABLE 8.1

Aetiology of Hypopituitarism

Pituitary tumours
Pituitary adenomas (chromophobe, eosinophil and basophil adenomas;
    oncocytoma; choristoma)
Intrasellar craniopharyngioma
Infarction of pituitary tumour
Pituitary carcinoma
Malignant disease
Secondary carcinomas, especially from breast and lung
Local cerebral tumours (e.g. meningioma, glioma of optic tract, chordoma)
Infectious diseases
Basal meningitis (e.g. tuberculosis)
Encephalitis
Syphilis
Granulomatous diseases
Sarcoidosis
Hand-Schüller-Christian disease (histiocytosis X)
Vascular disease
Post-partum infarction (Sheehan's syndrome)
Severe haemorrhage with hypotension
Diabetes mellitus
Cranial arteritis
Aneurysm of internal carotid artery
Pituitary apoplexy
Vascular malformations
Sickle cell disease
Trauma
head injury
Secondary to hypothalamic disease
Craniopharyngiomas and epidermoid cysts
Neural tumours
'Functional' (anorexia nervosa, starvation, malabsorption syndromes)
Iatrogenic
Surgical hypophysectomy for pituitary tumours, carcinoma of breast or for
    proliferative diabetic retinopathy
Intrasellar or external radiotherapy
TSH suppression after long-term thyroxine therapy
ACTH suppression after long-term corticosteroid therapy
Other
Pituitary cysts (arachnoid; Rathke's cleft cysts)
Autoimmune hypophysitis

---

resulting from direct extension of the tumour into the optic chiasm and optic nerves. Hypopituitarism and dementia with a histologically normal pituitary have been described as being due to microgliomatosis (Duchen and Treip, 1969). Seedlings from primary tumours of the brain, such as medulloblastoma and pinealoma, may grow within the cavity of the third ventricle.

A peculiar tumour reproducing some of the characteristic microvascular features of the tuber cinereum region is the infundibuloma (Wolman, 1959). Hypothalamic hamartoma, in the region of the tuber cinereum and mammillary bodies, may also affect hypothalamic–pituitary function (Davis and Hipkin, 1977). Suprasellar craniopharyngiomas, although often presenting in childhood or adolescence, may manifest later with endocrine effects. They are usually cystic or partly solid, and typically cholesterol crystals are numerous in the cyst fluid. Histological appearances of the craniopharyngioma are variable, ranging from groups of columnar cells on a basement membrane to squamous cells with cornified areas. They are often calcified and 70% show calcification on routine skull x-rays.

Endocrine evaluation has been undertaken by Kahana *et al.* (1962) in 14 patients with intracranial extrasellar lesions simulating primary pituitary disease. Two had aneurysms of the internal carotid artery, four had tumours involving the third ventricle, four had internal hydrocephalus due to a block in the aqueduct of Sylvius, and one each had a glioma of the optic chiasm, an arteriovenous anomaly of the left cerebrum, a meningioma of the floor of the anterior fossa and a mucocele of the sphenoid sinus. All but one had clinical and laboratory evidence of hypothalamic pituitary dysfunction. Abnormalities of gonadotropin secretion occurred in ten, of TSH secretion in six, of ACTH secretion in five, and four patients had diabetes insipidus. In a separate case study of a young man with a pineal tumour associated with internal hydrocephalus, diabetes insipidus, as well as anterior pituitary dysfunction, was found (Puschett and Goldberg, 1968).

Hypothalamic metastases, although not especially uncommon, have only been relatively rarely reported. Of six cases of carcinomatosis from breast primaries, three were described as showing direct hypothalamic involvement (Duchen, 1966). In the other three cases, the entire neural lobe and parts of the pituitary stalk and tuber cinereum had been destroyed by cancer, and degenerative changes were found in the supra-optic and paraventricular nuclei of the hypothalamus. A 1·5cm haemorrhagic metastasis was found at autopsy in the case of a 50-year-old man, who presented with the syndrome of inappropriate secretion of vasopressin and who also had clinical and biochemical hypopituitarism (Epstein *et al.*, 1973). Although there were no other cerebral metastases, there was also a centrally situated pituitary metasatic deposit from a primary undifferentiated small cell bronchogenic carcinoma. It is, therefore, impossible to ascertain which metastatic lesion was responsible for the patient's hypopituitarism. In a series of 88 cases of carcinoma metastatic to the pituitary, two patients were found to have lesions in the stalk and a further two patients had metastases in the capsule and stalk together (Teears and Silverman, 1975). Metastatic involvement of the hypothalamus was found in five out of 15 autopsies, performed on patients with diabetes insipidus and breast cancer (Yap *et al.*, 1979).

Hypopituitarism was suggested to have contributed to the documented adrenocortical failure in the case of a 59-year-old man with a primary squamous cell carcinoma of the bronchus (Modhi *et al.*, 1981). It had metastasised to the right adrenal gland, completely destroying it. The third ventricle was filled and distended with neoplastic tissue. Ventrally, the tumour was found to infiltrate the floor of the third ventricle, compressing the hypothalamus and completely destroying the infundibulum. The pituitary gland was histologically normal. The left adrenal was apparently normal, since it was referred to as showing a lack of gross atrophy. An important feature against the diagnosis of the patient's adrenocortical insufficiency being secondary hypopituitarism arising from the infundibular metastasis, is the fact that the patient was hyperpigmented. This is due to the melanin-stimulating action of the increased levels of ACTH found in patients with primary disease of the adrenal glands, causing adrenocortical failure.

Two earlier reports demonstrated that hypothalamic metastases could cause diabetes insipidus in the presence of unaffected normal pituitary gland (Elmer *et al.*, 1928; Futcher, 1929). Locally invasive tumours may also affect the hypothalamus. Thus, meningeal sarcomas, involving the basal dura mater and, more rarely, osteosarcoma or chondrosarcoma may invade the hypothalamus. Since these tumours are usually extensive and produce raised intracranial pressure, these aspects tend to manifest at a relatively early stage (Daniel and Treip, 1977).

In addition to local pressure effects on the visual pathway and disturbance of normal pituitary function, suprasellar lesions may produce abnormalities from pressure on various hypothalamic centres. Appetite may be affected in either direction, with gross hyperphagia and obesity (Wohlwill, 1928) or else with anorexia and emaciation. Disturbances of sleep such as somnolence, narcolepsy and cataplexy may also occur (Hall *et al.*, 1980).

HYPOPITUITARISM SECONDARY TO PITUITARY NEOPLASMS

Primary carcinoma of the pituitary gland is exceedingly rare. Two cases with hepatic metastases from carcinoma of the pituitary, associated with Cushing's syndrome, have been reported (Cohen and Dible, 1936; Forbes, 1947). Pituitary adenomas may give rise to hypopituitarism secondary to pressure effects, but this will not be discussed further. The most common cancers of the anterior pituitary are metastatic—mostly from breast and bronchus, and these will be analysed in more detail.

METASTATIC DISEASE OF THE PITUITARY GLAND

Metastases may reach the pituitary via a haematogenous route, by extension from juxtasellar and base of skull metastases or by invasion of the suprasellar cistern by leptomeningeal tumour (Max *et al.*, 1981). Table 8.2 shows the relative frequency of the incidental finding of pituitary metastases at post-mortem in cancer patients reported in the available literature. In no patient had the diagnosis of hypopituitarism been made before death. The incidence of pituitary metastases in the various series is reported to vary between 0 14 and 11·8%, with an overall mean value of 3·4%. The posterior lobe was generally reported to be more commonly involved by metastatic disease than the anterior lobe, with the exception of the series reported by Grabow and Schwesinger (1979). In all series where statistical evaluation had been applied, no significant difference could be detected between the incidence of metastatic disease in the two lobes.

There is general agreement that carcinoma of the breast is the commonest primary to metastasise to the pituitary, the next most common being primary bronchogenic carcinoma. An overall mean of 54% of all the patients who were found at post-mortem to have a pituitary metastasis had primary cancers of the breast. The frequency of bronchogenic carcinoma being the primary was three-fold less than that of breast cancer (16%). Hägerstrand and Schönebeck (1969), in their study of metastatic pituitary disease, found that secondaries from carcinoma of breast were significantly more common than all other malignancies.

The incidence of pituitary metastases in other cancers is relatively rare. Malignant melanoma was found to be the primary tumour in 6% and 17% in two recent series (Grabow and Schwesinger, 1979; Max *et al.*, 1981). Of the 18 cases of incidental pituitary metastases found at post-mortem reported by Kovacs (1973), two patients had intestinal primaries and a further two had prostatic cancers. Otherwise, single cases of pituitary metastasis have been reported from cancers of the cardia of the stomach and from Ewing's sarcoma (Walther, 1948), from carcinoma of the pharynx (Kovacs, 1973; Max *et al.*, 1981) and from primary cancers of colon, prostate, endometrium as well as from malignant lymphoma, acute lymphoblastic leukaemia and chronic lymphocytic leukaemia (Max *et al.*, 1981).

A number of studies have investigated the pituitary pathology in patients known to have metastatic disease. Kerkhoven and Hedinger (1967), in a series of 41 patients with secondary carcinoma of the pituitary gland, found 63% to originate from primaries of the breast, 21% from the bronchus and

TABLE 8.2

Incidence and Location of Pituitary Metastases and Principal Associated Primaries in Patients Dying from Cancer

Author	Total number of patients	Number of patients with pituitary metastases	(%)	Pituitary involvement (%)			Primary carcinoma			
				Anterior lobe	Posterior lobe	Both lobes	Breast	(%)	Bronchus	(%)
Simmonds, 1914	Not known	Not known	1·6				6/7	(86)	1/7	(14)
Wyeth, 1934	80	5	6·2				'Preferential inclination of breast cancer to metastasise in the hypophysis—could not be observed'			
Walther, 1948	3584	5	0·14				2/5	(40)	1/5	(20)
Abrams et al., 1950	1000	18	1·8				15/18	(83)	2/18	(11)
Willis, 1952	500	2—direct invasion 1—blood borne	0·6							
Simionescu, 1960	109 with solitary cerebral metastases	2	1·83							

Delarue *et al.*, 1964	280	33	11·8	18·2	51·5 (capsule 12·1)	18·2	23/33	(70)	4/33	(12)
Hägerstrand and Schönebeck, 1969	763	29	3·8	13·8	41·4	44·8				
Roessmann *et al* 1970	60	5	8·3				3/5	(60)	1/5	(20)
Schneider *et al* 1972	1000	40	4·0	Metastases more common in posterior lobe, but the difference in incidence from the anterior lobe was not statistically significant						
Kovacs, 1973	1857	18	1·0	22·2	33·3	44·4	7/18	(39)	5/18	(28)
Grabow and Schwesinger, 1979	1521	64	4·2	39·5	34·2	26·3	18/64	(28)	16/64	(25)
Max *et al.*, 1981	500	18	3·6				6/18	(33)	—	(0)
		Overall	3·8	23·4	40·1	33·4	—	55	—	16

10% to arise in the stomach. Of 11 patients with metastases in the posterior pituitary gland, seven had breast primaries (73%), one had both breast and pancreatic tumours, one had bronchogenic carcinoma, one had myelocytic leukaemia and another patient had erythroleukaemia (Houck *et al.*, 1970).

In a relatively large series of 88 cases of carcinoma metastatic to the pituitary gland, 61 (69%) had metastases localised either in the posterior lobe alone or in both anterior and posterior lobes (Teears and Silverman, 1975). In only 12 cases (14%) was there involvement of the anterior lobe alone. Of the 53 women, 35 (66%) had primary breast cancer, seven (13%) had lung cancer, four (7·5%) had stomach cancer and the remaining seven had primaries arising in the mouth, paranasal sinus, endometrium, ovary, tonsil, uterine cervix and colon. Of the 35 men, 22 (63%) had bronchogenic carcinoma, three (8·6%) had prostatic cancer, two had cancer of the bladder and the remaining seven men had primaries arising from ileum, pancreas, left vallecula, penis, paranasal sinus, skin (back) and soft palate (in one the primary was unknown).

CARCINOMA OF BREAST

In a specific study of patients with diabetes insipidus and breast cancer, not surprisingly, all 15 patients who underwent autopsy were found to have metastases in the posterior pituitary gland (Yap *et al.*, 1979). In six patients there was extension of the metastatic lesion to involve the anterior portion of the pituitary gland.

Another perspective on the incidence of pituitary metastases and their differential location in patients with breast cancer can be obtained both from post-mortem examination and from surgical hypophysectomy studies (Table 8.3). The incidence of coincident metastasis in hypophysectomy specimens removed surgically in the treatment of breast cancer patients (7·9%) is about half the mean incidence of pituitary metastases found at post-mortem in patients dying of breast cancer (17.7%). The reason for this discrepancy presumably lies in the fact that the cases coming to post-mortem will have had more advanced disease, since it is almost invariable to have multiple widespread metastases associated with pituitary metastases and the converse is presumably true. Thus, if a breast cancer has disseminated widely, there is a considerable likelihood that the pituitary may also be involved. In fact, in some series an incidence of one in four, or greater, of pituitary involvement has been reported (Gurling *et al.*, 1957; Smulders and Smets, 1960). The reported differential localisation of pituitary metastases in these breast cancer cases is very variable. In three series, metastases were found more commonly in the anterior lobe than in the posterior lobe (Gurling *et al.*, 1957; Smulders and Smets, 1960; Grisoli *et al.*, 1974).

TABLE 8.3

Breast Cancer Patients with Pituitary Metastases

Author	Source	Total number of patients	Number with pituitary metastases	%	Pituitary involvement (%)		
					Anterior lobe	Posterior lobe	Both lobes
Abrams, 1950	Post-mortem	167	15	9			
Gurling *et al.*, 1957	Post-mortem	44	11	25	90·9	9·1	
Smulders and Smets, 1960	Post-mortem	71	20	28·2	60	35	
Duchen, 1966	Hypophysectomy	155	12	7·7	5·4[a]	4·1	5·1
	Post-mortem	6	6	100	16·7	16·7	25
Hägerstrand and Schönebeck, 1969	Post-mortem	214	34	15·9			
Grisoli *et al.*, 1974	Hypophysectomy	160	13	8·1	55·6	33·3	11·1
	Post-mortem	205	19	9·3	10·5	36·8	52·6
Jänisch *et al.*, 1976	Post-mortem	97	19	19·6			
Cifuentes and Pickren, 1979	Post-mortem	704	117	16·6			

[a]Anterior pituitary tissue only identified in 36% of all specimens.

Since hypophysectomy may benefit some patients with breast cancer, then pituitary metastatic hypopituitarism might be considered beneficial. Brugge *et al.* (1965) reported 'spontaneous' remission in three cases of metastasised carcinoma of breast. They suggested that the remission might be attributable to 'autohypophysectomy', caused by metastatic growths in the pituitary gland. In one case, the diagnosis was confirmed by the autopsy findings.

CARCINOMA OF BRONCHUS

The incidence of pituitary metastases has also been ascertained in patients with bronchogenic carcinoma. Of 160 consecutive patients studied by Abrams *et al.* (1950), only two (1·3%) had pituitary metastases. Line and Deeley (1971) found pituitary metastases in 26 of 406 autopsies (6·4%), performed on cases with carcinoma of bronchus. In the great majority (23 out of 26, 88%), the pituitary metastasis was solitary. In only three patients were there multiple metastases in the brain as well as in the pituitary.

In another series, 18 of 55 patients (32·7%) with small cell bronchogenic carcinoma were found to have pituitary metastases at post-mortem (Nugent *et al.*, 1979). In six of these, the pituitary was the only site of metastatic spread. Metastatic involvement of the anterior pituitary was found in three (16·7%), the posterior pituitary gland was affected in 12 (66·7%) and another three patients (16·7%) had metastatic involvement of both lobes.

Most authors reporting an increased incidence of metastases involving the posterior rather than the anterior pituitary have ascribed this to differences in the blood supply to the two portions of the pituitary gland. Whereas the posterior lobe receives arterial blood from branches of the inferior hypophyseal artery, the bulk of the anterior lobe is supplied by sinusoidal blood of portal venous origin (Daniel and Prichard, 1975; Doniach, 1977; Ezrin *et al.*, 1978). The anterior pituitary does, however, receive a direct systemic arterial blood supply. Branches of the loral artery, of the inferior hypophyseal arterial ring and twigs of the inferior capsular artery are all reported to contribute a direct supply to the anterior lobe (Sheehan and Stanfield, 1961).

This direct arterial supply may explain the fact that metastases can occur in the anterior lobe, presumably blood-borne, without involvement of the posterior lobe. An early report stated that there was never involvement of the anterior lobe without posterior lobe involvement and that this was due to direct invasion (Duchen, 1966). This has not, however, been borne out by subsequent studies.

HYPOPITUITARISM IN METASTATIC DISEASE OF THE PITUITARY GLAND

Despite the relatively high frequency that metastases are discovered incidentally in the pituitary gland, only rarely has hypopituitarism been reported. Diabetes insipidus is the most common clinical manifestation of pituitary metastatic involvement, and this will be fully discussed in Chapter 11.

Table 8.4 lists ten cases where some reference has been made to anterior pituitary dysfunction in patients with pituitary metastases. In few cases have all the essential endocrine investigations been given. Furthermore, the case described by Epstein *et al.* (1973) was complicated by the fact that they had a hypothalamic metastasis in addition to that in the pituitary gland. This case was also described as having hyperpigmentation, which argues strongly against his having primary ACTH deficiency.

DIFFERENTIATION OF PITUITARY METASTASES FROM PITUITARY TUMOURS

It has been suggested that a pituitary tumour causing hypopituitarism would almost certainly cause expansion of the sella turcica, whereas metastatic carcinomatous lesions may destroy, but do not usually enlarge the sella (Doyle and McLachlan, 1977).

Skull radiology may, however, show a wide spectrum of changes in metastatic disease of the sella. Plain skull films, angiography, air encephalography and orbital venography were used in evaluating 11 patients with pituitary metastases (Kistler and Pribram, 1975). They found that the spectrum of changes included enlargement of the sella without evidence of destruction, sclerosis of the sphenoidal bone and destruction of the sella turcica and clivus. In an earlier study of sella metastases, x-ray examination of sella turcica specimens with the hypophysis *in situ* failed to detect the majority of the metastatic lesions (Roessmann *et al.*, 1970). Skull x-rays were performed on 49 specimens, eight of which were subsequently shown to have sella metastases. Only one was read as positive, with the other seven being regarded as normal. In addition, there were two 'false positive' evaluations with no abnormal histological findings. Metastases in the sella were only rarely associated with the presence of metastases within the pituitary gland itself.

In a recent series of cases with incidental pituitary pathology, radiological examination, including axial tomography and computerised tomography, was unable to distinguish reliably metastases from pituitary adenomas (Max *et al.*, 1981). Of 27 asymptomatic pituitary tumours, 18 were metastases and

TABLE 8.4

Hypothalamic–Pituitary Function in Patients with Pituitary Metastases

Author	Patient(s)	Clinical features	Primary/secondary tumours	Endocrine evaluation	Radiology
Houck *et al.*, 1970	6/11	Diabetes insipidus in nine No symptoms of anterior pituitary insufficiency	8 breast 1 lung 1 myelocytic leukaemia 1 erythroleukaemia	24-hour urinary hydroxycorticosteroid excretion: Low in one, but excellent response to metyrapone Normal in one Slightly elevated in two 24-hour urinary ketosteroid excretion: Low in two Normal in four Protein-bound iodine: Normal in seven Low in one but normal radioactive iodine uptake at 24 hours Authors conclude 'six patients had various studies of anterior pituitary function and all were normal.'	Abnormal sella in 2/8
Epstein *et al.*, 1973	Male, 50 years old	Hypogonadism Hyponatraemia	Small cell carcinoma of bronchus	Failure of cortisol and growth hormone	Normal pituitary fossa

		SIADH	Hypothalamic and pituitary metastases	responses to adequate insulin-induced hypoglycaemia Undetectable 24-hour urinary FSH excretion Normal protein-bound iodine Normal cortisol response to 'Synacthen'	
Teears and Silverman, 1975	Female, 62 years old	Diabetes insipidus	Adenocarcinoma of lung, metastases in anterior and posterior pituitary	Urinary 17-ketosteroids low on two occasions with good response to ACTH Low T_3	
Cox, 1979	Female, 42 years old	Bitemporal hemianopia Diabetes insipidus	Carcinoma of breast Pituitary metastases	Low cortisol, thyroxine, FSH and LH	Skull: Enlargement of sella turcica and erosion of sella floor CT: Enhancing sellar and suprasellar mass, deforming third ventricle
Nugent *et al.*, 1979	One patient	'Clinical symptoms of panhypopituitarism'	Small cell carcinoma of bronchus	'Laboratory evidence of panhypopituitarism'	CT: Metastases in the area of the pituitary.
Yap *et al.*, 1979	Two female patients	'Clinical evidence of anterior pituitary dysfunction' Diabetes insipidus	Carcinoma of breast Metastasis in anterior and posterior pituitary		

contd.

Rosen and Hasler, 1980	Post-menopausal female	Confusion, focal fits, right hemiparesis hypotension Diabetes insipidus	Small cell carcinoma of bronchus	Low normal thyroxine, free thyroxine index Low basal TSH with failure of response to TRH (but on dexamethasone therapy) Low gonadotropins No response of growth hormone to L-dopa Normoprolactinaemic	CT: Enhancing mass in suprasellar region
Leramo *et al.*, 1981	Male, 68 years old	Hypogonadal Hypopituitarism Diabetes insipidus	Carcinoma of colon Anterior and posterior pituitary metastases plus hypothalamic infarction	No TSH response to TRH No LH or FSH response to LHRH Hyperprolactinaemic	Skull: Enlarged sella CT: Suprasellar mass with parasellar extension
Bynke and Ottosson, 1982	Female, 37 years old	Amenorrhoea, fatigue weakness, weight loss Hyperthyroidism Diabetes insipidus Bitemporal hemianopia	Carcinoma of breast, anterior and posterior pituitary metastases with invasion of hypothalamus	Low 8 am plasma cortisol (off cortisone two days) Low 24-hour urinary cortisol excretion Moderate response of cortisol to corticotropin Low prolactin Low basal FSH Normal basal LH Water deprivation test—cranial diabetes insipidus	Skull: Erosion of the anterior wall and of the left part of the dorsum sellae Sella not enlarged CT: 15 mm intrasellar and suprasellar lesion

all were associated with widespread systemic metastases. These authors stressed that pituitary metastases tended to present with a different clinical manifestation from that associated with pituitary adenomas. The metastatic patients presented more often with diabetes insipidus, with or without the less common manifestation of oculomotor palsies, both being rare in patients with pituitary adenomas.

Another condition in which hypopituitarism may be associated with an abnormal sella on skull x-ray is autoimmune hypophysitis (Mayfield *et al.*, 1980). This is, as yet, a poorly understood condition. A number of patients have been described with symptoms and signs of hypopituitarism, often associated with severe hypoglycaemia. Subsequent histological examination has shown the anterior lobe of the pituitary to be infiltrated with lymphocytes (Goudie and Pinkerton, 1962; Hume and Roberts, 1967; Egloff *et al.*, 1969; Lack,1975; Gleason *et al.*, 1978). More recently, two such patients have been found to have circulating antibodies against pituitary cells (Ludwig and Schernthaner, 1978; Mayfield *et al.*, 1980).

INCIDENCE OF TUMOURS DEVELOPING IN HYPOPITUITARY PATIENTS

Hypophysectomy prevents or retards chemical carcinogenesis in several organs in hypophysectomised animals. Furthermore, hypophysectomy produces clinical remissions in some women with breast cancer. It might, therefore, be expected that patients with hypopituitarism would be less at risk from developing neoplasms. A number of case reports of tumours developing in hypopituitary patients have been recorded. In view of the claims, however, that there can be a very long latent period between the initiation of some tumours and the onset of symptoms, it could be argued that carcinogenesis in many of these cases had occurred before the hypopituitarism developed (Davis and Hipkin, 1977).

HYPOPITUITARISM—CLINICAL PICTURE

The clinical presentation, symptoms and signs of anterior pituitary dysfunction will depend on several factors:

1) Age and sex of patient.
2) Rate of onset, duration and progression of disease.
3) Degree of pituitary failure.
4) Differential loss of the various pituitary hormones.
5) The presence of symptoms and signs arising from increased tension in the sella or from a space-occupying lesion in the region of the pituitary.

Partial hypopituitarism is more common than total loss of all pituitary secretions. Luteinising hormone secretion is usually the earliest to be affected, followed by growth hormone, follicle stimulating hormone, ACTH and TSH secretion. The pattern of pituitary hormone loss may also be affected by the position of the metastasis within the gland as well as by generalised pressure effects. These hormonal deficiencies may be accompanied by hyperprolactinaemia if the normal dopaminergic inhibitory control has been damaged. It is, therefore, important to exclude hyperprolactinaemia as a cause of hypogonadism before diagnosing gonadotrophin deficiency.

If there is concomitant diabetes insipidus then the symptoms of polyuria and thirst may improve when anterior pituitary damage becomes sufficient to impair ACTH output. This may be due to a decrease in the glomerular filtration rate or to a diminished action of vasopressin on the renal tubules caused by cortisol deficiency. When treating such patients with adrenal corticosteroids the symptoms of diabetes insipidus may recur or may come to light for the first time.

The clinical diagnosis of hypopituitarism, especially if mild, may be easily missed unless symptoms and signs are specifically sought.

Gonadotrophin Deficiency

Decrease or loss of libido is a feature of gonadotrophin deficiency in both sexes. Premenopausal women may notice oligomenorrhoea or amenorrhoea, infertility, reduced body hair, and a reduction in breast size. Menopausal symptoms do not occur. Men may be impotent and infertile and have noticed decrease in facial hair growth and consequent reduction in shaving frequency. If the gonadotrophin deficiency has lasted several years (unlikely in most cases with cancer in the pituitary gland), then there may be a characteristic fineness and excessive wrinkling of the skin, especially of the face. There may be loss of body hair and atrophy of the genitalia. In men, a relatively objective assessment of testicular size may be derived using an orchidometer, comparing testicular volume against a series of calibrated standards. A decrease in testicular volume is usually associated with softening of the testes.

Thyrotrophin Deficiency

The symptoms of secondary hypothyroidism (due to pituitary failure of TSH secretion) and of tertiary hypothyroidism (due to hypothalamic failure of TRH secretion) are the same as those of primary thyroid insufficiency. Thus, the presence should be sought of lassitude, cold intolerance, dryness of the skin, hoarseness of the voice, constipation and poor cerebral function.

On examination the characteristic swelling of the subcutaneous tissues found in primary hypothyroidism is less prominent. Delay in the relaxation phase of the tendon reflexes is virtually pathognomonic and, if severe, there may be myotonia.

ACTH Deficiency

Early features of adrenocortical insufficiency include lassitude, asthenia, anorexia, nausea and weight loss. When more severe, there may be vomiting, symptoms of postural hypotension, hypoglycaemia, collapse and coma. On examination, there is a characteristic pallor of the skin which may be associated with depigmentation of the areolae of the breasts and decreased tanning after exposure to sunlight. The blood pressure should be checked lying and standing in order to detect any postural drop.

Prolactin

A history of spontaneous or expressible galactorrhoea should be sought and the breasts examined specifically for any secretion.

Visual fields

Plotting of the visual fields with red and/or white low intensity objects may give evidence of extrasellar extension of intrasellar pathology.

LABORATORY INVESTIGATIONS

General

Patients with hypopituitarism may have a mild to moderate normocytic normochromic anaemia, reflecting reduced bone marrow function. Hyponatraemia, if present, is more often due to relative water intoxication than to sodium loss, since aldosterone secretion by the adrenal glands is maintained.

Endocrine Evaluation

Basal levels of pituitary and target organ hormones in hypopituitary patients may in fact be within the lower limits of normal, unless there is gross failure of pituitary function. Only if dynamic tests of pituitary function are used will the impaired pituitary secretory reserve capacity become evident. Using specific drugs and releasing hormones (Fig. 8.1) it may be possible to ascertain whether there is a fundamental pituitary failure of secretion, or

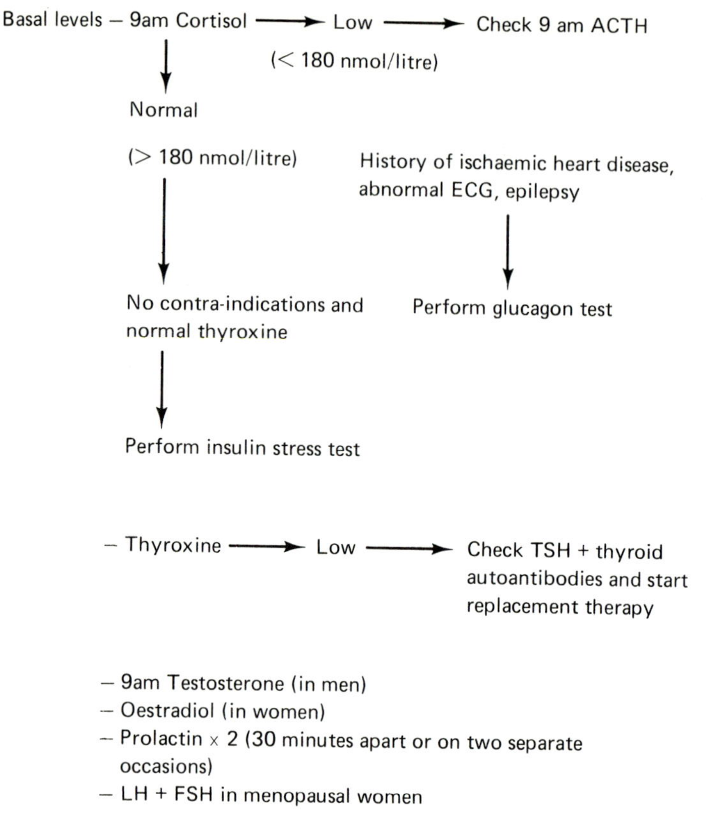

Fig. 8.1.   *Investigation plan in a patient with suspected hypopituitarism (Hall et al., 1980).*

whether this is secondary to hypothalamic disease (for precise details of tests see Hall *et al.*, 1980).

Although few district general hospitals will have the facilities to measure the necessary hormones, all departments of chemical pathology are able to send samples to the nearest appropriate endocrine laboratory via the supra-regional assay service. Precise details as to how specimens should be collected and handled are described in their handbook.

Combined test of pituitary function

With the patient fasted and lying recumbent, insert butterfly cannula into antecubital vein, explain nature and purpose of the test, warn of any possible effects and allow 30 minutes for acclimatisation. After taking basal blood samples (as below), intravenous bolus of soluble insulin

TABLE 8.5

Time (min)	Blood glucose	Cortisol	Growth hormone	TSH	LH	FSH
O (basal)	√	√	√	√	√	√
Intravenous soluble insulin + TRH + LHRH						
30	√	√	√	√	√	√
45	√	√	√			
60	√	√	√	√	√	√
90	√	√	√			
120	√	√	√			

(0·15 ∼ 0.10 units/kg), 200 m.c.g. TRH and 100 m.c.g. LHRH should be given and sampling continued indicated in Table 8.5.

At the end of the test oral glucose and breakfast should be given. If the initial bolus of insulin does not cause symptomatic and biochemical hypoglycaemia (monitored with blood glucose meter), then a further dose of soluble insulin at 45–60 minutes should be given, and sampling continued for longer. If severe hypoglycaemia is precipitated, intravenous dextrose (25 ml 25%, which should be drawn up ready) should be given and sampling continued. Then, 100 mg hydrocortisone i.v. is administered at the end of the test.

Gonadotrophin Deficiency

Post-menopausal women normally have elevated levels of both LH and FSH, so that in this particular instance measurement of the basal levels of these hormones may be sufficient. Normal levels of LH in a patient suspected of hypopituitarism should call into doubt this diagnosis if thought to be due to metastatic pituitary disease. Low levels of ovarian and testicular hormones in the blood or urine occur in hypopituitarism but rise in response to human menopausal gonadotrophin or human chorionic gonadotrophin. Unless there is suspicion of pre-existing gonadal disease, these tests should not be necessary.

Assessment may be made of whether the gonadotrophin deficiency, if present, is a pituitary or hypothalamic level. Administration of the hypothalamic releasing peptide, LHRH, may demonstrate a deficient rise in LH and FSH if the pituitary is involved, but a normal rise if there is hypothalamic disease. Estimation of the gonadotrophins following clomiphene administration may indicate a hypothalamic defect if there is no rise to clomiphene but a normal response to LHRH. Repetitive administration of LHRH may also help distinguish hypothalamic from pituitary hypo-gonadism (Snyder *et al.*, 1974).

Severe malnutrition and anorexia nervosa should be eliminated as these may mimic or even represent hypopituitarism.

Thyrotrophin Deficiency

If the basal thyroxine level is low in conjunction with a low free thyroxine index (steroid therapy may lower thyroid binding globulin and give a misleading figure for thyroxine), then it is essential to measure TSH. Primary hypothyroidism is common and may co-exist with hypopituitarism. In uncomplicated primary myxoedema the TSH is elevated and circulating thyroid autoantibodies may be present in significant titre.

The combination of a low serum thyroxine with a low level of TSH is suggestive of hypopituitarism. Since normal basal TSH levels are low, it is important to assess the TSH response to the stimulus of TRH adminis-tration. Dynamic tests of pituitary function should not be performed if the patient is chemically and biochemically hypothyroid. Only when they are stable on adequate thyroid replacement therapy should dynamic tests be undertaken. Although a failure of TRH to stimulate a normal rise in TSH is highly suggestive of hypopituitarism, it should be realised that other situations may also cause a flat TSH response. Thyrotoxicosis, multino-dular goitre and corticosteroids are but some of the causes of such a lack of response. A delayed rise in TSH with a 60-minute value greater than the 20-minute value may indicate hypothalamic pathology. There is, however, at present no accurate method to separate biochemically secondary (pituitary) from tertiary (hypothalamic) hypothyroidism (Snyder *et al.*, 1974).

When TSH assays are not available, it is possible to distinguish primary hypothyroidism from hypopituitarism by testing the response of the thyroid to TSH. Since some patients with long standing hypopituitarism are unable to respond to a singe injection of TSH, it is best to give at least three daily injections of ten units TSH before estimating the rise in serum thyroxine or 24-hour thyroid ^{131}I uptake.

ACTH Deficiency

Assessment of the hypothalamic–pituitary–adrenal axis must start with estimating the plasma cortisol at 9 am (when it should be near its maximum in the circadian cycle). If this is low and found to be associated with a low circulating level of ACTH, then this will distinguish hypothalamic or pituitary disease from primary adrenal disease. In this latter situation, ACTH levels are usually grossly elevated. It should be realised that an erroneously low plasma ACTH level may result from incorrect venesection and subsequent handling of blood and plasma. Adrenocorticotrophic hormone is unstable and adsorbs strongly to glass. Blood should be quickly spun in a refrigerated centrifuge and the separated plasma stored at −20° C, avoiding contact with glass. In practice, it is not usually necessary to measure ACTH in the diagnosis of hypopituitarism, unless the basal cortisol level is very low.

Plasma cortisol and ACTH levels may not, however, be low despite significant pituitary or hypothalamic disease, since ACTH secretion may be sufficient to maintain normal basal secretion but insufficient to increase adequately in response to stress. The best dynamic test of hypothalamic–pituitary–adrenocortical function is the insulin stress test. Providing there is no contra-indication (ischaemic heart disease, epilepsy, abnormal ECG), enough soluble insulin should be given as an intravenous bolus to cause symptomatic and actual hypoglycaemia (a nadir of blood glucose of less than 2.2 mmol/litre). It should be recorded whether or not the patient was sweating, had a tachycardia or felt sleepy. A normal dose consists of 0·15 units/kg body weight, but if ACTH deficiency is suspected then 0.10 unit/kg should be given. If the insulin test is contra-indicated, then 1 mg glucagon may be given subcutaneously.

In response to stress, ACTH levels should rise sufficiently to increase circulating cortisol levels to 580 nmol/litre or above. If this occurs, clinically significant ACTH deficiency is not present and replacement therapy is not required. Occasionally, some patients with normal basal 9 am cortisol levels have a somewhat obtunded response to adequate insulin-induced hypo-glycaemia. If such patients are not symptomatic, regular replacement therapy may not be necessary. They should, however, be given a supply of hydrocortisone tablets to take in the event of intercurrent illness or other stress.

Recently, one of the corticotrophin releasing factors (CRF) has been isolated, purified, sequenced and synthesised. It is a 41 amino acid peptide which specifically stimulates ACTH release and may help discriminate between hypothalamic and pituitary defects in ACTH secretion (Grossman *et al.*, 1982).

Growth Hormone Deficiency

It is useful, for the sake of completion, to assess the growth hormone response to insulin-induced hypoglycaemia, since it is one of the first pituitary hormones to suffer a failure of secretion in the presence of pituitary pathology. In adults, however, there are no clinical sequelae apart from increased insulin sensitivity.

RADIOLOGICAL ASSESSMENT

If a pituitary or hypothalamic neoplasm is suspected to be causing hypopituitarism, as much information should be sought concerning the precise anatomy as the clinical situation dictates. Thus, in some cases of carcinoma of the bronchus, the pituitary metastasis may be solitary and amenable to surgery, whereas in most cases of carcinoma of the breast, there may be widespread metastases. A straight lateral skull film, centred on the sella turcica, with good overlapping of the anterior clinoid processes, should be obtained (rotated films may give rise to erroneous conclusions). There may be a double-floor, enlargement, ballooning, local erosion of the floor of the dorsum sellae or of the anterior or posterior clinoid processes. Calcification in the region is often due to a craniopharyngioma or to previous tuberculous meningitis. An antero-posterior film may show the floor of the fossa to slope or to be eroded. Greater detail concerning the anterior and posterior aspects of the sella, as well as the floor, may be obtained using conventional lateral and antero-posterior tomography. If there is clinical suspicion of suprasellar pathology (bitemporal hemianopia, or abnormal visual evoked responses), it may be necessary to proceed to more detailed investigations.

The least invasive technique which gives great anatomical detail is the fourth generation CT head scanner, which is capable of reconstruction from serial axial scans in any plane required. When used to produce sagittal reconstructions of the suprasellar region, the precise anatomy of any lesion may be demonstrated. The availability of these CT scanners is very limited, and they are expensive. One of the earlier generation scanners may indicate the presence of a suprasellar mass, which may well enhance following injection of contrast medium. Another advantage of performing a CT head scan in these patients is in ascertaining whether or not the pituitary metastases is solitary or associated with other intracerebral metastases. The earlier CT scanners will not, however, give sufficient information concerning the superior aspects of a pituitary tumour. If the third ventricle appears involved, then an air encephalogram gives the best definition. Otherwise, metrizamide cisternography will allow sufficient delineation of the immediate suprasellar anatomy.

TREATMENT

The role of neurosurgery, chemotherapy and radiotherapy are outside the scope of this chapter, but are nevertheless of relevance.

Having performed a full endocrine assessment it should be evident whether or not the patient has partial or panhypopituitarism. If growth hormone deficiency is the only abnormality, no action is necessary apart from monitoring for the subsequent development of other pituitary hormone deficiency.

Panhypopituitarism

It is essential to give replacement therapy in the correct order in such patients. They should be started on hydrocortisone orally, usually twice daily, the first dose being taken on waking, beside the bed, before rising. The second dose of hydrocortisone is usually given at 6 pm. Cortisone acetate should be avoided, since its gut absorption is erratic and its subsequent conversion to cortisol, mainly in the liver, is also very variable. Even with hydrocortisone, blood levels often vary from patient to patient, and it is necessary to monitor the patient's cortisol levels (by the fluorimetric, Mattingley method) on any replacement hydrocortisone regimen. Most commonly, patients require 20 mg on waking and 10 mg at 6 pm. Plasma cortisol peaks 30–60 minutes after oral hydrocortisone and ideally the peak plasma concentration should reach between 700 and 1000 nmol/litre after the morning dose and then fall slowly to between 170 and 225 nmol/litre before the evening dose, after which a peak of 420 to 560 nmol/litre should be reached. The dose of hydrocortisone should be adjusted, sometimes adding a mid-day tablet, until these levels are obtained.

The patient should be told to increase the hydrocortisone in the event of minor stress to 20 mg orally, six to eight-hourly. In the event of major stress, 100 mg hydrocortisone hemisuccinate should be administered intramuscularly six-hourly. A 'steroid' card should always be carried by the patients, indicating full details of their therapy and they should also wear a bracelet or necklace giving the diagnosis of hypopituitarism and reference to the relevant hospital or consultant.

Thyroid Hormone Replacement

Once a patient with panhypopituitarism is established on hydrocortisone, it is then safe to start thyroid replacement therapy. The reverse order may precipitate a thyroid storm. L-Thyroxine may be given in a dose of 100 to 200 mcg orally once daily. Once established the serum thyroxine and free thyroxine index may be slightly raised without clinical evidence of overtreatment. Measurement of the serum level of triiodothyronine may, in fact, be more useful in monitoring the dose of replacement thyroxine.

In the advent of coma, continuing despite parenteral hydrocortisone, a naso-gastric tube should be passed and triiodothyronine given. A standard starting dose consists of 2·5 mcg eight-hourly, but this should be titrated against the patient's clinical and cardiovascular status. Once stabilised, the dose can be doubled every 48 hours until they are receiving 10–20 mcg eight-hourly, at which point L-thyroxine may be started. The triiodothyronine is continued for a further five day overlap period and then discontinued.

Sex Hormone Replacement

In the case of breast cancer the problem of oestrogen replacement may not arise or should be fully discussed with the oncologist or physician responsible.

If libido is relatively satisfactory and the principal symptom of oestrogen deficiency is of dyspareunia and lack of vaginal lubrication, this may respond to local oestrogen cream. If indicated in the case of breast cancer or if hypopituitarism has arisen from another malignancy, substitution therapy with cyclical oestrogens and progestogens (in the form of the oral contraceptive pill) can induce withdrawal bleeding and improve breast development, as well as conferring psychological benefit.

In men, testosterone may be given by intramuscular injection or orally. For a prompt initiation, testosterone proprionate 100 mg i.m. can be used, with long-term replacement (Primoteston, Sustanon), 500–750 mg every three to four weeks. A new oral form of testosterone, without the hepatotoxic side effects, is now available in the form of testosterone undecanoate (Restandol) 40–80 mg, either twice or three times daily.

Efficacy of treatment and the patient's personal preference to the method and frequency of administration should be of guidance in deciding the best form of therapy. Dose and frequency of administration should be titrated against the patient's response and no hormonal estimations are of relevance.

CONCLUSION

If a cancer patient presents with the rather non-specific symptoms which are typical of early hypopituitarism, they may well be dismissed as being secondary to the disease or to its treatment. A realisation of the relative frequency with which cancers of the breast and bronchus may metastasise to the pituitary may focus attention on the possibility of hypopituitarism contributing to their symptoms. The endocrine assessment of such patients is relatively simple and straightforward. Secretory failure of the anterior pituitary gland, often in association with that of the posterior lobe, producing diabetes insipidus, is easily treated and may contribute to a considerable improvement in well-being and quality of life.

EXAMPLE OF ENDOCRINE INVESTIGATION OF PRESUMED HYPOTHALAMIC AND POSTERIOR PITUITARY METASTASES

A 60-year-old lady presented with a six month history of dyspnoea with no associated cough or sputum production. She had smoked five cigarettes per day until ten years previously. She subsequently developed uncontrollable thirst, drinking 4 litres of fluid per day. This was associated with polyuria and a dry mouth. There were no abnormal findings on full physical examination. Transbronchial biopsy showed moderately differentiated squamous carcinoma. Serum calcium was normal. Tables 8.6 to 8.10 indicate the various investigations and tests which were performed. In addition, a skull x-ray showed the pituitary fossa to be expanded slightly at its postero-inferior angles.

TABLE 8.6
Endocrine Investigations : Basal Tests

		Normal range
Thyroxine	104 nmol/litre	(58–174)
Thyroid hormone uptake test	107	(92–118)
Free thyroxine index	102	(58–174)
9 am cortisol	550 nmol/litre	(180–700)
LH	> 50 U/litre	
FSH	> 25 U/litre	
Prolactin	377 mU/litre	(< 360)

TABLE 8.7
Water Deprivation Test

Time	Weight (kg)	Plasma Osmolality (mmol/kg)	Urine Osmolality (mmol/kg)	U/P ratio
0830	52·2	280	113	0·4
1130	51·65	279	246	0·88
1430	51·25	281	203	0·72
1530	51·05	282	256	0·91
1630	50·80	281	302	1·07
1730	—	286	351	1·23
DDAVP 2 mcg given i.m.				
1830			424	
1930			530	
2030			603	
2130			615	

TABLE 8.8
Insulin Tolerance Test

Time (min)	Blood glucose (mmol/litre)	Cortisol (nmol/litre)	Growth hormone (mU/litre)
0	3·7	370	10·6
Soluble insulin 0·15 μ/kg intravenously			
30	0·6	350	11·3
45	1·3	410	47·5
60	1·4	440	50·0
90	1·9	530	57·0
120	2·9	540	39·9

TABLE 8.9
CRF Test

Time (min)	Cortisol (nmol/litre)
0	331
CRF 100 mcg intravenously	
30	648
45	634
60	759
90	883
120	828

TABLE 8.10
TRH Test

Time (min)	TSH (mU/litre)
0	1·0
TRH 200 mcg intravenously	
20	13·0
60	9·7

INTERPRETATION OF ENDOCRINE DATA

Before a water deprivation test could be carried out, basal thyroid and adrenocortical function was checked and found to be normal. Both thyroxine and cortisol are necessary for the normal function of vasopressin. During the water deprivation test the patient lost almost 3% of her body weight. Although she did not become severely hypertonic (in severe diabetes insipidus the plasma osmolality often becomes greater than 300 mmol/kg), her urine to plasma osmolality ratios never exceeded 1·23. Normally this should be greater than 1·9 and often exceeds 2 (i.e. an urinary osmolality value more than twice that of the plasma osmolality). Following exogenous intramuscular DDAVP she achieved a significant further concentration of her urinary osmolality. On the basis of this test, a diagnosis of cranial diabetes insipidus was made and she subsequently derived considerable symptomatic benefit from intranasal DDAVP.

Subsequently the patient developed symptoms suggestive of adrenocortical deficiency, being tired and listless, lacking in energy, with anorexia. There was a mild postural drop in her blood pressure. Having checked that her basal 9 am cortisol was greater than 180 nmol/litre, an insulin tolerance test was performed. In response to the standard dose of soluble insulin (0·15 U/kg), she developed a very rapid and profound onset of hypoglycaemia, which was associated clinically with profuse sweating and tachycardia. She remained hypoglycaemic for the duration of the test, which in itself is unusual and tends to suggest a defect in the counter regulatory mechanisms (cortisol, growth hormone, pancreatic glucagon and catecholamine secretion). Although her basal cortisol was entirely within normal limits, there was a relatively poor rise in response to profound hypoglycaemia (normal > 580 nmol/litre). It is probable that this was due to a hypothalamic defect, since her cortisol response to corticotropin releasing factor was considerably greater.

She had a normal growth hormone response to insulin-induced hypoglycaemia, basal gonadotrophins were elevated (commensurate with her menopausal state), and she was only marginally hyperprolactinaemic.

She was treated with replacement hydrocortisone (20 mg on waking; 10 mg at 6 pm) with improvement in her symptoms. She became progressively more dyspnoeic and subsequently died at home. Unfortunately, no post-mortem was performed, so that the presumed hypothalamic with or without posterior pituitary metastases could not be verified as the cause of her endocrine problems.

REFERENCES

Abrams H.L., Spiro R., Goldstein N. (1950). Metastases in cancer—Analysis of 1000 autopsy cases. *Cancer*; **3**: 74–85.

Banna M. (1973). Craniopharyngioma in adults. *Surg. Neurol*; **1**: 202–204.

Brugge D.R.J., van Dongen J.A. Jr., Stofberg A.M.M. (1965). 'Spontane' remissie van een gemetastaseerd mammacarcinoom door metastasen in de hypofyse. *Nederlands tijdschrift voor geneeskunde*; **109**: 507–10.

Bynke O., Ottosson A.M. (1982). Is metastatic breast carcinoma in the pituitary a concealed manifestation? *Lancet*; **2**: 1336–7.

Cifuentes N., Pickren J.W. (1979). Metastases from carcinoma of mammary gland: An autopsy study. *J. Surg. Oncol*; **11**: 193–205.

Cohen H., Dible J.H. (1936). Pituitary basophilism associated with a basophil carcinoma of anterior lobe of the pituitary gland. *Brain*; **59**: 395–407.

Cox E.V. (1979). Chiasmal compression from metastatic cancer to the pituitary gland. *Surg. Neurol*; **11**: 49–50.

Daniel P.M., Prichard M.M.L. (1975). Studies of the hypothalamus and the pituitary gland with special reference to the effects of transection of the pituitary stalk. *Acta Endocrinol*; Suppl. **201**: 27–63.

Daniel P.M., Treip C.S. (1977). The pathology of the hypothalamus. *Clin. Endocrinol*; **6** (1): 3–19.

Davis J.C., Hipkin L.J. (1977). The pituitary. In *Clinical Endocrine Pathology*. pp. 11–91. Oxford: Blackwell Scientific Publications.

Delarue J., Chomette G., Pinaudeau Y., Brocheriou Cl., Auriol M. (1964). Les métastases hypophysaires. Fréquence. Etude histopathologique. Semaine des Hopitaux de Paris. *Arch. d'Anat. Pathol*; **12**: 179–82.

Doniach I. (1977). Histopathology of the anterior pituitary. *Clin. Endocrinol. Metab*; **6** (1): 21–52.

Doyle F., McLachlan M. (1977). Radiological aspects of pituitary–hypothalamic disease. *Clin. Endocrinol. Metab*; **6** (1): 53–81.

Duchen L.W. (1966). Metastatic carcinoma in the pituitary gland and hypothalamus. *J. Path. Bact*; **91**: 347–55.

Duchen L.W., Treip C.S. (1969). Microgliomatosis presenting with dementia and hypopituitarism. *J. Path*; **98**:143–6.

Egloff B., Fischbacher W., Von Goumoëns E. (1969). Lymphomatöse hypophysitis mit hypophysen-insuffizienz. *Schweizerische Medizinische Wochenschrift*; **99**: 1499–502.

Elmer A.W., Kedzierski J., Scheps M. (1928). Ein fall von diabetes insipidus verursacht durch eine metastase eines hypernephroms im zwischenhirn. *Wien. Klin. wochensch*; **41**: 591–4.

Epstein S., Ranchod M., Goldswain P.R.T. (1973). Pituitary insufficiency, inappropriate antiduretic hormone (ADH) secretion and carcinoma of the bronchus. *Cancer*; **32**: 476–81.

Ezrin C., Kovacs K., Horvath E. (1978). A functional anatomy of the endocrine hypothalamus and hypophysis. *Med. Clin. N. Am*; **62** (2): 229–33.

Forbes W. (1947). Carcinoma of the pituitary gland with metastases to the liver in a case of Cushing's syndrome. *J. Path. Bact*; **59**: 137–44.

Franks S., Nabarro J.D.N., Jacobs H.S. (1977). Prevalence and presentation of hyperprolactinaemia in patients with 'functionless' pituitary tumours. *Lancet*; **1**: 778–80.

Futcher T.B. (1929). Diabetes insipidus and lesions of the mid-brain: Report of a case due to a metastatic tumor of the hypothalamus. *Am. J. Med. Sci*; **178**: 837–52.

Gleason T.H., Stebbins P.L., Shanahan M.F. (1978). Lymphoid hypophysitis in a patient with hypoglycemic episodes. *Arch. Path. Lab. Med*; **102**: 46–8.

Goudie R.B., Pinkerton P.H. (1962). Anterior hypophysitis and Hashimoto's disease in a young woman. *J. Path. Bact*; **83**: 584–5.

Grabow Von D., Schwesinger G. (1979). Metastasen in der hypophyse. *Zentralblatt für neurochirurgie*; **40**: 29–34.

Grisoli F., Leclercq T.A., Robert F., Hardy J. (1974). Les métastases hypophysaires dans le cancer du sein. *Neuro-chirurgie*; **20**: 583–92.

Grossman A., Nieuwenhuyzen Kruseman A.C., Perry L. *et al.* (1982). New hypothalamic hormone, corticotropin-releasing factor, specifically stimulates the release of adrenocorticotropic hormone and cortisol in man. *Lancet*; **1**: 921–2.

Gurling K.J., Scott G.B.D., Baron D.N. (1957). Metastases in pituitary tissue removed at hypophysectomy in women with mammary carcinoma. *Br. J. Cancer*; **11**: 519–22.

Hägerstrand I., Schönebeck J. (1969). Metastases to the pituitary gland. *Acta Path. Microbiol. Scand*; **75**: 64–70.

Hall R., Anderson J., Smart G.A., Besser M. (1980). Hypopituitarism. In *Fundamentals of Clinical Endocrinology*, 3rd edn. London: Pitman Medical.

Von Hann F. (1918). Über die bedeutung der hypophysenveränderungen bei diabetes insipidus. *Frankfurter zeitschrift für pathologie*; **21**: 337–65.

Houck W.A., Olson K.B., Horton J. (1970). Clinical features of tumour metastasis to the pituitary. *Cancer*; **26**: 656–9.

Hume R., Roberts G.H. (1967). Hypophysitis and hypopituitarism: Report of a case. *Br. Med. J*; **2**: 548–50.

Jänisch W., Güthert H., Schreiber D. (1976). *Hypophysenmetastasen. Pathologie der Tumoren des Zentralnervensystems*, 399. Jena: G. Fischer.

Kahana L., Lebovitz H., Lusk W. *et al.* (1962). Endocrine manifestations of intracranial extrasellar lesions. *J. Clin. Endocrinol. Metab*; **22**: 304–24.

Kerkhoven P., Hedinger C. (1967). Hypophysenvorderlappennekrosen. *Schweizerische medizinische wochenschrift*; **97**: 263–73.

Kistler M., Pribram H.W. (1975). Metastatic disease of the sella turcica. *Am. J. Roentgenol*; **123**: 13–21.

Kovacs K. (1973). Metastatic cancer of the pituitary gland. *Oncology*; **27**: 533–42.

Lack E.E. (1975). Lymphoid 'hypophysitis' with end organ insufficiency. *Arch. Path*; **99**: 215–19.

Leramo O.B., Booth J.D., Zinman B., Bergeron C., Sima A.A.F., Morley T.P. (1981). Hyperprolactinemia, hypopituitarism, and chiasmal compression due to carcinoma metastatic to the pituitary. *Neurosurgery*; **8**: 477–80.

Line D.H., Deeley T.J. (1971). The necropsy findings in carcinoma of the bronchus. *Br. J. Dis. Chest*; **65**: 238–42.

Ludwig H., Schernthaner G. (1978). Multiorganspezifische autoimmunität bei idiopathischer Nebennierenrindeninsuffizienz. *Wiener Klinische wochenschrift*; **90**: 736–41.

Max M.B., Deck M.D.F., Rottenberg D.A. (1981). Pituitary metastasis: Incidence in cancer patients and clinical differentiation from pituitary adenoma. *Neurology (NY)*; **31**: 998–1002.

Mayfield R.K., Levine J.H., Gordon L., Powers J., Galbraith R.M., Rawe S.E. (1980). Lymphoid adenohypophysitis presenting as a pituitary tumor. *Am. J. Med*; **69**: 619–23.

Modhi G., Bauman W., Nicolis G. (1981). Adrenal failure associated with hypothalamic and adrenal metastases: A case report and review of the literature. *Cancer*; **47**: 2098–101.

Nugent J.L., Bunn P.A. Jr., Matthews M.J. *et al.* (1979). CNS metastases in small cell bronchogenic carcinoma: Increasing frequency and changing pattern with lengthening survival. *Cancer*; **44**: 1885–93.

Puschett J.B., Goldberg M. (1968). Endocrinopathy associated with pineal tumor. *Ann. Int. Med*; **69**: 203–19.

Roessmann V., Kaufman B., Friede R.L. (1970). Metastatic lesions in the sella turcica and pituitary gland. *Cancer*; **25**: 478–80.

Rosen C.J., Hasler G.R. (1980). Pituitary metastatic disease—Report of a case and review of the literature. *J. Maine Med. Assoc*; **71**: 238–40.

Schneider J., Jänisch W., Schreiber D. (1972). Zur häufigkeit von hypophysenmetastasen. *Zentralblatt für allgemeine pathologie und pathologische anatomie*; **115**: 74–7.

Sheehan H.L., Stanfield J.P. (1961). The pathogenesis of post-partum necrosis of the anterior lobe of the pituitary gland. *Acta Endocrinol*; **37**: 479–510.

Simionescu M.D. (1960). Metastatic tumors of the brain. A follow-up study of 195 patients with neurosurgical considerations. *J. Neurosurg*; **17**: 361–73.

Simmonds M. (1914). Ueber sekundäre Geschwülste des Hirnanhangs und ihre Beziehungen zum Diabetes insipidus. *Munch. med. Wschr*; **61**: 180–1.

Smulders J., Smets W. (1960). Les métastases des carcinomes mammaires. Fréquence des metastases hypophysaires. *Bulletin de l'association l'etude du cancer*; **47**: 434–56.

Snyder P.J., Jacobs L.S., Rabello M.M. *et al.* (1974). Diagnostic value of thyrotrophin-releasing hormone in pituitary and hypothalamic diseases. Assessment of thyrotrophin and prolactin secretion in 100 patients. *Ann. Int. Med*; **81**: 751–7.

Snyder P.J., Rudenstein R.S., Gardner D.F., Rothman J.G. (1979). Repetitive infusion of gonadotropin-releasing hormone distinguishes hypothalamic from pituitary hypogonadism. *J. Clin. Endocrinol. Metab*; **48**: 864–8.

Teears R.J., Silverman E.M. (1975). Clinicopathologic review of 88 cases of carcinoma metastatic to the pituitary gland. *Cancer*; **36**: 216–20.

Walther H.E. (1948). *Krebsmetastasen*. Basel: Schwabe.

Willis R.A. (1952). The spread of tumours in the human body. London: Butterworth & Co. Ltd.

Wohlwill F. (1928). Hypophyse und Zwischenhirn bei carcinom. *Dtsch Z. Nervenheilk*; **105**: 62–75.

Wolman L. (1959). Infundibuloma. *J. Path. Bact*; **77**: 283–96.

Wyeth G.A. (1934). The histological findings of the hypophysis in cancer. *Endocrinol*; **18**: 59–70.

Yap H.Y., Tashima C.K., Blumenschein G.R., Eckles N. (1979). Diabetes insipidus and breast cancer. *Arch. Int. Med*; **139**: 1009–1011.

Chapter 9

Peter H. Baylis

Disorders of Vasopressin Function

INTRODUCTION

The antidiuretic hormone in man and most mammalian species is arginine vasopressin, and it is well established that this hormone plays an important role in regulating water balance. Until a decade ago, it had proved difficult to define precisely the normal physiology of water regulation because the experimental methods were poor. In particular, the measurement of vasopressin in body fluids was very troublesome. But within the last few years, radioimmunoassay methodology has improved sufficiently to provide sensitive and specific methods capable of detecting the extremely low concentrations of vasopressin that circulate in blood under normal physiological conditions. Although numerous assays for the measurement of plasma arginine vasopressin have been described, it must be emphasised that these assays remain difficult to perform, are capricious and liable to non-specific interference, and the majority require extraction of vasopressin from plasma prior to assay.

Despite these methodological problems, there is remarkable agreement on the physiological control of vasopressin secretion and its function between most workers in this field (reviewed by Bie, 1980). In parallel with the increase in knowledge of the physiology of vasopressin function, a greater understanding of the disturbances in water balance and serum sodium concentration has developed. The pathophysiology of vasopressin secretion has been clearly and precisely defined in the two major clinical syndromes associated with water disturbances: cranial diabetes insipidus, and the syndrome of inappropriate antidiuresis. Both disorders are frequently, but not invariably, associated with neoplastic disease.

The following sections review the recent developments, information and ideas on vasopressin function in disturbances of water regulation associated with tumours, together with the most appropriate diagnostic methods and management of patients suffering from cranial diabetes insipidus and the syndrome of inappropriate antidiuresis. Before these are discussed, an outline of the physiological control of vasopressin secretion is presented.

PHYSIOLOGY OF VASOPRESSIN SECRETION

Arginine vasopressin is synthesised in the magnocellular neurones of the supraoptic and paraventricular nuclei in the hypothalamus. The hormone is transported as a vasopressin precursor–neurophysin complex in neurosecretory granules along nerve axons to at least four distinct areas of the brain. The major tract terminates in the neurohypophysis, while the others end at the median eminence of the hypothalamus, the floor of the third ventricle and the brain stem. Putative osmolality sensors (osmoreceptors) are located in the antero-lateral hypothalamus in close proximity to the thirst centre and the vasopressin-synthesising neurones.

Healthy adults maintain their plasma osmolality, determined mainly by the sodium concentration, within a remarkably narrow range. This stability is primarily achieved by the regulation of the excretion of solute-free water by the kidney. Under conditions of increasing osmolality, and after vasopressin has exerted its maximum antidiuretic effect, stability of plasma osmolality is attained by stimulation of thirst to encourage drinking, and in consequence plasma osmolality returns to normal.

The major physiological determinant of vasopressin secretion from minute-to-minute is plasma tonicity. The pioneering works of Verney

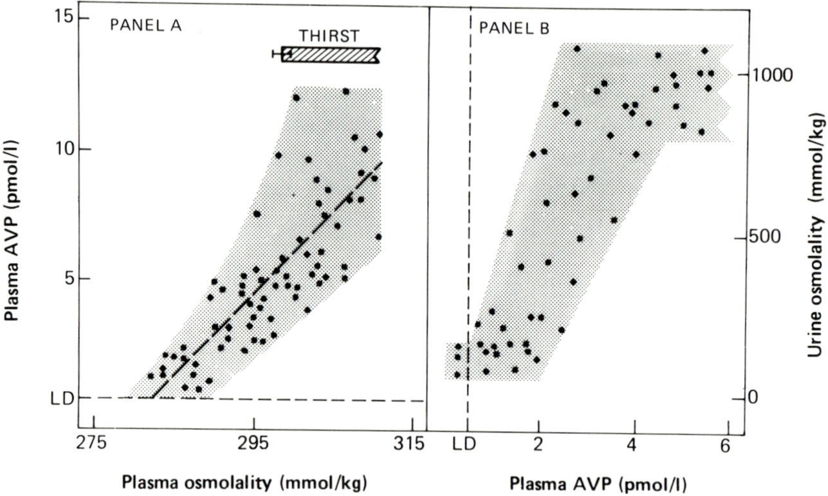

Fig. 9.1. *Panel A : The relationship between plasma arginine vasopressin (AVP) and osmolality during hypertonic saline infusion in healthy adults. LD is the limit of assay detection. Dashed line is the simple regression line of data points. Plasma osmolality at onset of thirst is 298 mmol/kg. Panel B : The relationship between urine osmolality and plasma AVP at various states of hydration in normal subjects.*

(1947) suggested this link, but the first direct confirmation that a rise in plasma osmolality caused an increase in circulating antidiuretic activity came from Baratz and Ingraham (1959). More recent studies (Robertson *et al.*, 1976; Baylis and Robertson, 1980) have defined the exquisitely sensitive relationship between plasma osmolality and vasopressin secretion. By infusing hypertonic saline into healthy adults to increase plasma osmolality, a direct correlation between these two variables was defined (Fig. 9.1, panel A). Simple linear regression analysis of these data, plasma vasopressin (pAVP) and plasma osmolality (pOs) defines the regression line,

$$pAVP = 0{\cdot}31\,(pOs - 281)$$
$$r = +0{\cdot}82, p < 0{\cdot}001$$

It will be immediately appreciated that the slope of the regression line is a measure of the sensitivity of the osmoreceptor and vasopressin releasing unit. Thus, for each mmol/kg increase in plasma osmolality, vasopressin concentration rises by 0·31 pmol/litre. The extraordinary sensitivity of the system is emphasised by the fact that rises in plasma osmolality of less than 1% are capable of causing vasopressin release sufficient to produce significant antidiuresis (*see* below). The abscissal intercept, 281 mmol/kg, defines the theoretical threshold for vasopressin secretion. Whether vasopressin secretion is ever completely suppressed at low plasma osmolalities remains controversial (Bie, 1980). The estimates of osmoreceptor sensitivity previously obtained by indirect methods (antidiuretic activity estimated from urine osmolality measurements) in acutely hydrated adults agree well with the above data (Moses and Miller, 1971).

Hyperosmolality produced by solutes other than sodium chloride may not cause a comparable rise in plasma vasopressin. Although Verney (1947) found little difference in the degree of antidiuresis induced by a variety of solutes, recent studies have clearly demonstrated that while sodium chloride and mannitol are very potent solutes stimulating the release of vasopressin, equimolar urea is less effective and glucose fails to stimulate vasopressin secretion (Robertson *et al.*, 1977; Milles and Baylis, 1981). Thus, the cells which sense the changes in solute concentration are not uniform in their response.

Although increasing plasma osmolality by hypertonic infusion causes a progressive linear rise in plasma vasopressin (Fig. 9.1, panel A), the antidiuretic activity of vasopressin does not continue to increase above plasma vasopressin concentrations of about 5 pmol/litre (Fig. 9.1, panel B). The data in the latter graph were obtained from hydrated and dehydrated healthy adults, and they agree with previous studies using indirect methods (Dashe *et al.*, 1963; Moses and Miller, 1971). Thus, the kidney is unable to continue concentrating urine and conserving free water despite rises in plasma vasopressin above 5 pmol/litre, a concentration which is obtained when plasma osmolality reaches 296 mmol/kg (Fig. 9.1, panel A). If the body becomes more dehydrated and plasma osmolality rises above this value, then the kidney which is producing maximally concentrated urine, cannot contribute further to correction of water balance, and another mechanism to maintain osmolality is required. That mechanism is, of course, thirst. At plasma osmolality values of the order of 298 mmol/kg and above, thirst sensation is switched on (Fig. 9.1, panel A). Healthy adults with free access to water will then start drinking with the consequence that plasma osmolality will fall again. In the converse situation, a falling plasma osmolality will suppress vasopressin secretion, allowing the kidney to excrete free water. As plasma osmolality falls below 280 mmol/kg, plasma vasopressin becomes undetectable ($<$0.5 pmol/litre) and the kidney is then capable of excreting 15–20 litres of urine per 24 hours. Thus, a healthy adult has to drink in excess of 20 litres to develop hypo-osmolality! It can now be appreciated how osmoregulation of vasopressin secretion and thirst controls water balance and maintains plasma osmolality within very narrow limits (281–296 mmol/kg).

Many other physiological factors that affect vasopressin secretion have been described (Scheiner, 1975), but the only two of physiological significance are the influence of blood pressure and blood volume (baroregulation). However, relatively large changes in these factors, of the order of 10%, are necessary to affect vasopressin secretion; if there are extreme falls in blood pressure or volume, as occurs in syncope, then there are enormous rises in hormone concentration (Baylis and Heath, 1977). Baroregulation probably plays only a minor role in the control of vasopressin secretion under physiological circumstances in healthy people.

In mammals, the major target organ of vasopressin is the nephron, and the collecting tubule the principal recognised site of action. Antidiuretic activity of vasopressin depends on the generation of a solute gradient across the tubular cell. This is achieved by the counter-current system, which generates a hyperosmolar interstitial renal medulla and allows hypo-osmolar urine to enter the distal nephron (Rector, 1977). In the presence of vasopressin, the permeability of the distal tubular cells to water is increased, thus allowing water to move from the tubular lumen into the medullary interstitial renal tissue, and consequently concentrating urine. Other actions of vasopressin, under physiological conditions, are minor in comparison to its renal effect (Scheiner, 1975).

CRANIAL DIABETES INSIPIDUS

Cranial diabetes insipidus, also known as hypothalamic or neurogenic diabetes insipidus, has been recognised as a clinical entity for two centuries. It may be defined as a disorder of urinary concentration which results from deficient secretion of vasopressin. Destruction of more than 80% of the neurohypophysis is necessary before the clinical features of polyuria and polydipsia appear.

Aetiology

Despite the occasional review on diabetes insipidus (Thomas, 1957; Hockaday, 1972; Maffly, 1977), there is little information on its prevalence. It is, however, generally agreed to be a rare disorder.

The causes may be divided into two major categories, familial and acquired (Table 9.1). The familial type is inherited as either a dominant or recessive trait, and occasionally becomes manifest late in life in association with optic atrophy, nerve deafness, diabetes mellitus and atonia of the

TABLE 9.1
Causes of Polyuria

Cranial diabetes insipidus	*Primary polydipsia*	*Nephrogenic diabetes insipidus*

A. *Familial*
  1. Dominant inheritance
  2. Recessive inheritance
  3. Associated with diabetes mellitus, optic atrophy, nerve deafness
	A. *Idiopathic*	A. *Hereditary*
		  1. Sex-linked recessive inheritance

B. *Acquired*
  1. Idiopathic
  2. Trauma (neurosurgery, head injury)
  3. Tumours (large pituitary tumours, metastases to hypothalamus, craniopharyngioma, pinealoma)
  4. Granuloma (sarcoidosis, histiocytosis X, eosinophilic granuloma)
  5. Infections (meningitis, encephalitis)
  6. Vascular (Sheehan's syndrome, aneurysms, sickle cell anaemia)
	B. *Associated with psychoses*	B. *Acquired*
		  1. Chronic renal disease (renal failure, polycystic disease, sickle cell disease)
		  2. Metabolic (hypokalaemia, hypercalcaemia, amyloid)
		  3. Drugs (lithium, demeclocycline, barbiturates)
		  4. Osmotic diuresis (diabetes mellitus, post-obstructive uropathy, mannitol)

bladder (Cremers *et al.*, 1977). The most common form of the disease is idiopathic, which accounted for 45% of cases in Blotner's series (Blotner, 1958).

Tumours of the anterior pituitary gland which are confined to the pituitary fossa rarely cause cranial diabetes insipidus. Even the large tumours which extend above the diaphragma sellae, as seen in the majority of acromegalic patients, usually produce no disturbance to vasopressin secretion. However, if tumour growth involves the pituitary stalk, particularly at a high anatomical level, then cranial diabetes may ensue. It is assumed that tumour pressure on a hypothalamo-neurohypophysial tract causes atrophy of the nerve axons and there is retrograde degeneration leading to neuronal cell death in the supraoptic and paraventricular nuclei. Consequently, there is a deficiency of vasopressin synthesis and release, either absolute or relative to plasma osmolality.

Tumours do not appear to spontaneously develop in the neurohypophysis, the hypothalamo-neurohypophysial tract, or the neurones that synthesise vasopressin. However, it is not uncommon for carcinoma of the breast or bronchus to metastasise to the hypothalamus. The major disturbance of hypothalamic function in these patients is cranial diabetes insipidus, although loss of thirst (adipsia) sometimes accompanies diabetes insipidus. The combination of adipsia and diabetes insipidus is catastrophic for the patient, because the usual signals to drink are lost and hypernatraemia with severe hypertonicity of extracellular body fluids can develop, which may lead to death. Other hypothalamic functions (e.g. temperature regulation, modulation of anterior pituitary hormone secretion) are usually not obviously deranged by metastatic disease. Similarly, the granulomatous disorders, such as sarcoid, that involve the hypothalamus tend not to involve functions other than those controlling water balance.

The other causes of cranial diabetes insipidus, infection and vascular abnormalities (Table 9.1), are rare. The only exception is diabetes secondary to neurosurgery to the pituitary and hypothalamic regions. Transfrontal craniotomy to remove large pituitary tumours is associated with a high incidence of permanent post-operative diabetes insipidus compared to the transphenoidal route which is approximately 10% (Tyrrell *et al.*, 1978; Nicola *et al.*, 1980). However, the latter route is only suitable for lesions with minimal suprasellar extension.

Differential Diagnosis

Patients with cranial diabetes with intact thirst sensation complain of polyuria and polydipsia, but those with only minor vasopressin deficiencies, i.e. partial cranial diabetes insipidus, may not emphasise their symptoms because they are so mild. A daily urine output of 3 litres may even go unnoticed by some patients. Complaints of a dry mouth must be differentiated from true thirst which is a compunction to drink, but is, of course, frequently associated with dryness of the mouth. Urinary frequency alone is easily distinguished from polyuria by the patient's realisation that only small volumes of urine are passed at a time and by the lack of thirst.

Once true polydipsia and polyuria have been recognised and confirmed by measurement of 24-hour urine volumes, then the cause must rest between one of three mechanisms; (i) cranial diabetes insipidus, (ii) nephrogenic diabetes insipidus, defined as complete or partial renal resistance to the antidiuretic activity of vasopressin, (iii) primary polydipsia or habitual fluid drinking. Table 9.1 outlines the major disorders associated with diabetes insipidus and primary polydipsia. Diagnostic problems occasionally occur in the patient who has disseminated malignant disease, polyuria and hypercalcaemia. In this instance, polyuria could be due to acquired nephrogenic diabetes insipidus, secondary to a metastatic deposit in the hypothalamus, or, very rarely, stimulation of the thirst centre by tumourous deposits. Investigations described in the following section should distinguish between the possibilities.

Investigations

The traditional method of investigation of the polyuric patient (24-hour urine output greater than 2 litres) has been some form of water deprivation test. Because of the problems of measuring vasopressin the demonstration of antidiuretic activity rested on indirect methods, but results from these tests may be difficult to interpret and occasionally lead to false conclusions (Zerbe and Robertson, 1981) During the past decade vasopressin assay methods have improved sufficiently to measure the hormone reliably, but they are not widely available to the clinician and tend to remain as research tools. In consequence, the indirect methods of testing antidiuretic activity are still commonly used.

The basis of the fluid deprivation test is simple. Urine and plasma osmolalities are measured at regular intervals during a period of dehydration, at the end of which vasopressin is administered and subsequent urine osmolalities recorded. Although a number of variations on this theme have been described (Dashe *et al.*, 1963; Price and Lauener, 1966; Miller *et al.*, 1970), all emphasise specific precautions. It is essential to allow the patient free access to water only during the 12 hours before the test; smoking must not be allowed; he must be weighed before and at hourly intervals during the test and, should he lose more than 5% of his intial body weight, dehydration *must* stop; and an observer should be present throughout the test to ensure that there is no surreptitious drinking. The test most frequently performed is a modification of that described by Dashe *et al.* (1963), the details of which are given in Table 9.2.

TABLE 9.2
Water Deprivation Test

A. *Preparation of patient:*
1. Water intake encouraged overnight
2. Light breakfast: no coffee, tea or smoking

B. *Dehydration period:*
1. No fluids for up to 8 hours. Dry food permitted
2. Supervision essential
3. Weigh patient hourly and stop dehydration if weight loss is greater than 5% of initial weight
4. Urine passed at hourly intervals to record volume and osmolality
5. Blood drawn at hourly intervals to measure plasma osmolality

C. *Response to vasopressin:*
1. After dehydration period, administer desmopressin (DDAVP) $2\,\mu g$ intramuscularly
2. Patient allowed to eat and drink normally
3. Urine passed at 1, 3, 5 and 12 hours after DDAVP to record volume and osmolality

Results from the Dashe test usually distinguish patients with severe cranial or nephrogenic diabetes insipidus from normals. A rising plasma osmolality during the dehydration period ensures that the patient has become sufficiently dehydrated and has not drunk during the test. If urine osmolality at the end of dehydration exceeds 750 mmol/kg, significant diabetes insipidus of either form is excluded. Hypotonic urine after dehydration, with subsequent urine osmolality greater than 650 mmol/kg after desmopressin strongly suggests cranial diabetes. If the urine remains hypotonic (urine osmolality <250 mmol/kg) throughout the test and following desmopressin administration, nephrogenic diabetes is suspected. Problems often occur in the interpretation of submaximal concentration of urine (osmolality 350–650 mmol/kg), particularly if there is little or no further concentration after desmopressin. Patients with primary polydipsia, partial cranial, or partial nephrogenic diabetes insipidus can have such results. A possible explanation for these anomalous results is that a mild state of nephrogenic diabetes insipidus occurs occasionally following a longstanding diuresis (DeWardener and Herxheimer, 1957).

In an attempt to overcome the difficulty of diagnosing partial abnormalities, prolonged dehydration tests have been recommended (Miller *et al.*, 1970). This method is extremely tedious for the patient and observer, since dehydration might exceed 24 hours.

Another approach to solve the problem came from the re-introduction of hypertonic saline infusion to rapidly increase plasma osmolality, stimulate vasopressin secretion and concentrate urine (Moses and Streeten, 1967).

This, too, is unsatisfactory because the natriuresis consequent to saline infusion spuriously raises urine osmolality. An accurate diagnosis can only be made by direct vasopressin measurements.

If facilities exist to measure plasma vasopressin reliably, this must be the method of choice to diagnose precisely the cause of polyuria, particularly the mild abnormalities. Isolated vasopressin measurements are difficult to interpret, but osmoregulation can be readily tested dynamically by infusion of 5% saline for 2 hours at a rate of 0·06 ml/kg/min, during which blood is drawn at regular intervals to measure plasma vasopressin and osmolality (Robertson *et al.*, 1976; Baylis and Robertson, 1980). When 5% saline is infused into polyuric patients, a clear pattern of responses emerges (Fig. 9.2). Patients who are deficient in vasopressin show absent or subnormal responses to osmotic stimulation (Fig. 9.2, panel B). There is some correlation between the degree of polyuria and the vasopressin response to hypertonic saline infusion. For example, patient I (panel B) who showed sub-optimal vasopressin secretion had a urine output of 4.4 litre/24 h, while all those who had undetectable vasopressin (patients E, F, J) had urine volumes of 11, 13 and 15 litre/24 h, respectively. In this series, four patients had normal osmoregulated vasopressin release (Fig. 9.1, panel A). Their results are compatible with either primary

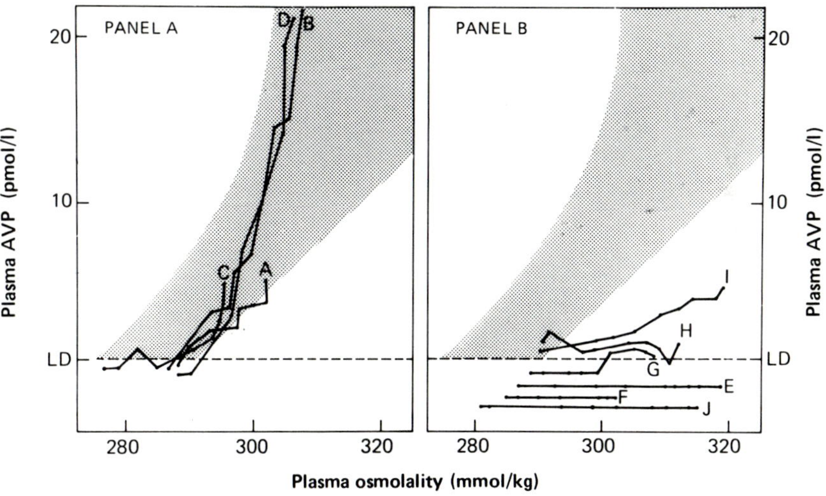

Fig. 9.2. *Plasma arginine vasopressin (AVP) response to infusion of hypertonic saline in a group of polyuric patients. LD is the limit of assay detection. Stippled areas are the normal ranges. Panel A: Four polyuric patients with normal AVP responses. Panel B: Six patients with absent or impaired responses (Baylis and Robertson, 1980; by kind permission of the Editor of Journal of the Royal Society of Medicine).*

polydipsia or nephrogenic diabetes insipidus, which can be readily differentiated by measuring plasma vasopressin in relation to urine osmolality after a
period of dehydration. Patients with nephrogenic diabetes insipidus have an
inappropriately high plasma concentration of vasopressin relative to urine
osmolality, while patients with primary polydipsia have low plasma
vasopressin levels (Fig. 9.3). Similar results demonstrating clear separation
between the different types of polyuria have been obtained in other series
(Robertson *et al.*, 1976; Baylis *et al.*, 1981; Zerbe and Robertson, 1981).

A recent comparison between indirect (water deprivation tests) and direct
(vasopressin measurement during hypertonic saline infusion) methods has
clearly shown the superiority of the direct approach (Zerbe and Robertson,
1981). In this series of 24 polyuric patients, five had discrepant results.
Three out of ten patients diagnosed as primary polydipsia by dehydration
tests had clear evidence of partial vasopressin deficiency (cranial diabetes
insipidus) using direct assay. A further two out of six patients with partial
cranial diabetes by indirect criteria had normal vasopressin responses to
osmotic stimulation; one had partial nephrogenic diabetes insipidus and the
other primary polydipsia.

It can now be appreciated that a major difficulty of indirect tests is
encountered in distinguishing primary polydipsia from partial diabetes
insipidus. If vasopressin measurement is not readily available, a therapeutic
trial of vasopressin may help identify primary polydipsia. Administration of

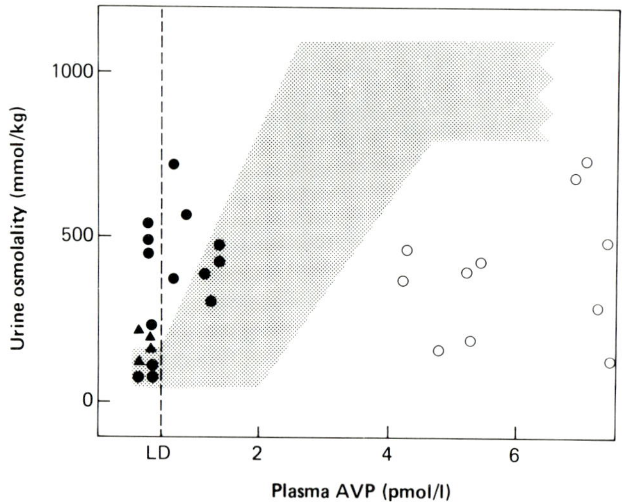

Fig. 9.3. *Urine osmolality related to plasma arginine vasopressin (AVP) of a
group of polyuric patients after dehydration (cranial diabetes insipidus, ● ;
primary polydipsia, ▲ ; nephrogenic diabetes insipidus, ○). LD is the limit of
assay detection and the stippled area is the normal range.*

desmopressin (DDAVP) 10 μg intra-nasally once daily for two weeks will cause progressive dilutional hyponatraemia in the primary polydipsic patient who continues to drink. Patients with partial nephrogenic diabetes insipidus will remain unaffected by the drug, while those with partial cranial diabetes will show improvement in thirst and polyuria.

In summary, patients with significant cranial diabetes insipidus can usually be identified by water deprivation tests, but those with mild disorders can only be reliably diagnosed by direct vasopressin measurements during osmotic stimulation. Unfortunately, the latter technique is available only in a few centres.

Treatment

A variety of methods are available for treating cranial diabetes insipidus, but it is always worthwhile first considering whether treatment is necessary. Undoubtedly, some patients with profound polyuria from birth, due to the rare familial disorders, may develop into normal adults showing no adverse affects and have minimal complaints (Baylis and Robertson, 1981). They rely on their thirst to maintain fluid intake and suffer from persistent urinary frequency day and night. Patients who acquire the disorder notice the inconvenience and demand treatment. A major difficulty occurs if an untreated patient is unable to gain access to fluid, loses thirst sensation or becomes unconscious, which may result in life-threatening dehydration. Other complications in untreated patients have been described. Longstanding severe diabetes insipidus can lead to distension and atonia of the bladder, hydroureter and hydronephrosis (Weller *et al.*, 1950), and has been associated with secondary nephrogenic diabetes (Friedland *et al.*, 1971). For these reasons, some form of therapy is advisable for patients with polyuria, particularly if the urine output exceeds 4 litre/24 h.

The most efficacious form of treatment is some type of vasopressin replacement. Arginine vasopressin itself is not suitable because it has a short biological half-life. However, the synthetic analogue desmopressin (DDAVP) introduced over a decade ago (Vavra *et al.*, 1968) appears to be an ideal agent. In this preparation the vasopressin molecule has been altered to decrease degradation and the pressor activity has been reduced to a minimum while antidiuretic potency has been increased. Unfortunately, like all vasopressins and analogues, it must be administered parenterally or by the intra-nasal route, as it is rapidly degraded in the gastrointestinal tract. It is the drug of choice for most patients although there is considerable individual variation in the dose required to control symptoms (Edwards *et al.*, 1973; Cobb *et al.*, 1978). The only significant side-effect of desmopressin is hyponatraemia due to water intoxication. This may result from persistent antidiuresis accompanied by normal social drinking. To avoid this complication, patients are advised to allow themselves to become polyuric by discontinuing the drug at least once each week. If desmopressin is not available or is too potent, then an alternative preparation, lysine vasopressin, may be suitable. It must also be administered intra-nasally, but doses need to be given at four-hourly intervals instead of twice a day as with desmopressin. Given in excess, lysine vasopressin will cause pressor effects, resulting in possible hypertension, cardiac ischaemia, and renal and intestinal colic. Pitressin tannate in oil, the extract from the posterior pituitary gland frequently used in the past, is no longer available.

Although desmopressin has revolutionised the treatment of cranial diabetes insipidus, some clinicians still prefer to use the well-tried oral agents. These are only useful in mild forms of cranial diabetes insipidus in which some vasopressin remains in the circulation. Chlorpropamide has been the most successful (Arduino *et al.*, 1966); it appears to potentiate the antidiuretic effect of vasopressin (Murase and Yoshida, 1973), reduces urine output by about 50% after several weeks therapy, but can cause significant hypoglycaemia. Although a number of other oral agents (thiazides, clofibrate, carbamazepine) reduce polyuria in cranial diabetes insipidus, they are less effective than chlorpropamide (Maffly, 1977).

The patient who has the combination of cranial diabetes insipidus and loss of thirst presents a particularly difficult management problem. These hypothalamic abnormalities are occasionally encountered in patients with metastatic disease (Robertson, 1979). Although the vasopressin deficiency can be readily treated, the major problem is maintaining an appropriate fluid input to avoid wide fluctuations in serum sodium and osmolality. One way to stabilise water balance is first to determine the dose of desmopressin and then to fix the intake of fluid to 1·5 litres provided the daily body weight remains constant. If the latter falls then an equivalent weight of fluid should be given, and if it rises the input must be reduced accordingly. Weekly measurements of serum sodium and osmolality ensure that this management is achieving satisfactory water regulation.

SYNDROME OF INAPPROPRIATE ANTIDIURESIS

Winkler and Crankshaw (1938) described a group of patients who had hypochloraemia and excessive urinary excretion of chloride. They deduced from indirect evidence that these abnormalities could be accounted for by persistent secretion of antidiuretic hormone. Similar findings together with hyponatraemia, urinary salt wasting and impaired urinary dilution in two patients with bronchogenic carcinoma led Schwartz *et al.* (1957) to propose the syndrome of inappropriate antidiuretic hormone secretion. The administration of exogenous vasopressin with persistent fluid intake, produced identical biochemical changes in healthy adults (Leaf *et al.*, 1952), lending support to the hypothesis. Despite the lack of methods to measure vasopressin, there was considerable indirect evidence confirming the underlying disorder. By 1967, Bartter and Schwartz had collected a large series of patients suffering from this syndrome and were able to define its cardinal features, which are as follows:

i) Hyponatraemia with appropriately low plasma osmolality.
ii) Urine osmolality greater than the concomitant plasma osmolality.
iii) Excessive renal excretion of sodium.
iv) Absence of hypotension, hypovolaemia, or oedema-forming states (e.g. cirrhosis, heart failure).
v) Normal renal and adrenal function.

If patients fulfil these criteria, they may be releasing vasopressin in quantities that are not appropriate for their plasma osmolalities (Fig. 9.1, panel A). Furthermore, not only do they have persistent secretion of vasopressin, but they must also continue to drink, albeit small amounts of fluid, to develop hypotonic hyponatraemia.

Aetiology

A large number of conditions have been described in association with the cardinal features of the syndrome of inappropriate antidiuresis (Table 9.3). In many cases, direct evidence of inappropriately elevated plasma vasopressin levels has not been obtained.

TABLE 9.3
Causes of the Syndrome of Inappropriate Antidiuresis

A. *Malignant disease*	C. *Chest disorders*
Carcinoma of bronchus, duodenum, pancreas, bladder, ureter, prostate	Pneumonia
	Tuberculosis
Thymoma	Empyema
Mesothelioma	Cystic fibrosis
Lymphoma, leukaemia	Pneumothorax
Ewing's sarcoma	Asthma
B. *Central nervous system disorders*	D. *Miscellaneous*
Meningitis, encephalitis	Drugs: vasopressin, oxytocin, chlorpropramide, vincristine, vinblastine, thiazides, phenothiazines, carbamazepine
Guillain–Barré syndrome	
Brain tumour, abscess	
Head injury	
Cerebral haemorrhage	Endocrine: hypothyroidism
Cavernous sinus thrombosis	Acute psychosis, delirium tremens
Hydrocephalus	
Cerebellar and cerebral atrophy	Idiopathic
Shy–Drager syndrome	
Porphyria	

The most common tumour to produce the syndrome is an oat cell carcinoma of the bronchus, but a wide variety of malignant tumours from different tissues and of diverse cell origins has been reported. It is frequently assumed that all these tumours synthesise vasopressin and release the hormone at random. Although some malignant cells are capable of synthesising vasopressin, and indeed many other peptides (Rees and Ratcliffe, 1974), it is probably not the only mechanism causing inappropriately elevated plasma vasopressin. Interestingly, in their original reports, Schwartz *et al.* (1957) proposed a non-ectopic mechanism for inappropriate secretion of antidiuretic hormone. However, direct evidence of large amounts of antidiuretic hormone activity has been found in bronchogenic carcinoma in patients fulfilling the diagnostic criteria (Amatruda *et al.*, 1963). Further studies have shown that bronchogenic carcinoma is capable of synthesising vasopressin *in vitro* (George *et al.*, 1972), which is immunologically and chromatographically identical to arginine vasopressin. These observations have led to the widespread erroneous belief that all cases of the syndrome of inappropriate antidiuresis associated with malignant disorders are due to ectopic production.

Another intriguing, but as yet unconfirmed observation was the demonstration of antidiuretic activity in a large proportion of bronchogenic carcinomas in patients who were not hyponatraemic (Morton *et al.*, 1978). It must be presumed that since these patients did not have the syndrome of inappropriate antidiuresis, their tumour cells were unable to release vasopressin from the tumours.

Pathophysiology

Within the past decade there has come confirmation of the hypothesis of Bartter and Schwartz. In many patients who fulfilled the criteria of the syndrome of inappropriate antidiuresis, vasopressin was detected in the circulation. The absolute levels of plasma vasopressin were often observed to be in the physiologic range but inappropriately high for the concomitant plasma osmolality. A few had extremely elevated plasma concentrations of vasopressin.

A considerable advance in the understanding of osmoregulation of vasopressin secretion in the syndrome of inappropriate antidiuresis came from a study of 79 hyponatraemic patients, all of whom filled the criteria (Zerbe *et al.*, 1980). Eighty per cent of their patients had plasma vasopressin levels in the range seen in normally hydrated adults. These workers studied osmoregulation by infusing hypertonic saline and/or water loading patients, and observed the response of plasma vasopressin and osmolality to define the threshold of vasopressin release and the sensitivity of the osmoreceptor mechanism. Four patterns of response were obtained (Fig. 9.4).

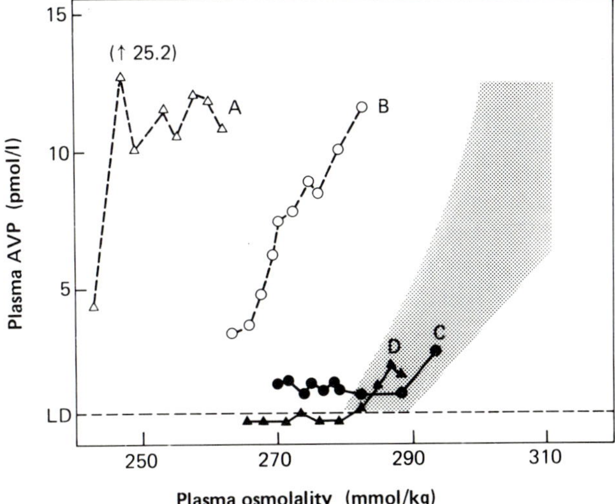

Fig. 9.4. *Four patterns (A,B,C,D) of plasma arginine vasopressin (AVP) response to infusion of hypertonic saline in a group of patients with the syndrome of inappropriate antidiuresis. LD is the limit of assay detection and the stippled area is the normal range (Zerbe et al., 1980; by kind permission of Annual Review of Medicine, Volume 31, 1980 by Annual Reviews Inc.).*

The first pattern (Fig. 9.4, type A) is characterised by wide erratic fluctuations in plasma vasopressin concentration, which are totally independent of plasma osmolality. This type accounts for approximately 37% of the patients. The precise mechanism of this type of abnormality is not known, although one might speculate that random ectopic release from tumours is a plausible cause. But patients with malignant disorders do not account for all those within this group. Since this pattern is observed in patients with non-tumourous disease, other mechanisms, possibly transient and erratic non-osmotic stimuli of vasopressin release, may play a role.

A second group of patients accounting for 33% of the total, demonstrate osmotically-sensitive vasopressin release (Fig. 9.4, type B). The vasopressin response of this group to hypertonic saline is very similar to normal individuals, with the exception that the regression line is shifted to the left of normal. The slopes and correlation coefficients of the lines are comparable to normals, but the osmotic thresholds for vasopressin release are lowered. Similar resetting of the 'osmostat' may be due to one of three mechanisms. The osmoregulatory line moves to the left under conditions of hypotension or hypovolaemia (Robertson and Athar, 1976), but these patients by definition cannot suffer from either of these disturbances. Resetting may occur as a result of interruption of the afferent baroregulatory pathways, leading to loss of normal tonic inhibition and thus providing false signals of volume or pressure depletion. A third possibility concerns the putative method of action of the osmoreceptor itself. It is believed that the osmoreceptor cells are stimulated by intracellular dehydration. Loss of intracellular solutes, as postulated in the 'sick cell syndrome' (Flear and Singh, 1973), would render the osmoreceptor responsive to fluctuations in osmolality at levels lower than normal. Irrespective of the mechanism, patients with type B abnormality may excrete maximally dilute urine if plasma osmolality falls sufficiently (DeFronzo *et al.*, 1976). This pattern of response may be observed in patients with both malignant and non-malignant disease.

The third pattern of response (Fig. 9.4, type C) accounts for 16% of patients. Osmoregulated vasopressin secretion is normal within the physiologic range of plasma osmolality, but as plasma osmolality is lowered vasopressin secretion cannot be suppressed completely. This 'leak' of vasopressin may be due to injury to the neurohypophysis, loss of inhibitory neurones, or hyperfunction of stimulatory neurones. This pattern has been observed in patients having meningitis, basilar skull fractures and rarely in patients with malignant disease.

The final group (14%) appear to have entirely normal osmoregulated vasopressin secretion (Fig. 9.4, type D). At low plasma osmolality their plasma vasopressin is undetectable, but nevertheless, they are unable to excrete a water load nor maximally dilute urine. Whether this abnormality is due to increased renal sensitivity, to very low plasma vasopressin concentrations, or to an antidiuretic substance other than arginine vasopressin, is unknown.

It can now be appreciated that patients with malignant disease and the syndrome of inappropriate antidiuresis may have many different abnormalities of vasopressin secretion, and do not all suffer from ectopic secretion.

Diagnosis

Any patient who has hypotonic hyponatraemia may have the syndrome of inappropriate antidiuresis. To make this diagnosis it is essential that the patient fulfils all the criteria described by Bartter and Schwartz (1967). Thus, adrenal and renal function must be evaluated, and hypotension and hypovolaemia excluded. Clearly, some patients who have dual pathologies, e.g. renal failure and ectopic vasopressin secretion from an oat cell bronchogenic carcinoma, will cause diagnostic difficulties. The demonstration of impaired excretion of a water load is not necessary to confirm the diagnosis.

Confirmation of the diagnosis can be obtained by measurement of plasma vasopressin during osmotic stimulation, but this is not essential, and clearly impractical for most clinicians, as vasopressin assays are not widely available. Thus, the diagnosis rests on the original criteria of Bartter and Schwartz (1967).

Management

The clinical features of hyponatraemia are varied; the most serious are due to cerebral oedema that is a direct consequence of the hypotonicity of body fluids (Arieff *et al.*, 1976). The severity of the symptoms which range from mild confusion, headaches and nausea to convulsions, coma and death, depend on both the degree and rate of development of hypo-osmolality.

Treatment of the syndrome of inappropriate antidiuresis will vary according to the individual patient. If at all possible, therapy directed at the cause of the syndrome is the most appropriate. Mild degrees of hyponatraemia (serum sodium > 125 mmol/litre) may not require treatment, particularly if the patient is symptom free.

For a patient who does require active therapy, the traditional method is fluid restriction, which is safe, rational and effective, although sometimes distressing for the patient (Schwartz *et al.*, 1957; Zerbe *et al.*, 1980). The aim of the treatment should be to raise serum sodium to about 130 mmol/litre. If fluid restriction fails, then drug therapy may prove necessary. One approach is to administer a drug that suppresses neurohypophysial vasopressin secretion, but this is only appropriate in patients with non-ectopic hormone secretion. Ethanol will inhibit vasopressin release but is impractical because the effects are inconsistent, short-lived, and require intoxicating doses (Helderman *et al.*, 1978). Oral phenytoin has met with only slightly greater success (Tanay *et al.*, 1979). Another method of correcting these patients' hyponatraemia is to inhibit the antidiuretic action of vasopressin, thus causing partial nephrogenic diabetes insipidus. Demeclocycline, a tetracycline derivative, is the most effective preparation and is relatively safe when 600–1200 mg per day are given in divided doses (Cherrill *et al.*, 1978). Potential side-effects include nausea, photosensitivity and renal failure. Less reliable at producing nephrogenic diabetes insipidus is lithium carbonate. Nevertheless, it has been advocated for the treatment of the syndrome, despite its rather toxic side-effects of cardiac dysrhythmias, thyroid dysfunction and neurological and gastrointestinal disturbances (Forrest *et al.*, 1978). A third method to correct the hyponatraemia involves the production of a natriuresis which, in turn, induces an osmotic diuresis and removes excess body water. Decaux *et al.* (1982) have recommended oral frusemide (40–80 mg), together with salt supplementation of up to 3 g per day. Their patients had a mean increase in serum sodium of 16 mmol/litre.

It is rarely necessary to correct hyponatraemia swiftly, but if the serum sodium is extremely low, of the order of 100 mmol/litre, and the patient's life is threatened, then more rapid means of improving hyponatraemia are advisable. This can be readily achieved by infusing 5% saline at a rate of 2 ml/min for 6 hours, which will raise the serum sodium by approximately 10 mmol/litre. It is important to realise the effects are short-lived and that too rapid a correction may cause convulsions and death.

CONCLUSIONS

Malignant disease can be associated with disorders of water regulation. Following the introduction of reliable and sensitive methods of measuring circulating vasopressin, those disorders have been defined more precisely. Partial defects of cranial diabetes insipidus can be easily distinguished from other causes of polyuria, and studies of osmoregulation in cranial diabetes insipidus have identified unexpected aspects of its pathophysiology. Similarly, more is understood about the syndrome of inappropriate antidiuresis. Tumourous disease with hypotonic hyponatraemia is not always due to ectopic vasopressin production by malignant cells, but frequently influences neurohypophysial vasopressin secretion in other more subtle ways. Precise definition of the osmoregulatory defects in the syndrome of inappropriate antidiuresis is leading to more accurate diagnosis and to more rational approaches to treatment.

REFERENCES

Amatruda T.T. Jr., Mulrow P.J., Gallagher J.C., Sawyer W.H. (1963). Carcinoma of the lung with inappropriate antidiuresis. *N. Engl. J. Med*; **269**: 544–9.

Arduino F., Ferraz F.P.J., Rodriguez J. (1966). Antidiuretic action of chlorpropamide in idiopathic diabetes insipidus. *J. Clin. Endocrinol*; **26**: 1325–8.

Arieff A.I., Llach F., Massry S.G. (1976). Neurological manifestations and morbidity of hyponatraemia: Correlation with brain water and electrolytes. *Medicine*; **55**: 121–9.

Baratz R.A., Ingraham R.C. (1959). Sensitive bioassay method for measuring antidiuretic hormone in mammalian plasma. *Proc. Soc. Exp. Biol. and Med*; **100**: 296–9.

Bartter F.C., Schwartz W.B. (1967). The syndrome of inappropriate secretion of antidiuretic hormone. *Am. J. Med*; **42**: 790–806.

Baylis P.H., Heath D.A. (1977). Influence of presyncope and postural change upon plasma arginine vasopressin concentration in hydrated and dehydrated man. *Clin. Endocrinol. (Oxf)*; **7**: 79–83.

Baylis P.H., Robertson G.L. (1980). Vasopressin response to hypertonic saline infusion to assess posterior pituitary function. *J. Roy. Soc. Med*; **73**: 255–60.

Baylis P.H., Robertson G.L. (1981). Vasopressin function in familial cranial diabetes insipidus. *Postgrad. Med. J*; **57**: 36–40.

Baylis P.H., Gaskill M.B., Robertson G.L. (1981). Vasopressin function in polyuric patients. *Quart. J. Med*; **50**: 345–58.

Bie P. (1980). Osmoreceptors, vasopressin, and control of renal water excretion. *Physiol. Rev*; **60**: 962–1048.

Blotner H. (1958). Primary or idiopathic diabetes insipidus: a system disease. *Metabolism*: **7**: 191–206.

Cherrill D.A., Stote R.M., Birge J.R., Singer I. (1975). Demeclocycline treatment in the syndrome of inappropriate antidiuretic hormone secretion. *Ann. Int. Med*; **83**: 654–6.

Cobb W.E., Spare S., Reichlin S. (1978). Neurogenic diabetes insipidus; Management with dDAVP (1-desamino-8-d-arginine vasopressin). *Ann. Int. Med*; **88**: 183–8.

Cremers C.W.R.J., Wijdeveld P.G.A.B., Pinker A.J.L.G. (1977). Juvenile diabetes mellitus, optic atrophy, hearing loss, diabetes insipidus, atonia of the urinary tract and bladder, and other abnormalities (Wolfram syndrome). *Acta Paed. Scand*; Supplement **264**: 1–16.

Dashe A.M., Cramm R.E., Crist C.A., Habener J.F., Solomon D.H. (1963). A water deprivation test for the differential diagnosis of polyuria. *J. Am. Med. Assoc*; **185**: 699–703.

Decaux G., Waterlot Y., Genette F., Hallemans R., Demanet J.C. (1982). Inappropriate secretion of antidiuretic hormone treated with frusemide. *Br. Med. J*; **2**: 89–90.

DeFronzo R.A., Goldberg M., Agus Z.S. (1976). Normal diluting capacity in hyponatraemia: Reset osmostat or a variant of SIADH. *Ann. Int. Med*; **84**: 538–42.

DeWardener H.E., Herxheimer A. (1957). The effect of a high water intake on the kidney's ability to concentrate the urine in man. *J. Physiol. (Lond)*; **139**: 42–52.

Edwards C.R.W., Kitau M.J., Chard T., Besser G.M. (1973). Vasopressin analogue DDAVP in diabetes insipidus: Clinical and laboratory studies. *Br. Med. J*; **3**: 375–8.

Flear C.T.G., Singh C.M. (1973). Hyponatraemia and sick cells. *Br. J. Anaesth*; **45**: 976–94.

Forrest J.N., Cox M., Hong C., Morrison G., Bia M., Singer I. (1978). Superiority of demeclocycline over lithium in the treatment of chronic syndrome of inappropriate secretion of antidiuretic hormone. *N. Engl. J. Med*; **298**: 173–7.

Friedland G.W., Axman M., Russi M.F., Fair W.R. (1971). Renal back pressure atrophy with compromised renal function. *Radiology*: **98**: 359–60.

George J.M., Capen C.C., Phillips A.S. (1972). Biosynthesis of vasopressin *in vitro* and ultrastructure of a bronchogenic carcinoma: Patient with syndrome of inappropriate secretion of antidiuretic hormone. *J. Clin. Invest*; **51**: 141–8.

Helderman J.H., Vestal R.E., Rowe J.W., Tobin J.D., Reubin A., Robertson G.L. (1978). The response of arginine vasopressin to intravenous ethanol and hypertonic saline in man: The impact of aging. *J. Geront*; **33**: 39–47.

Hockaday T.D.R. (1972). Diabetes insipidus. *Br. Med. J*; **2**: 210–3.

Leaf A., Bartter F.C., Santos R.F., Wrong O. (1952). Evidence in man that urinary electrolyte loss induced by pitressin is a function of water retention. *J. Clin. Invest*; **32**: 868–78.

Maffly R.H. (1977). Diabetes insipidus. In *Disturbances in Body Fluid Osmolality* (Andreoli T.E., Grantham J.J., Rector F.C. Jr., eds.) pp. 285–307. Bethesda: American Physiological Society.

Miller M., Dalakos T., Moses A.M., Fellerman H., Streeten D.H.P. (1970). Recognition of partial defects in antidiuretic hormone secretion. *Ann. Int. Med*; **73**: 721–9.

Milles J.J., Baylis P.H. (1981). Suppression of vasopressin release by hypertonic glucose infusion. *Clin. Sci*; **61**: 24–5p.

Morton J.J., Kelly P., Padfield P.L. (1978). Antidiuretic hormone in bronchogenic carcinoma. *Clin. Endocrinol. (Oxf)*; **9**: 357–70.

Moses A.M., Miller M. (1971). Osmotic threshold for vasopressin release as determined by hypertonic saline infusion and by dehydration. *Neuroendocrinology*; **7**: 219–26.

Moses A.M., Streeten D.H.P. (1967). Differentiation of polyuric states by measurement of responses to changes in plasma osmolality induced by hypertonic saline infusions. *Am. J. Med*; **42**: 368–77.

Murase T., Yoshida S. (1973). Mechanism of chlorpropamide action in patients with diabetes insipidus. *J. Clin. Endocrinol. Metab*; **36**: 174–7.

Nicola G.-C., Tonnarelli G.P., Griner A.C. (1980). Complications of transphenoidal surgery in pituitary adenomas. In *Pituitary Adenomas: Biology, Physiopathology and Treatment* (Bricaire H., Guiot G., Racadot J., ed.) pp. 237–40. France: Asclepios Publishers.

Price J.D.E., Lauener R.W. (1966). Serum and urine osmolalities in the differential diagnosis of polyuric states. *J. Clin. Endocrinol. Metab*; **26**: 143–8.

Rector F.C. Jr. (1977). Renal concentrating mechanisms. In *Disturbances in Body Fluid Osmolality* (Andreoli T.E., Grantham J.J., Rector F.C. Jr., ed.) pp. 179–96. Bethesda: American Physiological Society.

Rees L.H., Ratcliffe J.G. (1974). Ectopic hormone production by non-endocrine tumours. *Clin. Endocrinol. (Oxf)*; **3**: 263–99.

Robertson G.L. (1979). Physiopathology of ADH secretion. In *Clinical Neuroendocrinology* (Tolis G., Labrie F., Martin J.B., Naftolin F., ed.). pp. 247–60. New York: Raven Press.

Robertson G.L., Athar S. (1976). The interaction of blood osmolality and blood volume in regulating plasma vasopressin in man. *J. Clin. Endocrinol. Metab*; **42**: 613–20.

Robertson G.L., Shelton R.L., Athar S. (1976). The osmoregulation of vasopressin. *Kidney International*; **10**: 25–37.

Robertson G.L., Athar S., Shelton R.L., (1977). Osmotic control of vasopressin function. In *Disturbances of Body Fluid Osmolality* (Andreoli T.E., Grantham J.J., Rector F.C. Jr., ed.) pp. 125–48. Bethesda: American Physiological Society.

Scheiner E. (1975). The relationship of antidiuretic hormone to the control of volume and tonicity in the human. *Adv. Clin. Chem*; **17**: 1–52.

Schwartz W.B., Bennett W., Curelop S., Bartter F.C. (1957). A syndrome of renal sodium loss and hyponatraemia resulting from inappropriate secretion of antidiuretic hormone. *Am. J. Med*; **23**: 529–42.

Tanay A., Yust I., Peresecenschi G., Ambramov A.L., Aviram A. (1979). Long term treatment of the syndrome of inappropriate antidiuretic hormone secretion with phenyltoin. *Ann. Int. Med*; **90**: 50–2.

Thomas W.C. Jr. (1957). Diabetes insipidus. *J. Clin. Endocrinol. Metab*; **17**: 565–82.

Tyrrell J.B., Brooks R.M., Fitzgerald P.A., Cofoid P.B., Forsham P.H., Wilson C.B. (1978). Cushing's disease: Selective trans-sphenoidal resection of pituitary microadenomas. *N. Engl. J. Med*; **298**: 753–8.

Vavra I., Machova A., Holecek V., Cort J.H., Zaoral M., Sorm F. (1968). Effect of a synthetic analogue of vasopressin in animals and in patients with diabetes insipidus. *Lancet*; **1**: 948–52.

Verney E.B. (1947). The antidiuretic hormone and the factors which determine its release. *Proc. Roy. Soc. Lond. Series B*; **135**: 25–105.

Weller C.G., Elliott W., Gusman A.R. (1950). Hereditary diabetes insipidus: Unusual urinary tract changes. *J. Urol*; **64**: 716–21.

Winkler A.W., Crankshaw O.F. (1938). Chloride depletion in conditions other than Addison's disease. *J. Clin. Invest*; **17**: 1–6.

Zerbe R.L., Robertson G.L. (1981). A comparison of plasma vasopressin measurements with a standard indirect test in the differential diagnosis of polyuria. *N. Engl. J. Med*; **305**: 1539–46.

Zerbe R., Stropes L., Robertson G.L. (1980). Vasopressin function in the syndrome of inappropirate antidiuresis. *Ann. Rev. Med*; **31**: 315–27.

Chapter 10

Michael C. White

The Ectopic ACTH Syndrome

INTRODUCTION

The term ectopic ACTH syndrome is used in this context to refer to the clinical and metabolic features that are observed following the production of ACTH and related peptides by tumourous tissue, other than from an anterior pituitary corticotrophinoma (Meador *et al.*, 1962). It accounts for about 15% of all cases of Cushing's syndrome (Gold, 1979), and remains the most common and best documented of all the ectopic humoral syndromes.

While it was not until 1961 that a causal association between a malignant tumour and adrenocortical hyperfunction was clearly established (Christy, 1961), the earlier literature contained several reports of non-pituitary tumours associated with either the clinical, biochemical or pathological features of Cushing's syndrome. The first case, reported in 1896, was a thymic tumour (Gabcke, 1931), and the second in 1928 a probable bronchial carcinoid (Brown, 1928). Since then many different tumours have been firmly implicated in the aetiology of the syndrome. These are listed in order of frequency in Table 10.1. Approximately 50% of tumours responsible are small (oat) cell carcinomas of the bronchus (Liddle *et al.*, 1969; Imura, 1980). Benign and malignant carcinoids of the bronchus and thymus, islet cell tumours of the pancreas, medullary carcinomas of the thyroid, and phaeochromocytomas (functioning and non-functioning) make up most of the remainder, with all other tumours being exceedingly rare.

PATHOGENESIS

While there has been a considerable advance in our knowledge of the detailed histological and electron microscopic characteristics of tumours associated with the syndrome, their pathogenesis remains uncertain. The majority of tumours are found in tissue derived from the embryological foregut, where a number of cells with a probable local endocrine (paracrine) function are known to exist. Such cells have been found throughout the lungs (Bensch *et al.*, 1965), and are histologically similar to the Kultschitzky

TABLE 10.1
Tumours Associated with the Ectopic ACTH syndrome

Common	Small (oat) cell carcinoma of lung
Less common	Carcinoid tumour of lung
	Carcinoid tumour of thymus
	Islet cell tumour of pancreas
	Medullary carcinoma of thyroid
	Phaeochromocytoma and tumours of paraganglion system
Rare	Gastric and oesophageal carcinoids[a]
	Hepatic and gall bladder carcinoids[b]
	Appendiceal and ileal carcinoids[c]
	Ovarian tumours[d]
	Adenocarcinoma of lung, breast, colon and prostate[e]
	Nephroblastoma[f]
	Uterine carcinoid[g]
	Acute myeloid leukaemia[h]
	Malignant melanoma[i]
	Mixed salivary gland tumour[j]

N.B. References for the tumours comprising the common and less common groups are included in the text.
[a]Imura *et al.*, 1975; Hirata *et al.*, 1976*b*; Heitz *et al.*, 1981. [b]Spence and Burns-Cox, 1975; Himsworth *et al.*, 1977; Fuentes and Remis, 1979; Pullan *et al.*, 1980*b*. [c]O'Neal *et al.*, 1968; Gabrilove *et al.*, 1969; Johnson and Waisman, 1971; Davies *et al.*, 1982. [d]Parsons and Rigby, 1958; Nichols *et al.*, 1962; Brown and Lane, 1965. [e]Sachs *et al.*, 1970; Balsam *et al.*, 1972; Newmark *et al.*, 1973; Levern *et al.*, 1975; Suda *et al.*, 1977; Wenk *et al.*, 1977; Molland, 1978; Woodard *et al.*, 1981; Myers *et al.*, 1982. [f]Hashimoto *et al.*, 1980. [g]Lojek *et al.*, 1980. [h]Pfueger *et al.*, 1981. [i]Carey *et al.*, 1973. [j]Marks *et al.*, 1975.

cells of the gastrointestinal tract which relate to carcinoid tumours of the small bowel (Masson, 1924). Bronchial carcinoid tumours closely resemble the Kultschitzky cells found in the lungs, and small cell carcinomas also share several histological features including the presence of secretory granules and pseudopod cytoplasmic processes (Bensch *et al.*, 1968). Since ectopic ACTH-secreting thymic and thyroid tumours also share similar histological appearances (Gonzalez-Licea *et al.*, 1968; Salyer *et al.*, 1976), it has been proposed that all the above tumours belong to the carcinoid family, bronchial carcinoids representing the most benign and small cell carcinomas the most malignant end of the histological spectrum (Rosai *et al.*, 1976).

On the basis of certain cytochemical characteristics (amine precursor uptake and decarboxylation (APUD)), Pearse and Polak (1971) suggested that endocrine cells of the foregut, and probably also the mid- and hind-gut, had a common embryological origin from cells of the neuroectoderm. Since these cells were derived from a multipotential endocrine precursor, the production of any polypeptide hormone secreted ectopically following tumour development could thus be explained. This is an attractive hypothesis, but a number of other studies seem to show that at least some cells of the gastrointestinal tract and pancreas are derived from the endoderm (Pictet *et al.*, 1976; Larsson, 1981). A similar origin has been proposed for bronchial carcinoids and oat cell carcinomas of the lung (Sidhu, 1979). It thus seems unlikely that tumour production of ACTH can be explained on the basis of a single class of embryologically derived endocrine cells. Furthermore, the list of tumours associated with the ectopic ACTH syndrome has been considerably extended and cell types of differing embryological origins have been clearly documented including acute myeloid leukaemic cells and adenocarcinomas of the breast, lung, prostate and colon. An alternative explanation to the APUD concept is that all cells are pluripotential and may undergo divergent differentiation where random gene sequences may be expressed and result in the production of many cell products, including peptide hormones (Stevens and Moore, 1983).

Although this hypothesis is also attractive, it is perhaps surprising that ectopic hormone production is not more commonly associated with malignancy, and the fact remains that most ACTH secreting tumours are still situated within foregut derived tissues. Perhaps the frequency of their location in this area, and their histological similarities, reflect an origin from cells, which despite differing embryological backgrounds, have a common function to manufacture ACTH or related peptides with a local paracrine role in health or disease. The recent recognition of ACTH-LI within normal antropyloric cells provides evidence for such a possibility (Larsson, 1981), as may the same finding in the *normal* lung tissue of patients with lung tumours (Gerwitz and Yalow, 1974). In this circumstance, ACTH production may represent a physiological response to disease by cells with the capacity to manufacture the peptide, but which do not so in normal health; or only in concentrations so low that the peptide cannot be detected by current conventional techniques. ACTH-LI production from foregut tumours may therefore merely represent an inappropriate amplification of these mechanisms.

HISTOLOGY

Primary Tumour

As has been indicated in the preceding section, the majority of tumours share features suggestive of carcinoid tumours, but some of the rarer neoplasms, including adenocarcinoma of the breast, lung and colon, show the features of their primary cell type, with the additional ultrastructural finding on electron microscopy of the presence of neurosecretory granules.

Adrenal Glands

In contrast to the glands of patients with pituitary-dependent Cushing's disease, where each gland weight does not usually exceed 6–12 g (normal 4 g), there is marked adrenal hyperplasia in subjects with the ectopic ACTH syndrome, and the glands normally average between 14–16 g each (Neville and Mackay, 1972), not uncommonly exceeding 20–30 g (Singer *et al.*, 1977). The cortex of the glands is brown to the cut surface, indicating a considerable decrease in the lipid content, and this can be confirmed histologically. Hyperplasia affects cells in both the zona fasciculata and reticularis, often extending up to the fibrous capsule of the gland, leaving the unaffected zona glomerulosa cells as small islands in their midst.

Metastatic deposits from the primary tumour are frequently seen within the adrenals, especially from small cell carcinomas of the bronchus.

CLINICAL FEATURES

General Considerations

Almost all patients with evidence of the ectopic ACTH syndrome have a severe hypokalaemic alkalosis at the time of presentation ($K^+ < 3\cdot0$ mmol/litre; $HCO_3^- > 30$ mmol/litre), and hyperglycaemia or a diabetic glucose tolerance is common. Other features of Cushing's syndrome are very variable, or may be completely absent. Certain features are, however, characteristic of different tumour types and their anatomical location.

Small (Oat) Cell Carcinomas

These tumours account for approximately 25–33% of all bronchogenic carcinomas (Bensch *et al.*, 1968), and for about 50% of reported cases of the ectopic ACTH syndrome (Liddle *et al.*, 1969; Imura, 1980). All tumours thus studied contain abnormally elevated levels of immunoreactive or bioactive ACTH (Bloomfield *et al.*, 1977) and at post-mortem all cases demonstrate bilateral adrenal hyperplasia (Singer *et al.*, 1977). Paradoxically only a small percentage (2.8–7.2%) (Singer *et al.*, 1977; Kato *et al.*, 1969) are associated with the clinical or biochemical features of ACTH hypersecretion in life, and this has been ascribed to the rapidly progressive nature of the primary tumour. Affected patients are predominantly male, and over 50 years of age, although younger patients in their twenties have been reported (Kovach and Kyle, 1958). The typical habitus of Cushing's syndrome is almost always absent (Imura *et al.*, 1975). However, individual features such as pigmentation, myopathy and oedema may be present at the time of diagnosis or pre-terminally when there is evidence of widespread malignancy in about 30–50%. Hypertension may also occur, but just as often the blood pressure recording is normal or even low. Similarly, weight loss rather than weight gain may predominate.

The characteristic feature of adrenocortical hyperfunction in these patients is a metabolic alkalosis, noted at presentation or developing during the course of the disease. Abnormal glucose tolerance occurs in only one-third (Imura *et al.*, 1975). While the length of history is characteristically short, measurable in days or weeks, there are patients who have clinical evidence of Cushing's syndrome extending over as long as 12 months (Prunty *et al.*, 1963).

Until recently, the finding of adrenocortical hyperfunction was of academic rather than practical interest, since the prognosis of the primary disease was so poor. However, modern advances in chemotherapy are now extending the lifespan of this group of patients, so that recognition and control of the metabolic manifestations, with an associated increased risk of morbidity and mortality, may become more relevant.

Bronchial Carcinoid Tumours

After small cell carcinomas of the lung, benign and malignant carcinoids of the bronchus together account for the largest group of tumours responsible for the syndrome. Overall they account for the largest percentage of tumours in the third decade of life, are also common in the fourth decade, and are more frequent in males during these periods. Interestingly, in the sixth and seventh decades, bronchial carcinoids are more frequently found in women (Fig. 10.1). In about half of the tumours, the onset of illness is insidious and extends over 9–12 months, and while the clinical features of Cushing's syndrome may be incomplete even when the history extends over 5 years (Morse *et al.*, 1967), a classical cushingoid habitus is generally the rule at presentation (Mason *et al.*, 1972). Major neuropsychiatric manifestations including frank psychotic behaviour are extremely common, occurring in over 50% of patients, and significant hypertension (diastolic pressure $> 100\,\mathrm{mmHg}$) is found in a similar proportion. Pigmentation is a less constant clinical sign, present in about 25% of cases (Mason *et al.*, 1972). Severe hypokalaemia ($K^+ < 2\cdot0\,\mathrm{mmol/litre}$) is a common metabolic finding. These tumours are one of the most difficult of all ectopic tumours to locate by any investigative technique.

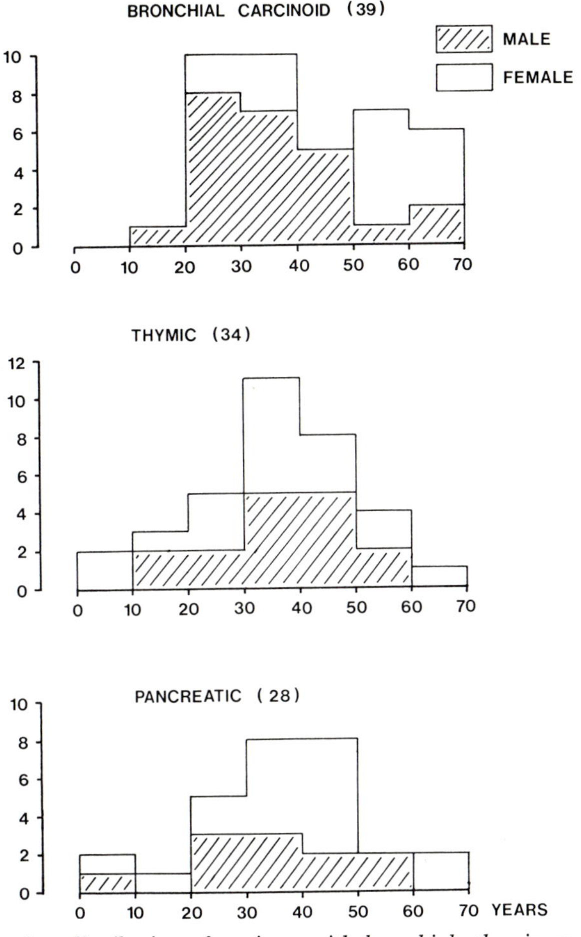

Fig. 10.1. *Sex distribution of patients with bronchial, thymic or pancreatic tumours associated with ectopic ACTH secretion, at age of presentation.*

Thymic Tumours

Excluding small cell carcinomas of the bronchus, these account for approximately one-fifth of all cases and are found equally in both sexes, being most common in the fourth decade of life (Fig. 10.1). They are one of the commoner tumours associated with cyclical Cushing's syndrome, and this may result in some confusion in the differential diagnosis from a pituitary corticotrophinoma. As with bronchial carcinoids, the time-course of symptomatology often exceeds 6–9 months, and the full clinical manifestations of Cushing's syndrome are usually apparent. Neuropsychiatric symptoms are not frequent, but significant hypertension is (diastolic pressure > 100 mmHg). Rarely, Cushing's syndrome may present some years after the removal of a primary thymic tumour, and is probably due to the ACTH activity contained within the developing metastases (Harris and El-Katib, 1968).

In view of the mediastinal location of these tumours, symptoms of superior venal caval obstruction have been reported (Scholz and Bahn, 1959), but this is rare, and in contrast to carcinoid tumours of the thymus not associated with the ectopic ACTH secretion (Rosai *et al.*, 1976; Wick *et al.*, 1980). Presumably the difference relates to the hormonal overactivity in the former which brings the patient to the attention of his physician at an earlier stage.

Early recognition of this source of ectopic ACTH is important since complete cure may follow surgical removal when there is no evidence of local or distant metastatic spread. However, the present mortality in this group at ten-year follow-up is 65% (Wick *et al.*, 1980). It is worth commenting that thymic carcinoids are also found in patients with the MEA I syndrome when they are exclusively confined to males and never associated with ectopic ACTH production (Wick *et al.*, 1980). In general, thymic carcinoids have a markedly different histology from conventional epithelial thymomas and are never associated with myasthenia gravis or red cell hypoplasia.

Pancreatic Tumours

There is a slight predominance of women over men, with the peak age of incidence occurring between 30–50 years (Fig. 10.1).

The classical features of Cushing's syndrome are often present in this group, even when the history is very short (three months); but just as with other causes of the syndrome, this is by no means a consistent feature, and the isolated development of pigmentation, hirsutism or weight gain may be the only signs of the underlying disorder. In general, the history is short (1–6 months), but may be as long as two years. Unfortunately, in many cases there is already evidence of widespread metastatic disease at the time of presentation. Some tumours are also associated with hormonal syndromes in addition to that of ACTH. In 1965, Geokas and colleagues (1965) described a patient with the classical features of the Zollinger-Ellison syndrome which was caused by an operable islet cell carcinoma. Five years later the patient presented with symptoms of excessive ACTH secretion including thirst, polyuria and severe hypokalaemic alkalosis. At post-mortem two months later there was evidence of widespread metastatic spread. Whether ACTH was present in the primary tumour was not established, but it seems likely that it became the predominant peptide secreted from the metastases and responsible for the symptoms at the time of death. Apart from gastrin (Kyriakides *et al.*, 1979; Belchetz *et al.*, 1973), insulin hypersecretion has also been found concomitantly with ACTH (Balls *et al.*, 1959; Marks *et al.*, 1965). Normo- rather than hyperglycaemia is the rule and clue to diagnosis in such cases. Subsequent treatment of the hypercortisolism, without regard for the hyperinsulinism, may result in intractable hypoglycaemia.

Phaeochromocytoma

Adrenocorticotrophic hormone secretion is also found in association with tumours of the adrenal medulla and very rarely the extra adrenal paraganglion system (Apple and Kreines, 1982). Nearly all affected subjects have been women, usually between the age of 40 to 60 years (Forman *et al.*, 1979). The adrenal tumours are unilateral and benign, although histological evidence of local invasion into the adrenal vein and vena cava has been observed (Schteingart *et al.*, 1972) and metastatic spread was suspected from a nasal paraganglioma (Apple and Kreines, 1982). In a number of cases the clinical features of Cushing's syndrome have been few or of short (<6 months) duration only, with neuropsychiatric symptoms often being the most prominent. Hypertension is also common but not invariable. Whilst most tumours are associated with excessive catecholamine secretion, in some cases, concentrations have been normal or low (Schteingart *et al.*, 1972; Drury *et al.*, 1982).

In at least two reports, the clinical symptoms of a phaeochromocytoma preceded those of Cushing's syndrome by several years (Davies *et al.*, 1982; Bourgoignie *et al*, 1964). This latter feature is of some considerable clinical significance, since failure to recognise the Cushing's component of the tumour may result in fatal adrenocortical insufficiency after an adrenalectomy. This is due to suppression of normal hypothalamo–pituitary ACTH by ectopically driven adrenal corticosteroids. All ACTH-secreting tumours of the adrenal medulla have been associated with a significant hypokalaemic alkalosis, a feature which is not normally present with a conventional phaeochromocytoma alone. This finding should therefore alert the physician to the possibility of the additional ACTH hypersecretion.

Other Causes of the Ectopic ACTH Syndrome

Of the other tumours, medullary carcinomas of the thyroid form the largest single group responsible for the syndrome. Of 18 cases collected by this author, 12 were female and the majority of cases presented in the fourth and fifth decades of life. The classical features of Cushing's syndrome are usually evident but may not develop until several years after the original thyroid diagnosis (Williams *et al.*, 1968; Keusch *et al.*, 1977). Increased secretion of calcitonin is commonly present together with the ACTH (Melvin *et al.*, 1970).

With most other causes, the development of Cushing's syndrome is usually rapid over a few months or weeks, and there are no specific distinguishing features of note. One rare tumour association, however, merits comment in this respect. Ectopic ACTH secreting prostatic tumours are associated with marked hypernatraemia and hyperchloraemia, together with an hypokalaemic alkalosis (Wenk *et al.*, 1977; Molland, 1978). The reason for this unusual biochemical feature is unclear, but appears to be specific. Lastly, it should be made clear that the secretion of ectopic ACTH from ovarian tumours, previously regarded as a common cause of the syndrome, is very rare.

THE PRODUCTION OF ECTOPIC ACTH AND RELATED PEPTIDES

From the foregoing paragraphs it must be evident that the clinical and metabolic manifestations of the ectopic ACTH syndrome are quite varied. On the one hand there are patients who have neither clinical nor metabolic manifestations of the disorder, and whose only feature is adrenal hyperplasia at post-mortem, while others have an hypokalaemic alkalosis, with or without the other clinical features of Cushing's syndrome. The rapidity of onset of ACTH hypersecretion may explain the lack of clinical features in many patients, but does not account for all, and other factors may be relevant. An understanding of the basic biochemistry and physiology of ACTH secretion is essential if the different clinical and metabolic manifestations are to be explained.

Human ACTH is a 39 amino acid peptide of which the first 24 amino acids are common to all species, and are essential for biological activity. Originally isolated as a separate peptide from anterior pituitary extracts, it is now known that ACTH is derived from a large precursor molecule termed pro-opiocortin (POC) and which in the mouse tumour model has a molecular weight of 31 000 (31K) (Mains *et al.*, 1977) (Fig. 10.2). In addition to

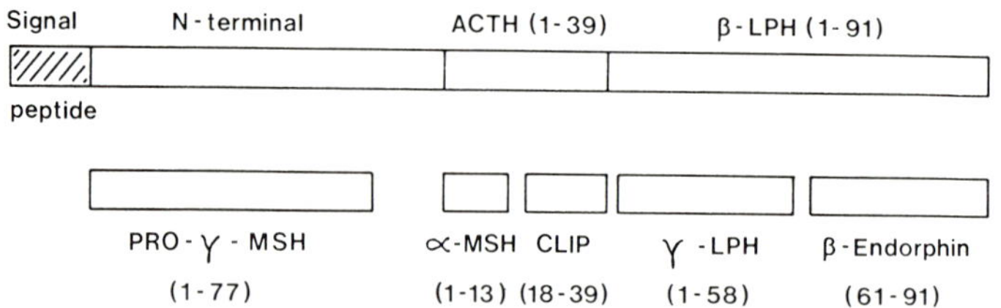

Fig. 10.2. *Proposed structure of pro-opiocortin showing the relationship between the N-terminal, ACTH, β-LPH and constituent peptides (after Nakanishi et al., 1979).*

ACTH, which occupies the central core of the molecule, POC gives rise to a large N (amino) terminal fragment. This contains a putative 12 amino acid peptide with homologous sequences to the melanotropic region of ACTH (ACTH 6–9), and β-LPH (50–53) and has thus been termed γ-MSH (Nakanishi *et al.*, 1979). While there is as yet no definitive evidence that the peptide exists independently, a large 77 amino acid glycoprotein containing the γ-MSH sequence has been isolated in anterior pituitary tissue and termed pro-γ-MSH (Estivariz *et al.*, 1980). At its C (carboxy) terminal, POC gives rise to β-LPH which in its turn may be processed to γ-LPH (β-LPH 1–53) and β-endorphin (β-LPH 61–91). This latter peptide also contains the sequence of metencephalin (β-LPH 61–65). In some species, but not normally in man, ACTH may be further processed to yield α-MSH (ACTH 1–13), and corticotropin-like intermediate lobe peptide (CLIP; ACTH 18–39).

There is little evidence that the different peptide products of POC are manufactured by peripheral enzymic cleavage of precursor peptide (and it appears are due to a strictly limited processing of POC which takes place within the cell at the point of exocytosis) (Ratter *et al.*, 1983). Thus, rat anterior pituitary corticotrophs produce equimolar concentrations of ACTH and β-LPH, but little α-MSH, CLIP or β-endorphin, whilst intermediate lobe cells (present in man during fetal life and pregnancy only) preferentially secrete α-MSH, CLIP and endorphins with little ACTH or β-LPH (Estivariz *et al.*, 1981).

In normal individuals and patients with a pituitary dependent tumour secreting ACTH, chromatographic profiles of their plasma reveal a single peak of N-terminal 1–39 ACTH. In patients with ectopic ACTH secretion a second and much larger (22K) peak may be found in addition (Ratter *et al.*, 1980). In some cases this may be the only form of ACTH present in the circulation. The existence of this larger molecular weight ACTH first recognised by Yalow and Berson (1971), and subsequently confirmed by other investigators, was found to have only 4% of the biological activity of normal 1–39 ACTH. However, after trypsinisation it released a molecule with the full steroidogenic activity of 1–39 ACTH (Yalow and Berson, 1973).

The preferential release of 'big' ACTH over 1–39 ACTH probably accounts for the relative lack of the classical features of Cushing's syndrome in many patients with ectopic ACTH secretion. Conversely, this or other fragments of POC not normally released into the circulation in patients with pituitary corticotrophinomas may account for those features which are more specific to the 'ectopic' group. Early observations in patients with small cell carcinomas indicated that their plasma contained an adrenal weight maintaining factor but which was devoid of steroidogenic activity (Nichols and Gourley, 1963). It seems probable that this factor is responsible for the marked adrenal hyperplasia of ectopically driven adrenal glands, though whether it is '22K' ACTH, currently remains unknown. In addition, it is likely the plasma of patients with the ectopic ACTH syndrome contains a POC-derived peptide which is responsible for the increased levels of desoxycorticosterone and corticosterone seen in this group, and believed to be the steriods predominantly responsible for the typical hypokalaemic alkalosis (Schambelan *et al.*, 1971). A potential candidate peptide might be pro-γ-MSH which in the rat model has no direct action on adrenal steroidogenesis alone, but is capable of potentiating the effects of 1–24 or 1–39 ACTH on corticosterone and to a lesser extent, aldosterone secretion, (Pedersen and Brownie, 1980; Al-Dujaili *et al.*, 1981). The excessive production of β-endorphin and metencephalins that has been found in both plasma and tumour extracts of a number of patients with the ectopic ACTH syndrome (Kleber *et al.*, 1980; Pullan *et al.*, 1980*a*; Pullan *et al.*, 1980*b*; Suda *et al.*, 1982) may account for the frequency of neuropsychiatric symptoms observed in this disorder.

It would thus appear that the intracellular enzymic cleavage of POC into its constituent peptides is quite varied in ectopic ACTH-secreting tumours. This process, and the subsequent bioactivity of the peptides produced, probably determines the specific clinical and metabolic features of any individual patient within the wide spectrum of the syndrome.

INVESTIGATION OF THE SYNDROME

General Consideration (Fig. 10.3)

Whatever the underlying aetiology, in an ill patient with Cushing's syndrome, the most immediate priority may be to alleviate life-threatening complications associated with the condition before an accurate diagnosis can be confirmed. However, since the management, and indeed the necessity for detailed investigation may be quite different in patients with an adrenocortical carcinoma or adenoma compared with those who have an ACTH-dependent cause, it is valuable to distinguish between the two at an early stage. Adrenocorticotrophic hormone measurements are clearly essential, but results may take some days or weeks to be processed. Measurements of cortisol and metabolites following dexamethasone or metyrapone are also time-consuming, and dependent on patient cooperation, a factor which may not be readily forthcoming if psychiatric symptoms predominate the clinical presentation.

Initial investigations should always include chest radiography, since this may demonstrate an obvious carcinoma or anterior mediastinal lesion, and an abdominal film, which may show calcification present in an adrenocortical carcinoma. The most useful investigation is, however, computerised tomography (CT) to delineate the adrenal glands. This radiological

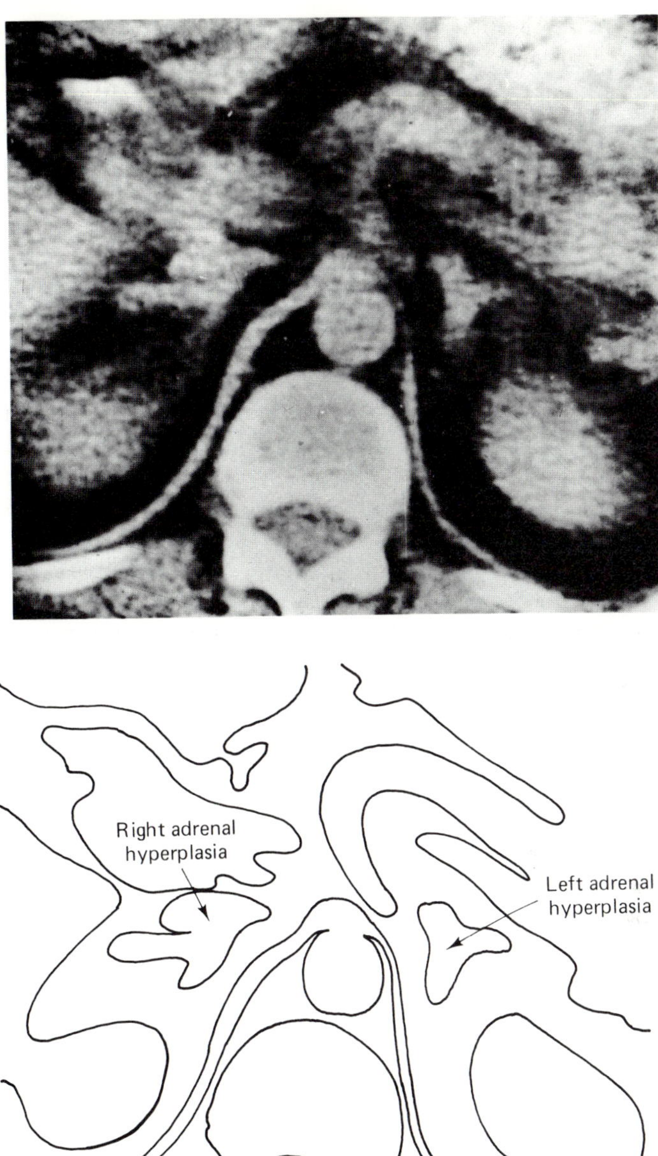

Fig. 10.3. *Bilateral adrenal hyperplasia in a patient with ectopic ACTH syndrome : CT scan through the adrenals shows diffuse enlargement of the glands whilst maintaining their normal shape. (Figure reproduced by courtesy of Dr F.E. White.)*

technique is a rapid and non-invasive means of visualising the normal or diseased adrenal in a severely ill patient (White *et al.*, 1982).

Computerised tomography seems able to detect 100% of adrenal tumours causing Cushing's syndrome, as they are usually 2 cm or more in diameter and clearly outlined by the increased retroperitoneal fat seen in most patients. In the absence of an adrenal mass on CT, a primary adenoma or carcinoma can be reliably excluded. The contralateral gland to a primary cortical tumour is not enlarged; indeed if the gland opposite an adrenal mass appears hyperplastic the possibility of nodular hyperplasia, an adrenal metastasis or even a primary adrenal ACTH-secreting tumour should be considered.

A useful pointer to the diagnosis of an ectopic ACTH-secreting tumour is the presence on CT of marked bilateral adrenal enlargement evident in over two-thirds of such cases, but not usually observed in pituitary-dependent Cushing's disease. This finding is not of course diagnostic but fits with the known pathological difference in adrenal gland size between the two conditions. It should be stressed, however, that treatment of patients with pituitary-dependent tumours using adrenal 11-β-hydroxylase inhibitors such as metyrapone, promote further adrenal hyperplasia, which should also be considered when marked gland enlargement is seen on CT.

Differential Diagnosis of Ectopic from Pituitary ACTH Hypersecretion

An hypokalaemic alkalosis is the rule in the ectopic syndrome but much less common in pituitary-dependent disease. Likewise, urinary-free cortisol or other adrenal steroid metabolites may be markedly elevated in ectopic disease, sometimes in excess of 10–20 times the upper limits of the normal range, but rarely over-reach these levels in Cushing's disease. Further distinguishing biochemical features include plasma immunoreactive ACTH levels greater than 200 pg/ml in ectopic disease, and levels often below 100 pg/ml in pituitary cases (Besser and Landon, 1968). Plasma immuno-reactive ACTH: β-LPH ratios are reversed in the two conditions, with higher levels of β-LPH than ACTH in the ectopic group (Gilkes *et al.*, 1977) who also demonstrate excess measurable levels in plasma and tissue of C-over N-terminal ACTH (Ratcliffe *et al.*, 1972). This latter finding is especially common when a bronchial carcinoid is the responsible tumour (Ratcliffe *et al.*, 1973).

Dynamic function tests include the use of dexamethasone (DXM) suppression and metyrapone stimulation of adrenal steroids. In a review of 100 patients with Cushing's syndrome, Liddle and colleagues found a reproducible 40% decrease in urinary 17-hydroxycorticosteroids levels in 98% of patients with a pituitary source of ACTH but in only 6% of those with an ectopic tumour (Liddle *et al.*, 1969). The minority of cases with

DXM suppression occurred in patients with bronchial or thymic carcinoids (O'Neal *et al.*, 1968; Mason *et al.*, 1972; Pfohl and Doe, 1963; Miura *et al.*, 1967; Nichols *et al.*, 1968; Strott *et al.*, 1968; Jones *et al.*, 1969; Horai *et al.*, 1973; Aron *et al.*, 1981). In some cases these results are not surprising since basal steroid values were within or only just exceeded, the upper limits of the normal range (O'Neal *et al.*, 1968; Miura *et al.*, 1967), and suppression of the hypothalamo–pituitary–adrenal axis as a result of ectopic ACTH secretion may not yet have taken place. In other cases a cyclical pattern of hormone was definite (Thorner *et al.*, 1982) and the observed fall in steroids was probably coincidental with the administration of DXM.

In those pituitary-dependent cases with an absence of DXM suppression, there is usually evidence of nodular adrenal hyperplasia (Aron *et al.*, 1981). However, an unusual pituitary corticotrophinoma with a plasma ACTH pattern chromatographically identical to other ectopic tumours has recently been described, and noted not to be suppressible with DXM (Ratter *et al.*, 1983).

Metyrapone administration has resulted in an increase in cortisol precursors typical of a pituitary tumour, but this is not usually associated with a positive DXM suppression test. There are, however, at least two cases in the literature where the adrenal hormone pattern following DXM and metyrapone has mimicked that of pituitary-dependent disease (Pfohl and Doe, 1963; Aron *et al.*, 1981). Thus, while both the high dose DXM and metyrapone tests are a helpful indicator in the differential diagnosis of ACTH hypersecretion, the results taken either alone or together cannot be regarded as diagnostic.

Localisation of Ectopic Tumours
(Table 10.2, Figs. 10.4 and 10.5)

Apart from its value in the preliminary differential diagnosis of Cushing's syndrome, CT would appear to be more accurate in the location of a primary ectopic source than any other radiological technique. It is particularly helpful in detecting small ($<1\cdot5$ cm) peripheral lung carcinoid tumours

TABLE 10.2

Localisation of Tumour

Clinical examination
Chest and mediastinal x-ray
Computerised tomography scan of abdomen, thorax (including mediastinum and
    neck)
Thyroid scan
Selective venous catheterisation with simultaneous peripheral sampling for
    ACTH

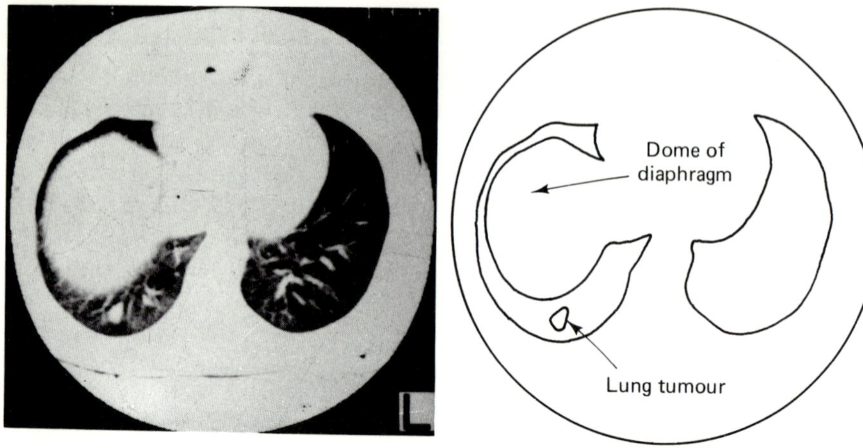

Fig. 10.4. *Computerised tomography scan through the lung bases shows a small nodule in the right costophrenic recess. At surgery this was a 4 mm bronchial carcinoid tumour, with microscopic deposits also present in the regional lymph nodes. All previous radiological investigations, including venous sampling, were negative. (Figure reproduced by courtesy of Dr F.E. White.)*

which may otherwise be undetectable, and is also valuable in identifying anterior mediastinal (thymic) lesions, pancreatic and liver tumours, including metastases. However, despite its superiority, in a recently published series the primary sites of only 5 out of 12 histologically confirmed ectopic tumours were demonstrable (White *et al.*, 1982). Further, while CT may clearly define an abnormal mass, it cannot determine whether this is responsible for ectopic hormone production. Finally, in those cases where no lesion is demonstrable, the suspicion will remain that the source of ACTH hypersecretion is in fact pituitary.

Selective venous catheterisation with simultaneous central and peripheral sampling for ACTH is a useful adjunctive investigation to CT in these circumstances, and especially in confirming the diagnosis of a pituitary dependent source. In two recently published series, 5 out of 6 and 9 out of 10 patients with a pituitary origin of ACTH hypersecretion were correctly diagnosed from the high levels of peptide found in the inferior petrosal sinus or jugular veins (Drury *et al.*, 1982; Findling *et al.*, 1981). Simultaneous peripheral sampling is essential since the secretion of ACTH may be episodic from both pituitary and ectopic tumours. With regard to the specific location of ectopic tumour sites, selective venous sampling has been of no value in detecting bronchial carcinoids, pancreatic and small bowel tumours, but has been helpful in detecting some adrenal medullary and thymic sources.

In cases where CT scanning has been unhelpful, but when a medullary carcinoma of the thyroid is suspected or needs to be excluded, a radioisotopic scan of the thyroid may be useful in the identification of a cold area.

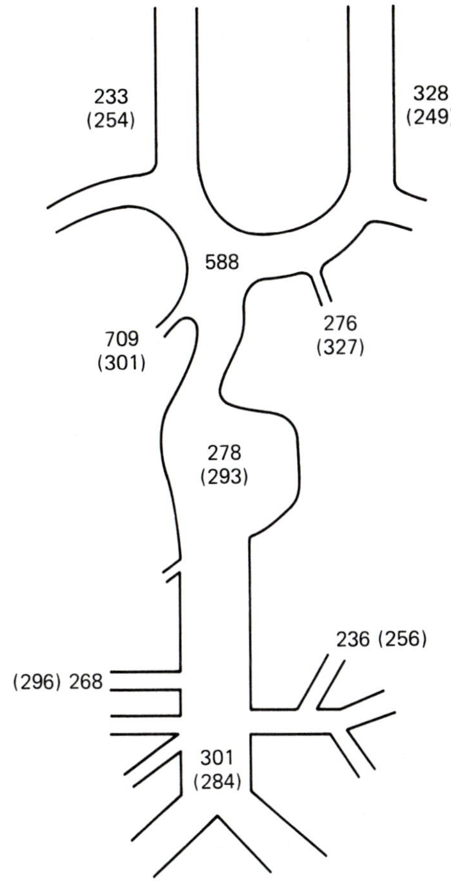

Fig. 10.5. *Immunoreactive ACTH levels during selective venous catheterisation procedure. High levels present in azygos vein. At surgery the patient was found to have an extensive thymic carcinoid tumour, with evidence of direct local spread to pericardium and involvement of lymph nodes. Figures within parentheses denote simultaneous peripheral venous sample.*

MANAGEMENT (Table 10.3)

Adrenal Blocking Drugs

The acute management of the ectopic ACTH syndrome may well include insulin to counteract the hyperglycaemia, and potassium replacement for the hypokalaemic alkalosis. Acute psychiatric symptoms can usually be managed with phenothiazine derivatives including thioridazine and chlorpromazine. Adrenal steroid blocking drugs include aminoglutethimide, which inhibits the conversion of adrenal cholesterol to pregnenolone; and

TABLE 10.3
Aims of Management

A. *Immediate*
   Control metabolic abnormalities, e.g. hypokalaemia,
     neuropsychiatric manifestations; others, i.e. diabetes
     mellitus, infection, etc.

B. *Intermediate*
   Control of hypercortisolism

C. *Definitive*
   Surgical removal of tumour
   Bilateral adrenalectomy
   Radiotherapy
   Chemotherapy

metyrapone, an 11-β-hydroxylase inhibitor preventing the conversion of deoxycortisol to cortisol. Both drugs are of value in the short- and long-term management of patients with the ectopic ACTH syndrome (Mason *et al.*, 1972; Miura *et al.*, 1967; Horai *et al.*, 1973; Steel *et al.*, 1967; Gordon *et al.*, 1968). This is particularly true for metyrapone which is often used in patients whose primary site of ectopic peptide secretion remains occult. It is necessary to give the drug every 4 hours because of its short half-life. The dose required has to be titrated against the urinary cortisol secretion of the affected patient, the aim being to maintain urinary cortisol levels within the normal range, or preferably to completely suppress adrenal cortisol secretion and replace the physiological requirements with DXM. The usual needs of metyrapone in the ectopic syndrome range between 250–750 mg four-hourly. Side-effects, predominantly of nausea and gastric irritation, are often present at the start of therapy, thus requiring a slow build-up of dosage, but are usually mild and disappear quickly. 2, 2-Bis (4-chlorophenyl, 2-chlorophenyl)-1, 1-dichloroethane (o,p'DDD), an adrenolytic agent, has been given in combination with metyrapone and/or aminoglutethimide with some success (Carey *et al.*, 1973; Apple and Kreines, 1982). However, it remains a drug with unpleasant and sometimes intolerable side-effects.

Surgery

Providing there is no evidence of metastatic spread from a tumour, surgical removal remains the prime aim of management as a permanent remission of symptoms can be expected. The subject has been recently reviewed (Davies *et al.*, 1982). Tumours which are readily amenable to this form of therapy include phaeochromocytomas, benign bronchial carcinoids (if they can be located) and solitary tumours of the gastrointestinal tract. Those tumours with a poorer prognosis include medullary carcinoma of the thyroid and islet cell tumours of the pancreas, usually because surgical removal of the tumour is incomplete or because metastatic spread has already occurred. Thymic carcinoid tumours have also been removed with complete success, but symptoms of the ectopic ACTH syndrome have still developed several years later from undetected metastases (*see* above). Carcinoma of the bronchus is usually so advanced at presentation that surgery cannot be contemplated. However, improvement and apparent cure have been reported in some cases (Liddle *et al.*, 1969; Sachs *et al.*, 1970; Ratcliffe *et al.*, 1972).

When extensive tumour growth or local metastatic spread makes primary surgical removal impracticable or dangerous, and palliative therapy is required, or the primary tumour remains occult, bilateral adrenalectomy is a valuable alternative to blocking drugs, resulting in cure of symptoms though not of the primary disease. However, in patients with widespread disease particularly that secondary to small cell carcinoma, it is doubtful if the quality of life can be sufficiently improved to justify the operation in many cases. Before any surgery is attempted, whether it be to remove the primary tumour or to perform a bilateral adrenalectomy, pre-operative medical therapy with aminoglutethimide or metyrapone should be instituted for 4–8 weeks if possible, to decrease the morbidity and mortality that are associated with surgery in a patient with active Cushing's syndrome (Scott *et al.*, 1977).

Very rarely, when patients are too ill for surgical adrenalectomy and unable to tolerate adrenal blocking or adrenolytic drugs, therapeutic infarction of the adrenals can be attempted under radiological control (Rosenstock *et al.*, 1981).

Radiotherapy

External radiotherapy directed at the tumour may be a useful adjunct to surgery both when complete resection of the tumour is impossible or if there is tumour recurrence at a later date.

Chemotherapy

The use of specific agents aimed at destroying malignant tumours which may be associated with the ectopic ACTH syndrome has been established for many years. The most important of these tumours is the small cell carcinoma of the lung. A number of drugs used singly and including cyclophosphamide, Methotrexate, vincristine and Adriamycin have all been reported to be of some value in this condition. However, the most effective regimens are those involving combination chemotherapy, with cyclophosphamide and vincristine together with either Methotrexate, or procarbazine and prednisone, or Adriamycin and bleomycin the most valuable (Weiss, 1978). In all cases, however, the long-term prognosis remains poor. Despite evidence for tumour regression, signs of the ectopic ACTH syndrome may develop whilst on chemotherapy, and this feature appears to coincide with a more aggressive phase of the tumour (Abeloff *et al.*, 1981).

If small cell carcinomas do reflect the most malignant end of the spectrum of carcinoid tumours, then the possibility of 5-fluorouracil and strepto-zotocin should be considered as chemotherapeutic agents since these agents are of value in the management of metastatic carcinoid disease (Moertel, 1975). Their use should perhaps also be considered for other malignant carcinoid tumours of foregut origin which are associated with ACTH secretion apart from primary pancreatic neoplasms.

OTHER CONSIDERATIONS OF THE ECTOPIC ACTH SYNDROME

Multiple Ectopic Hormone Production

Apart from the well known associations of calcitonin in medullary car-cinomas of the thyroid, and catecholamines in phaeochromocytomas, a number of other hormones have been found together with ectopic ACTH, and in at least one example both hormones were secreted from the same cell (Goltzman *et al.*, 1979). These other hormones (Himsworth *et al.*, 1977; O'Neal *et al.*, 1968; Suda *et al.*, 1977; Hashimoto *et al.*, 1980; Geokas *et al.*, 1965; Kyriakides *et al.*, 1979; Belchetz *et al.*, 1973; Balls *et al.*, 1959; Marks *et al.*, 1965; Upton and Amatruda, 1971; Rees *et al.*, 1974; Birkenhager *et al.*, 1976; Hirata *et al.*, 1976*a*; Coscia *et al.*, 1977; Baylin *et al.*, 1978; Hattori *et al.*, 1979; Krol and Wood, 1982) are listed in Table 10.4. It is likely that with regular screening, many more associations will be described, particularly from small cell carcinomas of the lung, in which other peptides such as bombesin and somatostatin have already been isolated (Wood *et al.*, 1981). The finding of corticotrophin releasing activity in some tumours is of special interest in Cushing's syndrome, since this presumed peptide may be acting to stimulate the pituitary corticotrophs at the same time as the ectopically driven adrenal corticosteroids are suppressing them. Clearly the secretion of both CRF and ACTH simultaneously may cause some diagnostic difficulty as to the likely aetiology of the Cushing's syndrome.

In Vitro Studies

Although *in vitro* cell culture systems have been widely employed to study hormonal release from endocrine cells, there are few reports which have examined ectopic ACTH release. Hirata and colleagues (1975, 1979) found that rat median eminence extract (SME) was a potent secretagogue of

TABLE 10.4
Ectopic ACTH-Secreting Tumours Associated with Other Hormones

Oat cell carcinoma of bronchus	Vasopressin
	Serotonin
	Corticotrophin-releasing factor (CRF)
	Calcitonin
	Prolactin
	Insulin
	HCG (α and β-subunits)
Bronchial carcinoids	Serotonin
Pancreatic islet cell tumours	Insulin
	Gastrin
	Glucagon
	Serotonin
	CRF
Medullary carcinoma of thyroid	Calcitonin
	CRF
	Prolactin-stimulating factor
Liver carcinoid	Calcitonin
	Bombesin
Phaeochromocytoma	Catecholamines
Ileal carcinoid	Serotonin
Nephroblastoma	CRF
Colonic carcinoma	CRF

ACTH release from five such tumours *in vitro*, and also elicited a rise in tissue levels of cyclic AMP. In contrast, Ratter and colleagues (1983) were unable to demonstrate a similar effect, and neither they nor Hirata showed any effect of vasopressin, a peptide with potent direct stimulatory activity on ACTH release from pituitary corticotrophinoma cells. Further studies by Hirata and colleagues (1979) have indicated that several amines and peptides including serotonin, TRH and nor-epinephrine, may be effective stimulators of ectopic ACTH release. This latter finding may be of some clinical relevance, since in patients with a mixed catecholamine and ACTH-secreting tumour, the former may have an important influence on the secretion of the latter.

Other recent *in vitro* data have been primarily concerned with factors which may inhibit ectopic ACTH release. Bromocriptine was ineffective in suppressing ectopic ACTH from a single tumour thus studied; while consistently inhibiting ACTH release from pituitary corticotrophinomas (Adams *et al.*, 1981). More recently, we have shown that DXM was unable to significantly suppress ACTH release from an ectopic bronchial carcinoid tumour at 1000 times the concentration needed to suppress ACTH release from a pituitary corticotrophinoma (Fig. 10.6). This difference between the two types of tumour to the direct feedback effect of corticosteroids may be one explanation for the rapid onset of clinical features in subjects with the

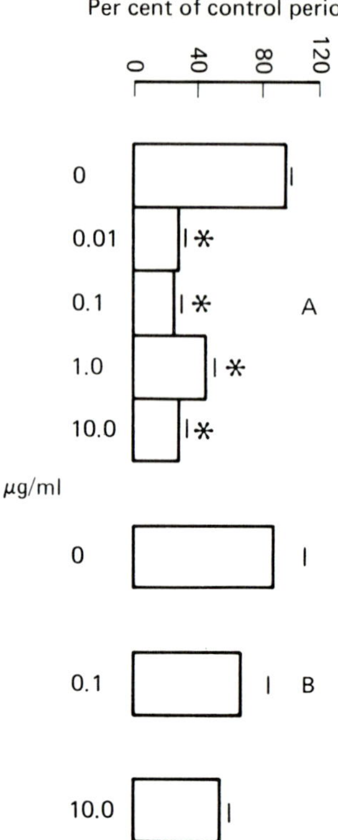

Fig. 10.6. *Effects of dexamethasone (µg/ml) on ACTH secretion from cells of human pituitary corticotrophinoma (A) or ectopic bronchial carcinoid (B) over 24 hours.(Secretion during 24-hour period of exposure to dexamethasone is expressed as a percentage(±SE) of basal secretion during preceding 24 hours, when cells are incubated with culture medium only.* Minimum of three cultures per group.)*
$p < 0.01$.

ectopic syndrome, and also concurs with the general lack of ACTH suppression after DXM *in vivo*. It seems that a lack of cytosol receptors for steroid translocation into the nucleus may explain this finding. The use of a cell culture system should continue to be of value for future studies of ectopic tumour pathophysiology.

REFERENCES

Abeloff M.D., Trump D.L., Baylin S.B. (1981). Ectopic adrenocorticotrophic (ACTH) syndrome and small cell carcinoma of the lung. Assessment of clinical implications in patients on combination chemotherapy. *Cancer*; **48**: 1082.

Adams E.F., Ashby M.J., Brown S.M., *et al.* (1981). Bromocriptine suppresses ACTH secretion from human pituitary tumour cells in culture by a dopaminergic mechanism. *Clin. Endocrinol*; **15**: 479.

Al-Dujaili E.A.S., Hope J., Estivariz F.E., Lowry P.J., Edwards C.R.W. (1981). Circulating human pituitary pro-γ-melanotropin enhances the adrenal response to ACTH. *Nature*; **291**: 156.

Apple D., Kreines K. (1982). Cushing's syndrome due to ectopic ACTH production by a nasal paraganglioma. *Am. J. Med. Sci*; **283**: 32.

Aron D.C., Tyrell J.B., Fitzgerald P.A., Findling J.W., Forsham P.H. (1981). Cushing's syndrome: Problems in diagnosis. *Medicine*; **60**: 25.

Balls K.F., Nicholson J.T.L., Goodman H.L., Touchstone J.C. (1959). Functioning islet cell carcinoma of the pancreas with Cushing's syndrome. *J. Clin. Endocrinol. Metab*; **19**: 1134.

Balsam A., Bernstein G., Goldman J., Sachs B.A., Rifkin H. (1972). Ectopic adrenocorticotropin syndrome associated with carcinoma of the colon. *Gastroenterol*; **62**: 636.

Baylin S.B., Weisburger W.R., Eggleston J.C. (1978). Variable content of histaminase, l-dopadecarboxylase and calcitonin in small cell carcinoma of the lung. *N. Engl. J. Med*; **299**: 105.

Belchetz P.E., Brown C.L., Makin H.L.T., *et al.* (1973). ACTH, glucagon and gastrin production by a pancreatic islet cell carcinoma and its treatment. *Clin. Endocrinol*; **2**: 307.

Bensch K.G., Gordon G.B., Miller L.R. (1965). Studies on the bronchial counterpart of the Kultschitzky (argentaffin) cell and innervation of bronchial glands. *J. Ultrastruct. Res*; **12**: 668.

Bensch K.G., Corrin B., Pariente R., Spencer H. (1968). Oat cell carcinoma of the lung. *Cancer*; **22**: 1163.

Besser G.M., Landon J. (1968). Plasma levels of immunoreactive corticotrophin in patients with Cushing's syndrome. *Brit. Med. J*; **4**: 552.

Birkenhager J.C., Upton V.G., Seldenrath J.H., Krieger D.T., Tashjian A.H. (1976). Medullary thyroid carcinoma: Ectopic production of peptides with ACTH-like, corticotrophin releasing factor-like and prolactin producing stimulating activities. *Acta Endocrinol*; **83**: 280.

Bloomfield G.A., Holdaway I.M., Corrin B., *et al.* (1977). Lung tumours and ACTH production. *Clin. Endocrinol*; **6**: 95.

Bourgoignie J., Dupont J.-Cl., Noiret R. (1964). Association d'un pheochromocytome et d'un hypercorticisme du type Cushing avec hyperaldosteronurie *Ann. Endocrinol*; **25**: 269.

Brown H., Lane M. (1965). Cushing's and malignant carcinoid syndrome from ovarian neoplasms. *Arch. Int. Med*; **115**: 490.

Brown W.H. (1928). A case of pluriglandular syndrome. *Lancet*; **2**: 1022.

Carey R.M., Orth D.N., Hartmann W.H. (1973). Malignant melanoma with ectopic production of adrenocorticotropic hormone: Palliative treatment with inhibitors of adrenal steroid biosynthesis. *J. Clin. Endocrinol. Metab*; **36**: 482.

Christy N.P. (1961). Adrenocorticotrophic activity in plasma of patients with Cushing's syndrome associated with pulmonary neoplasms. *Lancet*; **1**: 85.

Coscia M., Brown R.D., Miller M., *et al.* (1977). Ectopic production of antidiuretic hormone (ADH) adrenocorticotrophic hormone (ACTH) and beta-melanocyte stimulating hormone (β-MSH) by an oat cell carcinoma of the lung. *Am. J. Med*; **62**: 303.

Davies C.J., Joplin G.F., Welbourn R.B. (1982). Surgical management of the ectopic ACTH syndrome. *Ann. Surg*; **196**: 246.

Drury P.L., Ratter S., Tomlin S., *et al.* (1982). Experience with selective venous sampling in diagnosis of ACTH-dependent Cushing's syndrome. *Brit. Med. J*; **284**: 9.

Estivariz F.E., Hope J., McLean C., Lowry P.J. (1980). Purification and characterisation of a γ-melanotropin precursor from frozen human pituitary glands. *Biochem. J*; **191**: 125.

Estivariz F.E., Gillies G., Lowry P.J. (1981). Biosynthesis and control of secretion of corticotropic, lipotropic and melanotropic peptides. *Pharmacol. Ther*; **13**: 61.

Findling J.W., Aron D.C., Tyrell J.B., *et al.* (1981). Selective venous sampling for ACTH in Cushing's syndrome. *Ann. Int. Med*; **94**: 647.

Forman B.H., Marban E., Kayne R.D., *et al.* (1979). Ectopic ACTH syndrome due to pheochromocytoma: Case report and review of the literature. *Yale J. Biol. Med*; **52**: 181.

Fuentes J.A.G., Remis J.E.F. (1979). Syndrome de Cushing por ACTH ectopico y hepatocarcinoma. *Rev. Clin. Espan*; **155**: 77.

Gabcke C., quoted in Leyton O., Turnbull H.M., Bretton A.-B. (1931). Primary cancer of the thymus with pluriglandular disturbance. *J. Path. Bacteriol*; **34**: 635.

Gabrilove J.L., Nicolis G.L., Kirscher P.A. (1969). Cushing's syndrome in association with carcinoid tumor. *Ann. Surg*; **169**: 240.

Geokas M.C., Chun J.C., Dinan J.J., Beck I.T. (1965). Islet cell carcinoma (Zollinger–Ellison syndrome) with fulminating adrenocortical hyperfunction and hypokalaemia. *Can. Med. Ass. J*; **93**: 137.

Gerwitz G., Yalow R.S. (1974). Ectopic ACTH production in carcinoma of the lung. *J. Clin. Invest*; **53**: 1022.

Gilkes J.J., Rees L.H., Besser G.M. (1977). Plasma immunoreactive corticotrophin and lipotrophin in Cushing's syndrome and Addison's disease. *Brit. Med. J*; **1**: 996.

Gold E.M. (1979). The Cushing syndrome: Changing views of diagnosis and treatment. *Ann. Int. Med*; **90**: 829.

Goltzman D., Huang S.N., Broune C., *et al.* (1979). Adrenocorticotropin and calcitonin in medullary carcinoma: Frequency of occurrence and localization in the same cell type by immunocytochemistry. *J. Clin. Endocrinol. Metab*; **49**: 364.

Gonzalez-Licea A., Hartman W.H., Yardley J.H. (1968). Medullary carcinoma of the thyroid; Ultrastructural evidence of its origin from the parafollicular cell and its possible relation to carcinoid tumor. *Am. J. Clin. Pathol*; **49**: 512.

Gordon P., Becker C.E., Levey G.S., Roth J. (1968). Efficacy of aminogluthimide in the ectopic ACTH syndrome. *J. Clin. Endocrinol. Metab*; **27**: 921.

Harris P.W.R., El-Katib M.B. (1968). Cushing's syndrome and myelolipomatosis with carcinoma of the thymus. *Brit. J. Surg*; **55**: 472.

Hashimoto K., Takahara J., Ogawa N., *et al.* (1980). Adrenocorticotropin, β-lipotropin, β-endorphin, and corticotropin-releasing factor-like activity in an adrenocorticotropin-producing nephroblastoma. *J. Clin. Endocrinol. Metab*; **50**: 461.

Hattori M., Imura H., Matsukura S. (1979). Multiple hormone producing lung carcinoma. *Cancer*; **43**: 2429.

Heitz P.U., Kloppel G., Polak J.M., Straub J.J. (1981). Ectopic hormone production by endocrine tumours. *Cancer*; **48**: 2029.

Himsworth R.L., Bloomfield G.A., Coombes R.C., *et al.* (1977). 'Big' ACTH and calcitonin in an ectopic hormone secreting tumour of the liver. *Clin. Endocrinol*; **7**: 45.

Hirata Y., Yamamoto H., Matsukura S., Imura H. (1975). *In vitro* release and biosynthesis of tumor ACTH in ectopic ACTH producing tumors. *J. Clin. Endocrinol. Metab*; **41**: 106.

Hirata Y., Matsukura S., Imura H., *et al.* (1976a). Two cases of multiple hormone-producing small cell carcinoma of the lung. *Cancer*; **38**: 2575.

Hirata Y., Sakamoto N., Yamamoto H., Matsukura S., Imura H., Okada S. (1976b). Gastric carcinoid with ectopic production of ACTH and β-MSH. *Cancer*; **37**: 377.

Hirata Y., Yoshimi H., Matsukura S., Imura H. (1979). Effect of hypothalamic extract and other factors on release of adrenocorticotropin from adenosine 3'5'-monophosphate levels in dispersed non-pituitary tumor cells. *J. Clin. Endocrinol. Metab*; **49**: 317.

Horai J., Nishihara H., Tateishi R., Matsuda M., Hattori S. (1973). Oat cell carcinoma of the lung simultaneously producing ACTH and serotonin. *J. Clin. Endocrinol. Metab*; **37**: 212.

Imura H. (1980). Ectopic hormone syndromes. *Clin. Endocrinol. Metab*; **9**: 235.

Imura H., Matsukura S., Yamamoto H. *et al.* (1975). Studies on ectopic ACTH-producing tumors. *Cancer*; **35**: 1430.

Johnson W.H., Waisman J. (1971). Carcinoid tumour of the vermiform appendix with Cushing's syndrome. *Cancer*; **27**: 681.

Jones J.E., Shane S.R., Gilbert E., Flink E.B. (1969). Cushing's syndrome induced by the ectopic production of ACTH by a bronchial carcinoid. *J. Clin. Endocrinol. Metab*; **29**: 1.

Kato Y., Ferguson T.B., Bennett D.E., Burford T.H. (1969). Oat cell carcinoma of the lung: A review of 138 cases. *Cancer*; **23**: 517.

Keusch G., Binswanger U., Dambacher M.A., Fischer J.A. (1977). Ectopic ACTH syndrome and medullary carcinoma of the thyroid. *Acta Endocrinol*; **86**: 306.

Kleber G., Höllt V., Oelkers W., Quabbe H.J. (1980). Elevated plasma and tissue concentrations of β-endorphin and β-lipotropin associated with an ectopic ACTH-producing lung tumor. *Horm. Metab. Res*; **12**: 385.

Kovach R.D., Kyle L.H. (1958). Cushing's syndrome and bronchogenic carcinoma. *Am. J. Med*; **24**: 981.

Krol T.C., Wood W.S. (1982). Bronchogenic carcinoma and diabetes insipidus. *Cancer*. **49**: 596.

Kyriakides G.K., Silvis S.E., Ahmed M., Vennes J.A., Vogel S.B. (1979). Gastrinoma associated with common bile duct obstruction and the ectopic production of ACTH. *Amer. J. Surg*; **137**: 800.

Larsson L.I. (1981). Adrenocorticotropin-like and α-melanotropin-like peptides in a subpopulation of human gastrin cell granules: Bioassay, immunoassay, and immunocytochemical evidence. *Proc. Natl. Acad. Sci. USA*; **78**: 2990.

Le Dourain N.M. (1978). The embryological origin of the endocrine cells associated with the digestive tract. In *Gut Hormones* (Bloom S.R., ed.) pp. 49–56. Edinburgh: Churchill-Livingstone.

Levern W.J., Fariss B.L., Wettlanfor J.N., Hane S. (1975). Ectopic ACTH production in disseminated prostatic adenocarcinoma. *Urology*; **5**: 817.

Liddle G.W., Nicholson W.E. Island D.P., Orth D.N. Abe K., Lowder S.C. (1969). Clinical and laboratory studies of ectopic humoral syndromes. *Recent Progr. Hormone Res*; **25**: 283.

Lojek M.A., Fer M.F., Kasselberg A.G., *et al.* (1980). Cushing's syndrome with small cell carcinoma of the uterine cervix. *Amer J. Med*; **69**: 140.

Mains R.E., Eiper B.A., Ling N. (1977). Common precursor to corticotropins and endorphins. *Proc. Natl. Acad. Sci. USA*; **74**: 3014.

Marks V., Samols E., Bolton R. (1965). Hyperinsulinism and Cushing's syndrome. *Brit. Med. J*; **1**: 1419.

Marks A.D., Kim Y.N., Kroop H.S. (1975). Ectopic production by a minor salivary gland tumor. *Ann. Int. Med*; **83**: 521.

Mason A.M.S., Ratcliffe J.G., Buckle R.M., Stuart Mason A. (1972). ACTH secretion by bronchial carcinoid tumours. *Clin. Endocrinol*; **1**: 3.

Masson P. (1924). Appendicite neurogene et carcinoides. *Ann. Anat. Pathol*; **1**: 3.

Meador C.K., Liddle G.W., Island D.P. *et al.* (1962). Cause of Cushing's syndrome in patients with tumors arising from non-endocrine tissue. *J. Clin. Endocrinol. Metab*; **22**: 693.

Melvin K.E.W., Tashjian A.H., Cassidy C.E., Givens J.R. (1970). Cushing's syndrome caused by ACTH and calcitonin-secreting medullary carcinoma of the thyroid. *Metabolism*; **19**: 831.

Miura K., Sasaki C., Katsushima I. (1967). Pituitary adrenocortical studies in a patient with Cushing's syndrome induced by a thymoma. *J. Clin. Endocrinol. Metab*; **27**: 631.

Moertel C.S. (1975). Clinical management of advanced gastrointestinal cancer. *Cancer*; **36**: 675.

Molland E.A. (1978). Prostatic adenocarcinoma with ectopic ACTH production. *Brit. J. Urol*; **50**: 358.

Morse N.I., Kerenyi N., Nelson D.H. (1967). Prolonged hyperadrenocorticotrophism and pigmentation associated with a bronchial carcinoid tumour. *Can. Med. Ass. J*; **96**: 104.

Myers E.A., Hardman J.M., Worsham G.F., Eil C. (1982). Adenocarcinoma of the lung causing ectopic adrenocorticotropic hormone syndrome. *Arch. Intern. Med*; **142**: 1387.

Nakanishi S., Ingre A., Kita T., *et al.* (1979). Nucleotide sequence of a cloned cDNA for bovine corticotropin-β-lipotropin precursor. *Nature*; **278**: 423.

Neville A.M., Mackay A.M. (1972). The structure of the human adrenal cortex in health and disease. *Clin. Endocrinol. Metab*; **1**: 361.

Newmark S.R., Oluhy R.G., Bennett A.H. (1973). Ectopic adrenocorticotrophin syndrome with prostatic carcinoma. *Urology*; **2**: 668.

Nichols J., Gourley W. (1963). Adrenal weight-maintaining corticotropin in carcinoma of lung. *JAMA*; **185**: 696.

Nichols J., Warren J.C., Mantz F.A. (1962). ACTH-like excretion from carcinoma of the ovary. *JAMA*; **182**: 713.

Nichols T., Nugent C.A., Tyler F.H. (1968). Steroid laboratory tests in the diagnosis of Cushing's syndrome. *Am. J. Med*; **45**: 116.

O'Neal W.L., Kipnis D.M., Luse S.A., Lacy P.E., Jarrett L. (1968). Secretion of various endocrine substances by ACTH-secreting tumors—gastrin, melanotropin, norepinephrine, serotonin, parahormone, vasopressin, glucagon. *Cancer*; **21**: 1219.

Parsons V., Rigby B. (1958). Cushing's syndrome associated with adenocarcinoma of the ovary. *Lancet*; **2**: 992.

Pearse A.G.E., Polak J.M. (1971). Neural crest origin of the endocrine polypeptide (APUD) cells of the gastrointestinal tract and pancreas. *Gut*; **12**: 783.

Pedersen R.C., Brownie A.C. (1980). Pro-adrenocorticotropin/endorphin-derived peptides: Co-ordinate action on adrenal steroidogenesis. *Science*; **208**: 1044.

Pfohl R.A., Doe R.P. (1963). Adrenal-pituitary studies in a patient with bronchogenic carcinoma and Cushing's syndrome. *Ann. Int. Med*; **58**: 993.

Pfueger K.H., Gramse M., Gropp C., *et al.* (1981). Ectopic ACTH production with autoantibody formation in a patient with acute myeloblastic leukaemia. *N. Engl. J. Med*; **305**: 1632.

Pictet R.L., Rall L.B., Phelps P., Rutter W.J. (1976). The neural crest and the origin of the insulin-producing and other gastrointestinal hormone producing cells. *Science*; **191**: 191.

Prunty F.T.G., Brooks R.V., Dupre J., *et al.* (1963). Adrenocortical hyperfunction and potassium metabolism in patients with 'non-endocrine' tumors and Cushing's syndrome. *J. Clin. Endocrinol. Metab*; **23**: 737.

Pullan P.T., Clement-Jones V., Corder R. *et al.* (1980*a*). Ectopic production of methionine meophalin and beta endorphin. *Brit. Med. J*; **1**: 758.

Pullan P.T., Clement-Jones V., Corder R., Lowry P.J., Besser G.M., Rees L.H. (1980*b*). ACTH, LPH and related peptides in the ectopic ACTH syndrome. *Clin. Endocrinol*; **13**: 437.

Ratcliffe J.G., Knight R.A., Besser G.M., *et al.* (1972). Tumour and plasma ACTH concentrations in patients with or without the ectopic ACTH syndrome. *Clin. Endocrinol*; **1**: 27.

Ratcliffe J.G., Scott A.P., Bennett H.P.J., *et al.* (1973). Production of a corticotrophin-like intermediate lobe peptide and of corticotrophin by a bronchial carcinoid tumour. *Clin. Endocrinol*; **2**: 51.

Ratter S.J., Lowry P.J., Besser G.M., Rees L.H. (1980). Chromatographic characterization of adrenocorticotrophin in human plasma. *J. Endocrinol*; **85**: 359.

Ratter S.J., Gillies G., Hope J., *et al.* (1983). Pro-opiocortin related peptides in human pituitary and ectopic ACTH secreting tumours. *Clin. Endocrinol*; **18**: 211.

Rees L.H., Bloomfield G.A., Rees G.M., *et al.* (1974). Multiple hormones in a bronchial tumor. *J. Clin. endocrinol. Metab*; **38**: 1090.

Rosai J., Levine G., Weber W.R., Higa E. (1976). Carcinoid tumors and oat cell carcinomas of the thymus. *Pathol. Annu*; **11**: 201.

Rosenstock J., Allison D., Joplin G.F., *et al.* (1981). Therapeutic adrenal venous infarction in ACTH-dependent Cushing's syndrome. *Brit. J. Radiol*; **54**: 912.

Sachs B.A., Becker N., Bloomberg A.E., *et al.* (1970). 'Cure' of ectopic ACTH syndrome secondary to adrenocarcinoma of the lung. *J. Clin. Endocrinol. Metab*; **30**: 590.

Salyer W.R., Salyer D.C., Eccleston J.C. (1976). Carcinoid tumors of the thymus. *Cancer*; **37**: 958.

Schambelan M., Slaton P.E., Biglieri E.G. (1971). Mineralocorticoid production in hyperadrenocorticism. *Am. J. Med*; **51**: 299.

Schteingart D.E., Conn J.W., Orth D.N., *et al.* (1972). Secretion of ACTH and β-MSH by an adrenal medullary paraganglioma. *J. Clin. Endocrinol. Metab*; **34**: 676.

Scholz D.A., Bahn R.C. (1959). Thymic tumors associated with Cushing's syndrome: Review of three cases. *Mayo Clin. Proc*; **34**: 433.

Scott H.W., Liddle G.W., Mulhevin J.L., *et al.* (1977). Surgical experience with Cushing's disease. *Ann. Surg*; **185**: 524.

Sidhu G.S. (1979). The endodermal origin of digestive and respiratory tract APUD cells. *Am. J. Pathol*; **96**: 5.

Singer W., Kovacs K., Ryan N., Horvath E. (1977). Ectopic ACTH syndrome: Clinicopathological correlations. *J. Clin. Pathol*; **31**: 591.

Spence R.W. Burns-Cox C.J. (1975). ACTH secreting apendoma of gallbladder. *Gut*; **16**: 473.

Steel K., Baerg R.D., Adams D.O. (1967). Cushing's syndrome in association with a carcinoid tumor of the lung. *J. Clin. Endocrinol. Metab*; **27**: 1285.

Stevens R.E., Moore G.E. (1983). Inadequacy of APUD concept in explaining production of peptide hormones by tumours. *Lancet*; **1**: 118.

Strott C.A., Nugent C.A., Tyler F.H. (1968). Cushing's syndrome caused by bronchial adenomas. *Am. J. Med*; **44**: 97.

Suda T., Demura H., Demura R., *et al.* (1977). Corticotropin-releasing factor-like activity in ACTH producing tumors. *J. Clin. endocrinol. Metab*; **44**: 440.

Suda T., Tozawa F., Yamaguchi H., *et al.* (1982). Multiple forms of immunoreactive β-endorphin are present in an ectopic adrenocorticotropin-producing tumour but not in normal pituitary or pituitary adenomas. *J. Clin. Endocrinol. Metab*; **54**: 167.

Thorner M.O., Martin W.H., Ragan G.E., *et al.* (1982). A case of ectopic ACTH syndrome: Diagnostic difficulties caused by intermittent hormone secretion. *Acta Endocrinol*; **99**: 364.

Upton G.V., Amatruda T.T. (1971). Evidence for the presence of tumor peptides with corticotropin-releasing factor-like activity in the ectopic ACTH syndrome. *N. Engl. J. Med*; **285**: 419.

Weiss R.B. (1978). Small cell carcinoma of the lung: Therapeutic management. *Ann. Int. Med*; **88**: 522.

Wenk R.E., Bhagavan B.S., Levy R., Miller D., Weisburger W. (1977). Ectopic ACTH, prostatic oat cell carcinoma, and marked hypernatraemia. *Cancer*; **40**: 773.

White F.E., White M.C., Drury P.L. Kelsey Fry I., Besser G.M. (1982). Value of computed tomography of the abdomen and chest in investigation of Cushing's syndrome. *Brit. Med. J*; **284**: 771.

Wick M.R., Scott R.E., Li C.Y., Carner J.A. (1980). Carcinoid tumor of the thymus. *Mayo Clin. Proc*; **55**: 246.

Williams E.D., Morales A.M., Horn R.C. (1968). Thyroid carcinoma and Cushing's syndrome. *J. Clin. Path*; **21**: 129.

Wood S.M., Wood J.R., Ghatei M.A., *et al.* (1981). Bombesin, somatostatin and neurotensin-like immunoreactivity in bronchial carcinoma. *J. Clin. Endocrinol. Metab*; **53**: 1310.

Woodard B.H., Elsenbarth G., Wallace N.R., Mossler J.A., McCarty K.S. (1981). Adrenocorticotropin production by a mammary carcinoma. *Cancer*; **47**: 1823.

Yalow R.S., Berson S.A. (1971). Size heterogeneity of immunoreactive human ACTH in plasma and in extracts of pituitary glands and ACTH producing thymoma. *Biochem. Biophys. Res. Comm*; **44**: 439.

Yalow R.S., Berson S.A. (1973). Characteristics of 'big' ACTH in human plasma and pituitary extracts. *J. Clin. Endocrinol. Metab*; **36**: 415.

Chapter 11

L. Otto Uttenthal

Peptide-secreting Tumours of the Gut

INTRODUCTION

The advance in techniques of peptide purification and analysis that took place during the 1960s was paralleled by the development of very specific and sensitive immunochemical methods for quantitating and locating peptides in tissues. One consequence of this has been the realisation that the gut contains, in aggregate, the largest number of peptide-secreting endocrine cells in the body, dispersed throughout the mucosa, and in addition, has a rich intrinsic and extrinsic peptidergic innervation. This chapter deals with tumours arising from these peptide-secreting cells, including those of the pancreatic islets and ducts.

It will be apparent that for this complex endocrine, paracrine and neurocrine system, the concepts of ectopic and eutopic hormone production start to break down. The classification of hormone production by a tumour as ectopic depends on the demonstration of a negative, namely, that there are no cells in the adult elaborating that hormone at the site of the tumour. The confidence with which this can be stated varies from hormone to hormone, and is in a continuing state of flux as more sensitive localisation methods are deployed. Furthermore, it is impossible to make generalisations about the malignancy or otherwise of gut tumours according to whether their peptide production is currently classified as ectopic or eutopic. Irrespective of their present status within such a classification, the gut endocrine tumours tend to be malignant, but slow-growing, and most of them produce multiple molecular forms of the secreted peptides. The exception to this is provided by insulinomas, described in Chapter 5, but even here, the difference is only one of degree.

Any concept broad enough to provide a unifying classification of the wide range of cells secreting peptides with a proven or presumptive regulatory role must be broad indeed. Such a concept was provided by Pearse (1968), who noted certain cytochemical characteristics shared by many polypeptide-hormone-secreting cells. These characteristics (*a*mine and *p*recursor *u*ptake and *d*ecarboxylation, giving the acronym APUD) were originally associated with a proposed embryological origin from the endoderm, but subsequently a common origin from the neuroectoderm was postulated. While not all polypeptide-hormone-secreting cells share these characteristics (e.g. the parathyroid chief cells), and the endocrine cells of the gut mucosa are almost certainly of endodermal origin, the concept has been very useful in drawing attention to the fact that the same peptides could be elaborated by widely dispersed cells, and could thus be secreted by tumours arising in widely separated areas. As a consequence, such peptide- or amine-secreting tumours are often referred to as 'APUDomas'.

The majority of the gut endocrine tumours connected with the specific syndromes dealt with in this chapter arise from the endocrine pancreas. Earlier studies tended to focus on the single peptide products that could be related pathogenetically to the clinical features, but it is now apparent that the majority of these tumours contain multiple cell types, each secreting multiple molecular forms of individual peptide immunoreactivities. Very often, certain clinical features that might be expected from hypersecretion of some of these immunoreactivities are absent, suggesting that inactive molecular (perhaps precursor) forms are being secreted. The various syndromes are usually named after the peptide whose biological activities can be linked to the principal features of the case.

TYPES OF TUMOUR

Gastrinoma

Zollinger and Ellison (1955) first described a syndrome in which severe peptic ulceration and gastric acid hypersecretion were associated with a pancreatic tumour; hence the synonym Zollinger–Ellison syndrome or ZES. The demonstration that such tumours secreted gastrin occurred five years later (Gregory *et al.*, 1960). Gastrinomas represent the second most common pancreatic endocrine tumour after insulinomas, in that most immunocytochemists have been unable to demonstrate gastrin in the normal adult human pancreas, although it has been detected in fetal islet cells, pancreatic gastrinomas are at present classified as ectopic hormone-secreting tumours, possibly arising from fetal rests. Gastrinomas may also occur in the upper duodenum (where they would be regarded as eutopic), but only very rarely at other sites. Current figures suggest that at least 60% are malignant, mostly with multiple pancreatic primaries and hepatic metastases by the time of diagnosis, and it may well be that as follow-up is continued the malignancy rate will be seen to exceed 90%. Approximately one-third of patients have a family history of endocrinopathy, illustrating the frequent occurrence of gastrinomas as a component of multiple endocrine adenopathy (MEA) type 1. The majority of gastrinomas are of mixed cellular type and also secrete large amounts of pancreatic polypeptide, and there are a few cases of concurrence of gastrinoma and other tumour syndromes, e.g. glucagonoma. In those cases where chromatographic studies have been carried out on gastrinoma tumour extracts or plasma samples, there have been varying ratios of gastrin-17 and gastrin-34, in sulphated and unsulphated forms, without evident correlation with clinical features.

Since the original description of the syndrome, it has become apparent that symptoms of peptic ulceration need not be severe. More recent experience has been reviewed by Stage and Stadil (1979). The history of dyspepsia may be intermittent, and may stretch back to over a decade before the first operation is needed. In some cases, peptic ulceration has been asymptomatic, and intermittent or chronic diarrhoea, sometimes with features of steatorrhoea, may be the only symptom in 10% of cases. The mechanism of diarrhoea includes gastric fluid hypersecretion, upper intestinal mucosal damage with partial villous atrophy, inactivation of pancreatic enzymes and precipitation of bile acids by the excess of gastric acid reaching the duodenum.

No single clinical test is diagnostic of a gastrinoma. All patients with gastrinomas have an elevated fasting plasma gastrin concentration (greater than 40 pmol/litre), but major elevations of plasma gastrin are also found in atrophic gastritis (the most common cause of raised plasma gastrin concentrations) with or without pernicious anaemia, in the rare syndrome of G-cell hyperplasia, and in occasional individuals in whom no other abnormality is found. Lesser degrees of elevation may be found in peptic ulcer disease not associated with tumour, during treatment with H_2-receptor antagonists, after vagotomy, in hypercalcaemia, or in uraemia. For this reason, plasma gastrin determinations should be supplemented with estimation of basal and pentagastrin-stimulated gastric acid output (as well as plasma calcium and urea estimations). Although a basal acid output above 20 mmol H^+ per hour, without further rise with pentagastrin, is regarded as diagnostic, about 20% of patients may have basal acid secretion of 5 mmol/h, and the ratio of basal to maximally stimulated acid output may not differentiate these from normal (Aoyagi and Summerskill, 1966). Thus, even with acid studies, a definite diagnosis will not be reached in a proportion of cases. For such cases, various supplementary diagnostic tests have been proposed, such as measuring gastrin responses to food or protein hydrolysates, to intravenous injection of secretin, or to intravenous infusion of calcium or bombesin. In general, tumour secretion of gastrin is not subject to normal control mechanisms, so that those agents which normally stimulate gastrin secretion have a lesser effect on tumour-related output. In the case of secretin, many gastrinomas show a paradoxical release of gastrin, not usually seen in conventional peptic ulcer disease or in G-cell hyperplasia. However, for all these tests there is some overlap between tumour and non-tumour responses, and no single test is of proven reliability.

Endoscopy findings may span a whole range of possibilities, from multiple to single ulcers or even no ulcers at all. Nevertheless, multiple gastric or duodenal ulcers or ulcers distal to the duodenal bulb will suggest the possibility of a gastrinoma. The trophic effects of gastrin may produce giant gastric mucosal folds. Radiological findings, in addition to ulcers, may include a rapid transit time, fluid levels and signs of upper small intestinal mucosal damage.

VIPoma

Verner and Morrison (1958) described two cases of refractory watery diarrhoea with hypokalaemia in whom post-mortem examination revealed pancreatic islet cell tumours. Subsequent descriptions of similar cases showed a fairly regular constellation of *w*atery *d*iarrhoea, *h*ypokalaemia and *a*chlorhydria, so that the syndrome has been called WDHA syndrome, Verner–Morrison syndrome, or pancreatic cholera. Compared with gastrinomas, VIPomas are rare. The neuropeptide VIP (vasoactive intestinal polypeptide) has been found in raised concentrations in the plasma and tumours of many patients with this syndrome (reviewed by Long *et al.*, 1981). As this peptide is a potent stimulator of intestinal fluid and electrolyte secretion, and an inhibitor of gastric acid secretion, it seems probable that the secretion of VIP from the tumour is a principal pathogenic mechanism of the syndrome. However, other peptides may also be involved. A proportion of tumours may also secrete neurotensin (Blackburn *et al.*, 1981), a brain–gut peptide with rather similar pharmacological activities to those of VIP; recently, the newly discovered VIP-like peptide PHI has been found in tumour extracts and plasma from VIPoma patients (Bloom *et al.*, 1983). The relative contribution of these peptides to the clinical features has not been elucidated. As with most gut-hormone-secreting tumours, pancreatic polypeptide is often secreted as well, but does not contribute to the pathogenesis of the syndrome. Insulin and somatostatin have also been found in isolated cases. Chromatographic analysis of the tumour or plasma VIP-like immunoreactivity often reveals the presence of larger cross-reacting molecular forms which may not have the biological activity of VIP.

Most VIPomas are malignant pancreatic tumours, but VIP may also be secreted from ganglioneuroblastomas, usually presenting in childhood. In the former case, peptide production would be regarded as ectopic, in the latter as eutopic. Profuse watery diarrhoea, whether intermittent or continuous, is a universal feature, with hypokalaemia and weight loss as a regular consequence. Achlorhydria or hypochlorhydria is less common (70% of patients), while episodes of flushing may occur in 20% of patients, and hypercalcaemia is relatively rare, either associated with the hyperpara-thyroidism of MEA type 1, or as a direct effect of VIP on bone resorption (Hohmann *et al.*, 1983).

Diagnosis of a VIPoma depends on finding an elevated plasma VIP concentration (greater than 30 pmol/litre) in a patient with the relevant clinical features. It must be remembered, however, that VIP is by no means the only peptide implicated in tumour-related diarrhoeal syndromes. As mentioned above, diarrhoea may be the main presenting feature of a gastrinoma, and it may be a prominent feature in medullary carcinoma of the thyroid, and in the glucagonoma and carcinoid syndromes. Thus, appropriate marker substances for other types of tumour should be looked for. Occasionally, an apparently elevated VIP concentration is found in plasma from patients without diarrhoea, or with an atypical history. In such cases, chromatography may reveal the presence of higher molecular weight cross-reacting substances without elevation of true VIP. The origin of the higher molecular weight substances in these cases is not known, and in the absence of further evidence cannot be regarded as diagnostic of a tumour.

Glucagonoma

Pancreatic tumours secreting glucagon are relatively rare; the first case with documented hyperglucagonaemia was reported by McGavran *et al.* (1966), and the classical description of the glucagonoma syndrome was given by Mallinson *et al.* (1974). Subsequently, Stacpoole (1981) has reviewed 84 proven and probable cases. The majority (two-thirds) of proven gluca-gonomas are malignant, but case histories suggest that they are slow-growing, and are usually only detected after metastatic spread to the liver has occurred. Thus, most patients present in middle age, often with a long history of mild diabetes, and a glucagonoma is only suspected after the appearance of the characteristic skin rash. The rash is the distinctive feature of the syndrome, and is described as a necrolytic migratory erythema. This appears as a figurate erythema with a migratory edge over the trunk, usually lesser involvement of the extremities, and an eczematous symmetrical rash of the perineum and buttocks. The erythematous areas may develop a psoriatiform scaling, or progress to bullae, which break down with crust formation or secondary infection. Healing occurs with brown pigmentation, and patients will usually show the various stages of evolution and resolution of the rash in different areas. Histological examination of the edge of a developing lesion may show superficial epidermal spongiosis and necrosis, with subcorneal and mid-epidermal clefts.

The rash has some features in common with acrodermatitis enteropathica and the cutaneous manifestations of malabsorption syndromes, and may be related to a deficiency of zinc and plasma amino acids. Part of the zinc deficiency may be explained by the sequestration of zinc by the tumour, and the increased gluconeogenesis stimulated by the excessive glucagon secretion may explain the reduced levels of plasma amino acids. Remissions of the rash have been obtained with oral and topical zinc, intravenous amino acids and with somatostatin infusions, or with combinations of these therapies. Parenteral somatostatin is effective in reducing plasma levels of glucagon, but it may also act via other mechanisms, as there are isolated reports of its benefit in psoriasis.

As might be expected from the relationship of the glucagonoma rash with those of nutritional deficiencies and other protein hypercatabolic states, there are further cutaneous manifestations; these include angular stomatitis, glossitis, thinning of hair, dystrophy of the nails and occasionally, purpura.

The excessive glucagon secretion from the tumour and its metastases produces a variety of other effects, some of which can be deduced from the metabolic actions of glucagon. Mild diabetes is present in about 95% of proven cases, and patients will show an impaired or frankly diabetic glucose tolerance. Because of wide individual variation in insulin secretion and sensitivity, there is only a poor relationship between the degree of hyperglycaemia and the plasma glucagon concentration. The reduced plasma amino acid levels have already been referred to, and the plasma albumin concentration may also be low. There is regularly a normochromic, normocytic anaemia. Weight loss is common, and diarrhoea has been reported in about 15% of cases. There is a high incidence of thrombotic phenomena, and pulmonary embolism is a significant cause of mortality. The mechanism underlying the increased tendency to thrombosis is poorly understood. It is a speculative possibility that both this and some of the zinc deficiency could be related to disturbances of prostaglandin biosynthetic pathways.

Glucagonomas secrete an excess of pancreatic glucagon, but as with the other pancreatic tumours described, chromatographic analysis usually reveals varying quantities of larger molecular species cross-reacting with the antisera used in the radioimmunoassays. 'Void volume' glucagon immunoreactivity, referring to gel filtration analysis (molecular weight greater than 150 000), is a normal finding, the amount detected depending on the glucagon antiserum used. This cross-reactivity has been attributed to the Fc region of IgG. Intermediate molecular species (molecular weight 8000–12 000) are frequently seen in plasmas from glucagonoma patients, but also have a rare familial occurrence, and are seen in uraemia and cirrhosis of the liver, where presumably the small amounts normally secreted can accumulate in the circulation. The biological activities of these intermediate forms are not known. The recently reported sequence of hamster preproglucagon (Bell *et al.*, 1983) shows that proglucagon contains two further glucagon-like peptide sequences, and it seems likely that glucagonomas may also be secreting large amounts of these hitherto unsuspected peptides, which may not be detected in current assays.

Glucagonomas commonly secrete pancreatic polypeptide in addition to glucagon and glucagon-like peptides. There are also reports of glucagonoma–insulinoma, glucagonoma–gastrinoma, and even glucagonoma–insulinoma–gastrinoma combinations. These are rarer, but of greater interest in that the additional hormones have contributed to the symptomatology. There seems to be no reason why further constellations of peptide secretion may not also be expected.

Diagnosis of a glucagonoma is supported by the demonstration of a raised fasting plasma pancreatic glucagon level in a patient with the relevant clinical features. It will be apparent from the above discussion that chromatographic analysis of the plasma immunoreactivity is desirable to demonstrate which molecular forms are present; this is especially important when the glucagon antiserum is sensitive to the 'void volume' cross-reactivity. Even so, the hyperglucagonaemia of diabetes mellitus, pancreatitis, trauma, severe illness and impaired glucagon metabolism in uraemia and cirrhosis of the liver must be excluded. Various functional tests have been proposed that might demonstrate autonomous or paradoxical glucagon secretory responses from the tumour. Intravenous glucose may not suppress plasma glucagon concentrations in glucagonoma patients, but the same may be true in diabetes or uraemia. Oral glucose or test meals may produce a paradoxical release of glucagon. However, glucagonomas frequently maintain a normal secretory response to arginine, and secretion is suppressed normally by somatostatin. It is evident that while these research procedures have provided interesting information on the behaviour of proven glucagonomas, they are unlikely to contribute to the diagnosis of individual cases.

The rarity of glucagonomas, the late presentation of the rash, and the lack of specificity of the other clinical features make early diagnosis difficult. Attempts at early detection by screening all diabetic outpatients for grossly elevated plasma glucagon levels are unlikely to be fruitful.

PPomas (Pancreatic-Polypeptide-Secreting Tumours)

Pancreatic polypeptide (PP) is secreted from a majority (60%) of pancreatic endocrine tumours, and has occasionally been detected in carcinoid tumours (Polak *et al.*, 1976; Öberg *et al.*, 1981). For pancreatic endocrine tumours there seems to be a fairly good agreement between elevated plasma concentrations of PP and the detection of PP in the tumour, but this is only occasionally true for other types of tumour, where in most cases the elevation of plasma PP would seem not to be of tumour origin. Plasma PP concentrations rise with age and, in addition to the physiological postprandial elevation, may be elevated by stress, acute illness, chronic inflammatory diseases, chronic pancreatitis, cirrhosis of the liver and renal failure. Consequently, some care is needed in the interpretation of a raised plasma

PP level as a tumour marker. One test which may be of value in differentiating between PP secreted under normal cholinergic control and autonomous secretion from a tumour is the atropine suppression test (Adrian *et al.*, 1982). In patients with tumours subsequently shown to contain PP, intravenous atropine has failed to suppress the elevated plasma concentrations, whereas substantial reductions in plasma PP occur in patients where no tumour has been demonstrated. However, failure of suppression may also be expected in circumstances where elimination of PP in the circulation is impaired, such as in renal failure. When the above considerations are borne in mind, elevated plasma PP levels may provide additional evidence of a pancreatic endocrine tumour in suspected cases. Its value as a tumour marker when taken in isolation is limited by the very high rate of false positive and false negative findings.

There are only a few reports of tumours in which PP has been the only product known to have been secreted into the blood-stream. Such tumours have been detected sporadically in patients presenting with non-specific symptoms such as anorexia and weight loss, or as a result of screening members of families with MEA type I. Although PP has an inhibitory effect on gall bladder contraction and pancreatic exocrine secretion in man, effects related to these possible actions have been absent, as have other specific clinical features.

Somatostatinoma

The first case reports of pancreatic tumours secreting somatostatin appeared in 1977 (Ganda *et al.*, 1977; Larsson *et al.*, 1977), and there are now about a dozen cases recorded in the literature. In addition, there are reports of tumours at other sites (including thymic and bronchial carcinoids and oat cell bronchial carcinomas) secreting substantial amounts of somatostatin. In so far as generalisations are possible from the limited number of reports, somatostatinomas seem to fall into two groups: one of these consists of pancreatic tumours, usually relatively large at the time of resection, with hepatic metastases and very high plasma immunoreactive somatostatin levels, where these have been measured. Most commonly, these tumours have been found at cholecystectomy, pointing to the lack of specificity of the other clinical features. Because of this mode of presentation it is hardly surprising that gall stones figure prominently in the manifestations of a presumed 'somatostatinoma syndrome'. The other group comprises usually smaller tumours, in the pancreas or elsewhere, which present in a variety of ways, often with syndromes of tumour secretion of other hormones such as ACTH or insulin. In these cases, the finding of somatostatin secretion has been incidental, following screening for many peptide hormones. For the first group of cases, clinical features, apart from gall stones, have included diabetes mellitus and steatorrhoea (Krejs *et al.*, 1979). Although it is possible to relate these features to excessive somatostatin secretion, the fact that they are not characteristic of somatostatinomas at other sites suggests either that they reflect local effects of the tumour or possibly that very high plasma levels of somatostatin are required. There remain considerable discrepancies between the pharmacological effects of infused somatostatin and the biochemical findings in these patients. For example, far from being diabetogenic, somatostatin usually produces a slight fall in blood glucose concentrations when infused into normal volunteers, and reduces insulin requirements in diabetics. It has been postulated that tissue resistance to somatostatin may develop after long exposure, and in any case, the molecular forms of most of the somatostatin-like immunoreactivity may not be biologically active. It is remarkable that most patients with raised plasma somatostatin levels of tumour origin have shown only relatively slight metabolic or endocrine disturbances.

Evidence of up to four molecular forms of somatostatin-like immunoreactivity has been reported for these patients. The two smaller forms may correspond to somatostatin-14 and somatostatin-28, while the larger forms could either be precursors or larger molecules with somatostatin linked via disulphide bridges. Findings vary in different patients; in some, but not all cases, somatostatin can be dissociated from larger molecular forms by reduction of disulphide links. In addition to somatostatin, other peptides such as ACTH, insulin and calcitonin have been found, and all recent reports are of mixed tumours.

It will be apparent from the non-specificity of the clinical features that pre-operative diagnosis of a somatostatinoma will depend on screening of plasma for multiple peptide hormones in cases where there are other grounds for suspecting an endocrine or pancreatic tumour.

Carcinoid Tumours

Carcinoid tumours are derived from the argentaffin and argyrophil cells found in tissues of endodermal origin; principally the gastrointestinal, respiratory and urogenital tracts. Two-thirds to three-quarters of the tumours originate from the mid-gut, the appendix being the most common site, and about equal portions of the remainder from the foregut (including the respiratory tract) and the hindgut. Relatively few derive from ovarian teratomas, the urinary tract and the testis.

The occurrence and characteristics of the carcinoid syndrome in individual patients would seem to depend on: (1) the capacity of the tumour and/or metastases to secrete sufficient quantities of biologically active substances to cause symptoms, (2) whether the majority of the secreting tissue is upstream or downstream from the liver and lungs (the principal sites of degradation of serotonin), and (3) on the nature and activities of the secreted substances.

The classical carcinoid syndrome, due to argentaffin mid-gut carcinoids with liver metastases or to primary tumours such as ovarian carcinoids with direct drainage into the systemic circulation, consists of attacks of skin flushing, diarrhoea, and less frequently, bronchoconstriction, with right-sided endocardial fibrosis in long-standing cases. These features vary between patients, and are the subject of detailed textbook descriptions (Kaplan, 1978). The two secretory products of the neoplastic tissue that have been implicated in the causation of the classical syndrome are the monoamine serotonin (5-hydroxytryptamine) and the enzyme kallikrein. The latter generates the potent vasodilator peptide bradykinin from kininogen in the plasma. The short-term and long-term direct and indirect biological effects of serotonin and bradykinin probably account for the major part of the clinical features. Other secretory products may include prostaglandins, histamine (more common in foregut carcinoids), calcitonin, substance P and motilin. These may contribute to the symptomatology, but assessment of this in individual patients has been sporadic, beyond the therapeutic trial of different monoamine receptor or biosynthetic blocking agents.

The atypical or variant carcinoid syndromes are more characteristic of the argyrophil carcinoids of foregut origin, i.e. those of the bronchus, stomach and the so-called carcinoid islet cell tumours of the pancreas and duodenum. Many of these tumours do not secrete sufficient quantities of monoamines into the circulation to cause a carcinoid syndrome, but declare themselves through their secretion of one or more of the whole range of peptides secreted by APUD cells. Peptides that appear relatively often are gastrin, insulin, calcitonin, glucagon, ACTH and other pro-opiomelanocortin-derived peptides; growth hormone releasing factor (GRF) and VIP have also been reported. In fact, the recently determined structure of GRF depended on its isolation from human pancreatic tumours causing acromegaly (Guillemin *et al.*, 1982).

When foregut carcinoids do cause skin flushing, the episodes may be prolonged for up to three or four days, with periorbital oedema, lachrymation and considerable systemic and often neuropsychiatric disturbance. This variant syndrome is particularly associated with bronchial carcinoids. Gastric carcinoids may produce a sharply delineated blotchy red flush, triggered by meals. Foregut carcinoids may lack the decarboxylase necessary to produce serotonin from 5-hydroxytryptophan, so that the latter substance rather than serotonin is released into the circulation. The variant syndromes associated with bronchial and gastric carcinoids have thus been attributed to release of histamine and kallikrein, rather than serotonin.

Hindgut carcinoids most commonly occur in the rectum, but only account for about 1% of cases of carcinoid syndrome. The majority are endocrinologically 'silent', and they are often found incidentally at proctoscopy or sigmoidoscopy, without obvious relationship between the patient's complaints and the presence of the tumour. However, many can be shown by immunocytochemistry to contain a variety of peptides; thus, in one series of 25 tumours, 21 contained identifiable peptide immunoreactivities including pancreatic polypeptide, glucagon, somatostatin, insulin, substance P, leu-enkephalin, and beta-endorphin. Only four of those tumours contained serotonin, and in no case could the patient's symptoms be related to excessive secretion of these peptides (Alumets *et al.*, 1981).

Diagnosis of carcinoid tumours causing endocrine or pharmacological symptoms depends on the physician's awareness of the very wide spectrum of endocrine effects that may occur. Measurement of 24-hour urinary 5-hydroxyindoleacetic acid remains a very useful test, most likely to give elevated values in classical carcinoid syndrome. Serotonin-containing foods (e.g. bananas, tomatoes, avocadoes, aubergines) and some drugs (e.g. phenacetin, now withdrawn) may give falsely high values, and other drugs (phenothiazines, monoamine-oxidase inhibitors, methyldopa and alcohol) may cause low values. Such substances should be avoided before and during urine collections. The test may need to be supplemented by urinary 5-hydroxytryptophan estimations if a decarboxylase-deficient tumour is suspected. Depending on the clinical features, plasma levels of appropriate peptide hormones can be estimated by a specialist laboratory. Provocative tests are not usually necessary, but both oral alcohol and intravenous calcium infusion may produce a severe carcinoid reaction in many patients. So will intravenous adrenaline, but this procedure seems unnecessarily dangerous.

Tumours Producing Other Peptides

It will probably only be a question of time before tumours elaborating any known pharmacologically active, intracellularly produced, mammalian peptide are described. Carcinoid tumours and oat cell bronchial carcinomas are already known to display a particularly wide range. In the latter case, this includes the mammalian bombesin-like peptides found in the brain and intrinsic nervous system of the gut, and in the human fetal lung. Bombesin stimulates the release of a wide range of other regulatory peptides, while apparently suppressing parathyroid hormone release (Ghatei *et al.*, 1982). However, although bombesin-like immunoreactivity has been found in the plasma of a number of patients with oat cell carcinomas, no clinical or biochemical features have related to this with any certainty. Similarly, neurotensin may be secreted by oat cell carcinomas as well as by pancreatic VIPomas, again without obvious clinical correlates. By contrast, pancreatic tumours secreting other active peptides not yet found in the gut (such as antidiuretic hormone, parathyroid hormone and CRF bioactivity) often declare themselves by the appropriate clinical and biochemical findings.

LOCALISATION OF TUMOURS

The non-invasive techniques of ultrasonic and isotope scanning of liver and pancreas, and computerised axial tomography, are used precisely because they are non-invasive. They only detect pancreatic endocrine tumours in about one-third of subsequently confirmed cases (Dunnick *et al.*, 1980), chiefly the minority of larger tumours, and there are often difficulties in interpreting appearances, producing unhelpful or even misleading 'maybe' results. As the planning of treatment will depend on knowledge of whether there are single or multiple tumours, their precise location and whether metastases are present, a more reliable assessment will be required. In practice, this means selective pancreatic and hepatic arteriography. These procedures (with oblique views and magnified subtraction films) currently provide the best chance of accurate pre-operative localisation, but are very dependent on the skill and experience of the radiologist. Even in the best hands, a small proportion of tumours may not be detected. In such cases, help has been sought from percutaneous transhepatic portal and splenic venous sampling, with radioimmunoassay of the appropriate peptides. This difficult and hazardous technique opens up a rich field of possible misinterpretations. There is little information on normal portal venous peptide levels, and tumour secretion may fluctuate during the procedure. Thus, the portal venous concentrations must be compared with simultaneous systemic concentrations for each sampling site. The venous drainage may be anomalous and give an incorrect location for the tumour, even if a definite upward step in the peptide level is detected. Apparent steps in peptide concentration may also occur in the absence of a tumour, or may only reveal one tumour when there are in fact multiple tumours. Because of these difficulties, many clinicians may choose to make their therapeutic decisions without the dubious assistance of this investigation, but their choice will be influenced by the local experience of their clinical centre. Other localisation techniques, including nuclear magnetic resonance scanning, are currently under assessment.

TREATMENT

Curative
Surgical excision offers the only chance of curative therapy for the gut endocrine tumours. However, because of the malignancy of the majority of

the tumours mentioned (insulinomas, discussed in Chapter 5, are the notable exception), the chances of a permanent cure are low. In general, surgery is attempted when symptoms are due to a single (occasionally multiple) resectable primary tumour, without evidence of metastases. This remains the most commonly adopted policy even in the controversial case of gastrinomas, where the high rate of appearance of further primaries or metastases leads to an overall surgical cure rate as low as 5%. Surgical cure rates for pancreatic VIPomas and glucagonomas may be somewhat better, approaching one-third of cases.

Palliative

Because of the slow growth of most of the gut endocrine tumours, palliative treatment is particularly important, and effective palliation can give the patient many years of useful life.

Surgery

Debulking of secretory tumour mass (primary and metastatic) has produced worthwhile symptomatic improvement in cases of gastrinomas, glucagonomas and carcinoid syndrome, and may still be considered when medical means of palliation are failing. However, improved control of symptoms by pharmacological means, particularly in the case of gastrinomas, is reducing the need for this type of surgery. In addition, arterial embolisation of hepatic metastases provides an alternative debulking procedure which can also be used in many cases where surgery would not be attempted.

In the specific case of gastrinomas, vagotomy and drainage may improve the response to H_2-receptor blockade, but the former standard method of palliation by total gastrectomy (a procedure of considerable morbidity and mortality) is now unnecessary in the vast majority of cases because of the very effective control of gastric acid secretion obtained pharmacologically.

Hepatic artery embolisation

Embolisation of hepatic metastases through their arterial supply provides a very effective means of reducing secreting tumour mass, and may be used in cases where surgery or chemotherapy are unsuitable, without precluding subsequent chemotherapy when necessary (Allison, 1978). The technique is carried out under sedation and local anaesthesia, with broad-spectrum antibiotic cover (including metronidazole). Patency of the portal vein is, of course, essential to ensure an adequate blood supply to the liver. Significant symptomatic improvement lasting many months is commonly obtained, and the procedure may be repeated as revascularisation of the metastases occurs. Complications are infrequent, but may include massive release of tumour secretions (usually only a problem in the carcinoid syndrome, where cover with pharmacological blocking agents may be used), or hepatic abscess formation.

Cytotoxic chemotherapy

Although cytotoxic therapy has not, as far as the author knows, been demonstrated to improve survival in patients adequately palliated by surgical or other medical means, cytotoxic chemotherapy should be considered in all persistently symptomatic patients that are beyond hope of surgical cure. Cytotoxic chemotherapy offers the hope of extended remissions, with symptomatic improvement in a significant proportion of patients, sufficiently, in the author's opinion, to justify the immediate toxic effects. The most frequently used agent is streptozotocin, a toxic nitrosourea antibiotic from *Streptomyces achromogenes*. Because this has a specific islet cell toxicity in experimental animals (e.g. producing insulin-dependent diabetes in rats), it was tried in advanced human islet cell carcinomas. Fortunately, it does not seem to produce diabetes in man. The most extensive study reported has been carried out by the Eastern Cooperative Oncology Group in the USA (Moertel *et al.*, 1980). Effects of streptozotocin alone or in combination with 5-fluorouracil were evaluated in 84 patients with a variety of islet cell carcinomas, randomised between the two treatments. Streptozotocin alone produced a 36% overall response rate with 12% complete responses (disappearance of all clinical and laboratory evidence of malignant disease), with significantly better response rates of 63% overall, and 33% complete for streptozotocin plus 5-fluorouracil. The median duration of responses was 17 months (24 months for complete responses), and median survival times were $16\frac{1}{2}$ months with streptozotocin alone and 26 months with the combination; these differences were not statistically significant. With small numbers of each functional type of tumour in the study, no evidence was obtained of a preferential response according to tumour type. The most frequent toxic effects were nausea and vomiting (83–85% of patients), renal toxicity (21–31% of patients), and bone marrow depression (rare with streptozotocin alone). One patient died of acute hepatotoxicity, and one of acute renal failure, but the latter patient had also received renal irradiation. Renal toxicity from streptozotocin (proteinuria, Fanconi syndrome, nephrogenic diabetes insipidus) is usually mild and reversible if a close watch is kept on proteinuria and creatinine clearance, and the dosage reduced or stopped promptly. Streptozotocin was given by rapid intravenous injection of 500 mg/m² daily for five days, these courses being repeated at six-weekly intervals. 5-Fluorouracil was given intravenously at 400 mg/m² with each streptozotocin injection, when used in combination. Close monitoring of haematology, renal and hepatic function is, of course, mandatory; response is assessed clinically, by radiological or scanning measurements of tumour size, and by biochemical measurements including plasma peptide concentrations. Other streptozotocin treatment regimens (e.g. weekly injections) may be equally effective, but may allow the patient little respite from nausea. The five streptozotocin doses constituting one course may be given on alternate days to permit a quicker reaction to the appearance of proteinuria, for which results are not available until the following day.

Although the Eastern Cooperative Oncology Group study did not provide evidence of a selective effect of streptozotocin on different types of pancreatic endocrine tumour, there is evidence from the Hammersmith Hospital (London) of a particularly high response rate of VIPomas to this type of treatment. In a retrospective survey, seven of eight such cases had satisfactory responses to streptozotocin alone (Long *et al.*, 1981).

There are isolated reports of good responses of glucagonomas to dacarbazine (dimethyltriazenoimidazole carboximide, DTIC) when no response to streptozotocin has been obtained. Other agents under trial include chlorozotocin (similar to streptozotocin, but said to induce less nausea), doxorubicin, and for carcinoid syndrome, additional cytotoxic drugs such as cyclophosphamide and methotrexate.

Other palliative measures

Palliation of the biochemical effects of gut endocrine tumours by pharmacological means can often be very effective and skilful manipulation of this type of therapy makes all the difference to the patient's well-being, while definitive treatment is being planned. In some cases it may be the only effective treatment that can be offered.

Gastrinoma: The advent of H_2-receptor blocking agents has been the major advance in treatment of the Zollinger–Ellison syndrome. Those patients that are not controlled by normal or high dosage cimetidine may respond to ranitidine in doses up to 900 mg daily. The latter drug may be preferred because it can be given twice rather than four times daily, and has given rise to fewer reports of side effects such as mental confusion and gynaecomastia. If control is unsatisfactory with ranitidine, an anticholinergic agent may be added. Currently, the most fashionable of these is pirenzepine, at doses of 50 mg twice or thrice daily. This drug is related to the tricyclic antidepressants but has little central nervous effect because of its hydrophilic nature, and offers a degree of specificity for gastric muscarinic receptors. A new drug under trial is omeprazole (H 168/68, Hässle/Astra), a long-acting inhibitor of the H^+/K^+-ATPase of gastric oxyntic cells, which can produce a nearly total inhibition of gastric acid secretion with a single daily dose. Further possibilities include the use of long-acting somatostatin analogues to suppress gastrin secretion; eventually it may be possible to give such analogues orally.

Note that although blockers of gastric acid secretion will produce some elevation of plasma gastrin levels, it is dangerous to withdraw these drugs during the investigation of possible gastrinomas. The hormone assay laboratory should be consulted about the interpretation of results obtained with the patient on therapy.

VIPoma: Intravenous fluid and electrolyte replacement will be required in cases with severe diarrhoea. Antidiarrhoeal agents such as codeine, loperamide and diphenoxylate may have some effect, but this is usually short-lived. Sometimes dopamine antagonists, such as metoclopramide or trifluoperazine, and occasionally prostaglandin synthetase inhibitors, may be effective; sometimes corticosteroids give short-term relief. Here again, long-acting somatostatin analogues are under trial. In general, the poor response of the diarrhoea to pharmacological manipulations but the good response to streptozotocin will incline the physician to early cytotoxic streptozotocin therapy in inoperable cases.

Glucagonoma: Although the diabetes can be treated with oral hypoglycaemic agents in most cases, the possible gastrointestinal side effects of these treatments favour the substitution of insulin. The rash may respond well to oral and topical zinc, intravenous amino acids and parenteral somatostatin. Antibiotics may well have been used before the rash was correctly diagnosed, but these are only appropriate in cases of secondary infection. Aspirin and dipyridamole may be used in an attempt to prevent thrombotic complications.

Carcinoid Tumours: The diarrhoea may be relieved by opiate antidiarrhoeal agents and by the serotonin antagonist methysergide, 2 mg thrice daily. Retroperitoneal fibrosis, which may in any case result from high serotonin levels, is a possible danger with prolonged use of the latter. Parachlorophenylalanine can be used to block serotonin biosynthesis (by inhibiting tryptophan hydroxylase), but may be associated with mental changes. Various pharmacological blocking agents can be tried to relieve skin flushing. Phenoxybenzamine may block flushing in-so-far as this is mediated by adrenergic influences on the tumour, and for forgut carcinoids producing 5-hydroxytryptophan, methyldopa may reduce flushing by blocking peripheral production of serotonin by decarboxylation. Histamine-related flushing may respond to a combination of H_1 and H_2-receptor blockade and prednisolone may be effective in bradykinin mediated flushing from bronchial carcinoids. Bronchoconstriction may respond to β_2-adrenoceptor stimulant inhalations. Patients with carcinoid syndrome may suffer from pellagra due to the diversion of dietary tryptophan to serotonin production, and nicotinamide supplementation 50 mg daily should be given.

CONCLUSION

Gut endocrine tumours have assumed an importance that is quite disproportionate to their low incidence. This is because of their illustration of many of the recent concepts of the molecular mechanisms in peptide hormone production and because study of them has contributed directly to advances in this field. Over the next few years we may expect further advances, for example, from sequencing of cDNA derived from gut tumour mRNA, to give further amino acid sequences of peptide precursors, and greater understanding of post-translational processing of peptide hormones. For this reason, every case should be treated not only as a therapeutic challenge, but also as of great potential scientific importance. This merits very thorough initial investigation in liaison with laboratory colleagues working in the relevant basic sciences, and wherever possible, the delivery of tumour specimens for subsequent biochemical study.

ACKNOWLEDGEMENT

I am very grateful to Dr S.M. Wood for helpful discussions during the planning of this chapter.

REFERENCES

Adrian T.E., Wood S.M., Bloom S.R. (1982). Atropine suppression of pancreatic polypeptide (PP) completely distinguishes tumour PP production from other rises. *Gut*; **23**: A905.

Allison D.J. (1978). Therapeutic embolization. *Br. J. Hosp. Med*; **20**: 707–15.

Alumets J., Alm P., Falkner S. *et al.* (1981). Immunohistochemical evidence of peptide hormones in endocrine tumours of the rectum. *Cancer*; **48**: 2409–15.

Aoyagi T., Summerskill W.H.J. (1966). Gastric secretion with ulcerogenic islet cell tumour. *Arch. Intern. Med*; **117**: 667–72.

Bell G.I., Santerre R.F., Mullenbach G.T. (1983). Hamster preproglucagon contains the sequence of glucagon and two related peptides. *Nature*; **302**: 716–18.

Blackburn A.M., Bryant M.G., Adrian T.E., Bloom S.R. (1981). Pancreatic tumours produce neurotensin. *J. Clin. Endocrinol. Metab*; **52**: 820–2.

Bloom S.R., Christofides N.D., Yiangou Y., Blank M.A., Tatemoto K., Polak J.M. (1983). Peptide histidine isoleucine (PHI) and the Verner–Morrison syndrome. *Gut*; **24**: A473.

Dunnick N.R., Doppman J.L., Mills S.R., McCarthy D.M. (1980). Computed tomographic detection of nonbeta pancreatic islet cell tumours. *Radiology*; **135**: 117–20.

Ganda O.P., Weir G.C., Soeldner J.S. *et al.* (1977). 'Somatostatinoma': A somatostatin-containing tumour of the endocrine pancreas. *N. Engl. J. Med*; **296**: 963–7.

Ghatei M.A., Jung R.T., Stevenson J.C. *et al.* (1982). Bombesin: Action on gut hormones and calcium in man. *J. Clin. Endocrinol. Metab*; **54**: 980–5.

Gregory R.A., Tracy H.J., French J.M., Sircus W. (1960). Extraction of a gastrin-like substance from a pancreatic tumour in a case of Zollinger–Ellison syndrome. *Lancet*; **1**: 1045–8.

Guillemin R., Brazeau P., Böhlen P., Esch F., Ling N., Wehrenberg W.B. (1982). Growth hormone-releasing factor from a human pancreatic tumour that caused acromegaly. *Science*; **218**: 585–7.

Hohmann E.L., Levine L., Tashjian A.H. (1983). Vasoactive intestinal peptide stimulates bones resorption via a cyclic adenosine 3′, 5′-monophosphate-dependent mechanism. *Endocrinology*; **112**: 1233–9.

Kaplan E.L. (1978). The carcinoid syndromes. In *Surgical Endocrinology : Clinical Syndromes* (Friessen S.R., Bolinger R.E., eds.) pp. 120–47. Philadelphia: J.B. Lippincott Company.

Krejs G.J., Orci L., Conlon J.M. *et al.* (1979). Somatostatinoma syndrome: Biochemical, morphologic and clinical features. *N. Engl. J. Med*; **301**: 285–92.

Larsson L.-I., Hirsch M.A., Holst J.J. *et al.* (1977). Pancreatic somatostatinoma: Clinical features and physiological implications. *Lancet*; **1**: 666–8.

Long R.G., Bryant M.G., Mitchell S.J., Adrian T.E., Polak J.M., Bloom S.R. (1981). Clinicopathological study of pancreatic and ganglioneuroblastoma tumours secreting vasoactive intestinal polypeptide (VIPomas). *Br. Med. J*; **282**: 1767–71.

Mallinson C.N., Bloom S.R., Warin A.P., Salmon P.R., Cox B. (1974). A glucagonoma syndrome. *Lancet*; **2**: 1–5.

McGavran M.H., Unger R.H., Recant L., Polk H.C., Kilo C., Levin M.E. (1966). A glucagon-secreting alpha-cell carcinoma of the pancreas. *N. Engl. J. Med*; **274**: 1408–13.

Moertel C.G., Hanley J.A., Johnson L.A. (1980). Streptozotocin alone compared with streptozotocin plus fluorouracil in the treatment of advanced islet-cell carcinoma. *N. Engl. J. Med*; **303**: 1189–94.

Öberg K., Grimelius L., Lundqvist G., Lörelius L.-E. (1981). Update on pancreatic polypeptide as a specific marker for endocrine tumours of the pancreas and gut. *Acta Med. Scand*; **210**: 145–52.

Pearse A.G.E. (1968). Common cytochemical and ultrastructural characteristics of cells producing polypeptide hormones (the *APUD* series) and their relevance to thyroid and ultimobranchial C cells and calcitonin. *Proc. R. Soc. Lond. [Biol]*; **170**: 71–80.

Polak J.M., Bloom S.R., Adrian T.E., Heitz P. Bryant M.G., Pearse A.G.E. (1976). Pancreatic polypeptide in insulinomas, gastrinomas, vipomas, and gluca-gonomas. *Lancet*; **1**: 328–30.

Stacpoole P.W. (1981). The glucagonoma syndrome: Clinical features, diagnosis, and treatment. *Endocrine Rev*; **2**: 347–61.

Stage J.G., Stadil F. (1979). The clinical diagnosis of the Zollinger–Ellison syndrome. *Scand. J. Gastroenterol*; **14**: Suppl 53: 79–91.

Verner J.V., Morrison A.B. (1958). Islet cell tumour and a syndrome of refractory watery diarrhea and hypokalemia. *Am. J. Med*; **25**: 375–80.

Zollinger R.M., Ellison E.H. (1955). Primary peptic ulcerations of the jejunum associated with islet cell tumours of the pancreas. *Ann. Surg*; **142**: 709–23.

Chapter 12

R. Timothy D. Oliver & Jonathan H. Waxman

Gonadal and Genito-urinary Cancer

Endocrine problems in the context of the management of genito-urinary malignancies arise both from the tumour and its cure. Cancers originating from genito-urinary tumours may cause endocrine effects due to excessive production of either normal or ectopic hormones. In addition, because tumour induction and treatment damages the normal gonad, expertise is required in the recognition and treatment of the gonadal failure that results.

This chapter will review the endocrine problems seen in patients with ovarian, testicular, prostatic, renal and bladder tumours, ending with a discussion of the frequency of the clinical problem of inappropriate hormone production in this group of malignancies.

OVARIAN CANCER

Introduction

Ovarian cancer is the second most frequent malignancy of women and caused 3784 deaths in England and Wales in 1978 (Mortality Statistics: Cause). The WHO classification defines adult tumours according to their cellular origin, i.e. epithelial, sex cord stromal tissue, germ cells and lipid cells. Ovarian epithelial tumours constitute 80–90% of all cases. The limited success of current conventional therapy is striking, with less than 10% of patients surviving four years (Cancer Statistics: Registrations, 1974, 1982), predominantly because only 30% have localised disease at presentation (Julian and Woodruff, 1969). Treatment mainly involves a combination of chemotherapy and surgical debulking of the residual tumour masses. Despite the encouragingly frequent initial response to chemotherapy, this approach has been associated with no real improvement in survival (Tobias and Griffiths, 1976). The frequency of publications on the use of chemotherapy contrasts with relative paucity of information regarding the hormonal therapy of this tumour of an endocrine organ.

Epidemiology

The epidemiology of ovarian cancer shows a striking parallel to that of breast cancer, which would support the idea that there might be similar endocrine factors involved in causation of both tumours. Breast cancer predisposes to a two-fold increased risk of the development of ovarian cancer, whilst carcinoma of the ovary increases the chance of breast cancer by three to four times (Lingeman, 1974). The incidence of cancer of the ovary increases with age, apart from a decrease at 50–54 years and this is a feature of breast cancer in those countries with a high incidence of the disease. Ovarian cancer exhibits a similar racial variation to that of breast cancer, occurring with the greatest frequency in Caucasians and with the least frequency in Japanese (Haenszel and Kurihara, 1967). In both malignancies an environmental factor is suggested by the increased incidence, respectively, of ovarian and breast cancer in Japanese migrants to Hawaii and California (Buell and Dunn, 1965). Carcinoma of the ovary is classically described in nulliparous women and, just as is described for breast cancer, there is an inverse relationship between parity and the risk of development of ovarian cancer (Newhouse *et al.*, 1977). It is not obvious whether an ambience of low fertility predisposes to ovarian cancer, or that women with ovarian cancer are less fertile than matched control groups. Although the association between parity and ovarian cancer suggests that oestrogen deficiency predisposes to this malignancy, this approach is simplistic as there is a suggestion that non-contraceptive oestrogen usage is associated with an increase in the incidence of a rare subgroup (endometriod) of epithelial carcinoma of the ovary (Weiss *et al.*, 1982).

Hormone Receptors

The parallel with breast cancer continues with the finding of hormone receptors within the cytosols of ovarian tumour cells. Ovarian carcinoma contains high affinity, low capacity receptors for oestradiol, progesterone, dihydrotestosterone, follicle stimulating hormone, luteinising hormone, and human chorionic gonadotrophin. The frequency of occurrence of hormone receptors is less in secondary than in primary tumours. Fifty per cent of ovarian adenocarcinoma primary tumours contain receptors for both oestradiol and progesterone, whilst 33% of secondary tumours contain oestradiol receptors (Holt *et al.*, 1979). Androgen receptors are common and, in a series of ovarian malignancies of varied histology, 88% contained receptors for dihydrotestosterone (Hamilton *et al.*, 1981). Binding of both oestradiol and dihydrotestosterone may occur within the same tumour, and has no correlation with histological differentiation. Receptors for the pituitary gonadotrophins have been demonstrated in a variety of histological subtypes; receptors for follicle stimulating hormone occur in epithelial tumours as well as in sex cord-stromal tumours (Kammerman *et al.*, 1981). *In vitro*, follicle stimulating hormone and human chorionic gonadotrophin have both been shown to bind to ovarian adenocarcinoma cell receptors, promoting cyclic AMP production within them. Human chorionic gonadotrophin was found to promote testosterone production by a thecoma (Givens *et al.*, 1975). It is of interest that these hormones, in addition to their ability to regulate cellular steroidogenesis from tumour cells, are able to regulate their receptor number within these cells. Prolonged exposure of cultured Leydig tumour cells to human chorionic gonadotrophin, results in a decrease in hormone binding because of a reduction in receptor numbers (Freeman and Ascoli, 1981). The observation of hormone receptors in these tumours raises the possibility of using hormones therapeutically.

Hormone Production by Ovarian Tumours

The dramatic clinical effects produced by excessive normal hormone production, seen in the rare virilising and feminising ovarian sex cord tumours, are well known. Steroid metabolism has been examined in these tumours and found to depend upon an identical metabolic pathway. The difference in clinical effect, results from different peripheral conversion of the pathway's product (Mandel *et al.*, 1981). The epithelial ovarian carcinoma constitutes 80–90% of all ovarian tumours. It is rare for them to be associated with normal or ectopic hormone production, though occasional tumours produce clinically evident endocrine effects. The Zollinger–Ellison syndrome has been described, resulting from gastrin production by a cystadenocarcinoma (Bollen *et al.*, 1981). These rare presentations have diverted attention from the hormonal features of the commoner ovarian epithelial carcinomas. In one study, there were significantly higher serum concentrations of oestrone and oestradiol in patients with cancer than in matched control groups (Heinonen *et al.*, 1982). That oestrogenic steroid production is a function of tumour activity was noted in a prospective study, where urinary steroid excretion was observed pre- and post-operatively. High 24-hour urinary oestrogen excretion was noted in 70% of patients with mucinous tumours and 4% of patients with serous ovarian carcinoma. Post-operatively, oestrogen excretion fell in 13 of 16 patients. Two patients in whom oestrogen excretion remained elevated post-operatively were demonstrated to have residual tumour (Rome *et al.*, 1981).

Pituitary and Hypothalamic Interactions with Ovarian Tumours

Only in a few patients has the relationship between higher hormonal controlling centres and ovarian cancer been investigated. Normal basal and dynamic gonadotrophin levels have been observed in two patients with ovarian cancer and nine patients with serous cystadenoma (Ylikorkala *et al.*, 1974). Normal sensitivity to hypothalamic control has been demonstrated in the rare 'functioning' tumours. Isolated androblastoma cells exhibit a diminution in testosterone synthesis when a gonadotrophin-hormone releasing-hormone agonist is added to the culture medium (Lamberts *et al.*, 1982).

The Endocrine Treatment of Ovarian Cancer

Apart from the preceding epidemiological and hormone receptor studies, data from *in vitro* studies support the hypothesis that these tumours may be hormone responsive. The effect of oestradiol and progesterone upon DNA synthesis by ovarian cancer cells was assessed following exposure to combinations of different concentrations of these adrenal steroids. Deoxyribonucleic acid synthesis was inhibited by these hormones and the inhibition was maximal when the tumour cells were incubated with any mixture containing both 17β-oestradiol and progesterone (Darwish, 1978). In one early study of the use of oestrogens, approximately 15% of patients with advanced disease were observed to respond to diethylstilboestrol (Long and Evans, 1963). Recent interest has been directed towards progesterone therapy; an overview in 1976 suggested a cumulative response rate of 38% in 60 patients (Tobias and Griffiths, 1976). However, this order of response has not been found in recent programmes, where medroxyprogesterone acetate is given in high dosages intramuscularly, initially daily, then weekly. With this type of regimen, remission occurs at best, in 15% of patients (Mangioni *et al.*, 1981) but may only be in 5% (Slayton *et al.*, 1981).

The presence in ovarian cancer of cytoplasmic hormone receptors, particularly that for 17β-oestradiol, suggests that an approach using anti-oestrogens might be more effective than progesterone therapy. The report of significant tumour regression in three patients with advanced serous cystadenocarcinoma treated with tamoxifen (Myers *et al.*, 1981), suggests that this approach requires further investigation.

Future Prospects

Because of the parallels demonstrated with breast cancer, one might expect that the hormonal therapy of ovarian cancer might be as successful. So far it has not been so, though the best approach suggested by *in vitro* studies, i.e. using a combination of oestrogen and progestogen has, at the time of writing, not been tested. Equally important will be larger scale investigations using tamoxifen to attempt to confirm an earlier encouraging result. The presence of gonadotrophin receptors is of interest, and their relevance as in breast and prostatic cancer may be to the future use of gonadotrophin-hormone releasing-hormone analogues in the management of ovarian cancer.

PROSTATIC CANCER

Prostatic cancer is very common in Western society. At post-mortem, depending on the number of sections examined, it can be demonstrated in up to 40% of all prostates, though only one-third of these were clinically evident (Catalona and Scoff, 1978). In the UK in 1976 it affected 7510 men (Cancer Statistics, 1982) and caused the death of 4611 (Mortality Statistics, 1978). That carcinoma of the prostate is responsive to endocrine manipulation has been known since 1941, when Charles Huggins reported evidence of tumour response after orchidectomy in 80–90% of patients. The rationale for this response remains obscure, as the simplistic interpretation of the effect of endocrine manipulation (i.e. that it is simply a question of lack of testosterone drive which causes tumour regression) is not supported by the observation that the lowest dose of diethylstilboestrol known to produce response in this condition (1 mg/day) does not suppress testosterone levels.

Endocrine Studies in Patients with Carcinoma of the Prostate

Patients presenting with prostatic cancer do not have any consistent endocrine abnormality. Gross measurements of serum prolactin, follicle stimulating hormone, luteinising hormone, growth hormone, testosterone and 17β-oestradiol reveal no difference between age matched controls and patients with carcinoma of the prostate. The only possible significant observation from these studies is that patients with advanced metastatic prostatic cancer, show increased levels of growth hormone in comparison with normal men, and men whose cancer is confined to the prostate (British Prostate Study Group, 1979). In the hypophysectomised rat, growth hormone has been shown to act synergistically with testosterone to promote prostatic growth (Chase *et al.*, 1957). This synergy, if it occurred in man, might explain the above observation and provide a more compelling justification for the use of hypophysectomy at an early stage in the management of patients with prostatic cancer than at present.

Hormonal factors involved in normal prostate growth are equally poorly understood. In the rat, androstenedione induces hypertrophic change; on its own 17β-oestradiol does not, though it does potentiate the effect of androstenedione (Walsh *et al.*, 1976). Such a mechanism may explain the aetiology of benign hypertrophy in man, but not carcinoma. More relevant might be a study of hormone production rates and tissue concentration. However, when androstenedione and testosterone levels are studied in both normal and hypertrophic glands they show similar tissue concentrations and, in addition, conversion rates of testosterone to dihydrotestosterone are equal. Although assessment of hormone concentrations and conversion rates have not been performed in carcinomatous tissue, reduced urinary androgen and increased urinary oestrogen metabolites have been demonstrated in patients with prostatic cancer, despite plasma hormone levels similar to the control group (Shteri *et al.*, 1970).

Even production rates do not reflect the true state of the prostate, as the presence of cytoplasmic receptor proteins in the prostate makes these turnover studies and plasma hormone levels irrelevant to the situation in the gland. These receptor proteins are for dihydrotestosterone and 17β-oestradiol. They are located in the stromal rather than the epithelial compartment of the prostate (Chassiri and Pierrepoint, 1979). Perhaps the most important observation as far as management of patients is concerned is the suggestion from a preliminary study of the androgen receptor that the levels of this receptor can be used to predict the chance of response to endocrine manipulation (Ekman *et al.*, 1979).

Endocrine Effect of Therapy in Carcinoma of the Prostate

Orchidectomy

Although the short-term effects of orchidectomy upon carcinoma of the prostate are dramatic, and prolonged as compared to the remission achieved by chemotherapy, the duration of response is limited. There is no evidence that orchidectomy produces indefinite control of metastases by destruction of tumour stem cells. The five-year survival of stage IV patients remains at 20%, and of stage III patients at 50% (Resnick and Grayhack, 1975). Both total and subcapsular orchidectomy are equally effective in reducing concentrations of testosterone, and result in equivalent elevations of pituitary gonadotrophins (Clark and Houghton, 1977). With both procedures testosterone falls by 95%. The remaining source of production is the adrenal, and it is thought that an increase in adrenal production of testosterone may be a principal cause of tumour escape from endocrine control.

Diethyl stilboestrol

Seventy to eighty per cent of patients with stage IV disease, respond to diethylstilboestrol. Its effects are not clearly related to changes in plasma hormone levels. At dosages higher than 3 mg daily, in both responding and non-responsive patients, testosterone levels fall to castrate range, growth hormone and prolactin rise, whilst follicle stimulating hormone and luteinising hormone fall (Boyne *et al.*, 1974). At lower doses of diethylstilboestrol (1 mg/day) the response rate is equivalent to that seen with higher dose regimens, though at these lower levels, the changes in plasma hormone concentrations, although they occur, are not nearly so marked, and responding patients may have testosterone levels within the normal range (Catalona and Scott, 1978). The importance of changes in gonadotrophin levels to response is uncertain because chlorotrianisene, a synthetic oral oestrogen which suppresses testosterone levels without affecting gonadotrophins, can induce a response (Baker *et al.*, 1973). Diethylstilboestrol is thought to act by direct suppression of gonadotrophin production at a hypothalamic level (Franchimont, 1977). There is still debate whether even at the proper dose level diethylstilboestrol does influence overall survival or is more effective than orchidectomy. In early studies comparing orchidectomy and high dose diethylstilboestrol there were cardiovascular deaths with high dose regimens, leading to a decreased survival in the diethylstilboestrol group (Veterans Administration Cooperative Urological Research Group, 1967). As cardiovascular deaths are lower in the low dose diethylstilboestrol regimen it is possible that this may be more effective than orchidectomy. The question as to whether treatment should be employed before or with the onset of symptoms is still unresolved.

Secondary Endocrine Manipulation

Relapse from primary endocrine control may represent the selection and overgrowth of cell lines that are hormonally independent, whilst hormone dependent clones remain controlled. This hypothesis is supported by the observation that relapse occurs despite 'adequate' suppression of testosterone. However, relapsed prostatic cancer is sensitive to secondary hormonal manipulation, as demonstrated below. Until recently, routine endocrine investigation of such patients to establish adequate suppression of testosterone was not the rule, and reports on more detailed endocrine investigation of relapsed patients and their response to secondary treatment are urgently needed.

Adrenalectomy

Although the testis is the major source of testosterone, some 5% of circulating testosterone is derived from the adrenal. It is in an attempt to completely eliminate extratesticular production of androgen that adrenalectomy is performed to control the advance of prostatic cancer.

Surgical adrenalectomy

Surgical adrenalectomy is a major operative procedure with a significant mortality and morbidity. Because of these risks in a population frequently not in prime surgical condition, this procedure is not widely practised.

Although surgical adrenalectomy produces no advantage in terms of prolongation of life, as a secondary salvage procedure it is effective. It was first introduced as a treatment for carcinoma of the prostate by Charles Huggins in the 1940s. The hormonal basis for response remains unknown, and in those 30% of patients objectively responding, no changes in testosterone levels are observed. Pain relief may be seen in up to 86% of patients, whilst mean survival post-adrenalectomy ranges between six months and one year (Bhanalaph *et al.*, 1974; Brendler, 1973).

Medical adrenalectomy

Aminoglutethimide was originally introduced as an anti-epileptic, and observed to be a selective adrenal poison. Its effect upon the adrenal is cumulative, occurring two to three months after initial use. It is ineffective in producing complete adrenal suppression. Aminoglutethimide has two main modes of action. It blocks adrenal cortical synthesis of steroids at the level of conversion of cholesterol to 5-pregnenolone, and peripheral aromatisation of androstenedione to oestrone (Santen *et al.*, 1978). A high incidence of subjective response has been observed with up to 60% of patients having some relief of bone pain, though objective response with reduction in acid phosphatase and healing of bone secondaries is less usual (Sanford *et al.*, 1976; Worgul *et al.*, 1983). At the higher doses used initially the frequency of side effects (nausea, drowsiness, skin rash and hypotension) outweighed the clinical benefit. Currently, studies are in progress using a lower dosage schedule (125 mg b.d.) and comparing its activity with the use of replacement corticosteroid alone, which also suppresses adrenal steroid synthesis.

Hypophysectomy

Hypophysectomy, whether performed as an open procedure, by the transphenoidal route, by cryosurgery or by interstitial irradiation, may provide useful palliation of symptoms in up to 75% of patients with disseminated disease (Silverberg, 1977). Though remission is usually short, it occurs in both endocrine non-responders and relapsed endocrine responders (Brendler, 1973).

Testosterone

Remarkably, one patient with advanced disease showed prolonged response to androgen administration though for the majority, testosterone induces rapid deterioration (Prout and Brewers, 1967).

Cyproterone acetate

This compound has four main modes of action. It is a progestogen and inhibits the release of the pituitary gonadotrophins, it inhibits the formation of the nuclear androgen complex, diminishes testosterone synthesis by Leydig cells, and displaces testosterone from its cytoplasmic receptor (Neumann, 1977). By these means, testosterone levels fall and its peripheral actions are suppressed. There is no evidence that cyproterone acetate is more effective than diethylstilboestrol in the management of carcinoma of the prostate (Tunn *et al.*, 1983), though in the EORTC and British Prostate Group trials the lower incidence of cardiovascular complications and gynaecomastia makes it an important though expensive alternative to diethylstilboestrol or orchidectomy. The combination of orchidectomy plus cyproterone acetate has been widely used in Italy. There is no evidence that its routine use after orchidectomy improves on what can be achieved by using cyproterone acetate as salvage treatment for patients who fail to respond or progress after initial response to orchidectomy.

Tamoxifen

This compound, of use in the management of breast cancer, acts by displacing oestrogen from its cytoplasmic receptor. The presence of oestrogen receptors in prostatic cancer therefore prompted a study of tamoxifen in this disease. Though 23% of patients responded to therapy with either an objective or good partial response, the duration of remission was short, ranging from 6 to 23 weeks (Glick *et al.*, 1980).

Gonadotrophin-releasing hormone analogues

Approximately 700 analogues of gonadotrophin-releasing hormone have been elaborated (Coy and Schally, 1978). Analogues with activity greater than the parent compound, i.e. superactive, were produced by substitution at positions six or ten of the basic molecule. These compounds were originally applied to the hypogonadal in the hope that puberty would be induced; this failed (Brook and Dombey, 1979). With their repeated administration to animals, puberty was observed to be suppressed and sexual maturity reversed (Tcholakian *et al.*, 1978). The effect is at the level of the pituitary where gonadotrophin receptors respond to the pulsatile release of endogenous gonadotrophin-releasing hormone (Belchetz *et al.*, 1978). The so-called superactive gonadotrophin-releasing hormone analogues have extended half-lives, and their prolonged binding renders the pituitary unresponsive (Smith and Crighton, 1978). Thus, after initial stimulation there is down regulation of the gonadotrophins and gonadal hormones (Bergquist *et al.*, 1979). Most experience using these analogues in

Europe has been with Buserelin (d ser⁶TBU GnRH ethylamine). Although there is interest in this compound as a contraceptive, and its use is under investigation, its role as an alternative to diethylstilboestrol or orchidectomy in patients with metastatic carcinoma of the prostate is also under investigation. Evidence of profound suppression of testosterone in such patients receiving intranasal Buserelin has been established, and a response rate similar to conventional treatment has been demonstrated, though follow-up is too short to establish the duration of response (Waxman *et al.*, 1983).

Future Prospects

There has been no change in the prognosis of patients with advanced metastatic carcinoma of the prostate in the 38 years since Huggins first demonstrated the effects of endocrine manipulation in patients with this tumour. However, recent research and clinical trials have given a better understanding of the disease and enabled more reasoned strategy in the use of endocrine manipulation. The recent development of cyproterone acetate and gonadotrophin-releasing hormone analogues offers the prospects of further reduction in the side effects of treatment.

TESTICULAR TUMOURS

In contrast to the ovary, where 80–90% of tumours are epithelial and 5–10% germ cell, 90% of testicular tumours are of germ cell origin. Though undoubtedly rarer than ovarian epithelial tumours, germ cell tumours of the testis are the most frequent malignant disease in males in the age range of 15–40 (Registrar General, 1968–1970), and their incidence has been increasing continuously since the beginning of this century (Davies, 1981).

Epidemiology

The only established risk factor for this disease is cryptorchidism, with the risk for patients with maldescent as far as the inguinal canal being 15 times the risk of an individual with normally descended testicles, but for an individual with an abdominal undescended testicles, the risk is 40 times increased (Whitaker, 1980).

Prematurity and maternal ingestion of oestrogen during gestation are two factors increasingly recognised as important in the aetiology of maldescent and recent reports are also suggesting that they may be a factor in the aetiology of testicular tumours (Henderson *et al.*, 1979).

The risk of tumour is also increased for the normally descended testis in individuals with unilaterally descended testicle and descent of the testis into the scrotum by the age of 10 does not protect from the risk of malignancy (Whitaker, 1980). This has led to attempts to get the testis into the scrotum at increasingly earlier age, such that it is now routine to suggest that it should be attempted by the age of 5. There has been some success by giving courses of hormone treatment at this age (Happ *et al.*, 1974; Athanasio *et al.*, 1974), but the majority still require surgical intervention. The recognition that surgical trauma can abrogate any advantage of early surgery, because of the small size of the vessels at this age, has led to increasing use of microsurgical techniques to enable transplantation of the testis to the scrotum with anastomosis to a neighbouring blood vessel.

It will take another 20 years before it will be clear whether early surgical intervention has had any influence on the incidence of tumours. However, an early indicator of success will be elimination of the 50% incidence of azoospermia seen in individuals with unilateral undescended testicle at puberty (Hecker and Heinz, 1967).

From the above discussion it is clear that prenatal influences are obviously important in the aetiology of testis tumours. Whether the increased risk of tumours in undescended testis is purely a mechanical problem is far from clear, because of the high incidence of tumours in the contralateral testis in patients with unilateral maldescent. However, the demonstration that unilateral damage can produce autoimmune destruction of the contralateral testis (Harrison *et al.*, 1981), and the anecdotal suggestion that trauma may be an aetiological factor in man, do not entirely exclude a mechanical factor. Our own retrospective study of patients and casualty department controls, however, showed no difference in incidence of severe trauma (Oliver *et al.*, 1984). The only possibly new aetiological factor discovered in this study was the observation of a 9% incidence of relapsing herpes genitalis in patient population, compared to 0.8% in the control population. The knowledge that this class of virus is important in other malignancies (Galloway and McDougall, 1983) does justify more detailed serological and DNA biochemical investigation of patients with this type of tumour for evidence of infection with herpes genitalis.

Endocrine Changes in Patients with Germ Cell Tumours

The observation that at presentation two-thirds of patients with testicular germ cell tumours have lower than normal sperm counts, and nearly a quarter azoospermia (Fig. 12.1), associated with altered endocrine profiles (Table 12.1), has prompted speculation that a factor causing widespread damage to the germinal epithelium could be a precursor of testicular tumours. This hypothesis is supported by the observation that the incidence of testicular tumours is higher in males investigated for infertility, and the discovery the between 0.1 and 0.5% of biopsies from infertile men have atypical germ cells, thought to represent *in situ* carcinoma (Krabbe *et al.*,

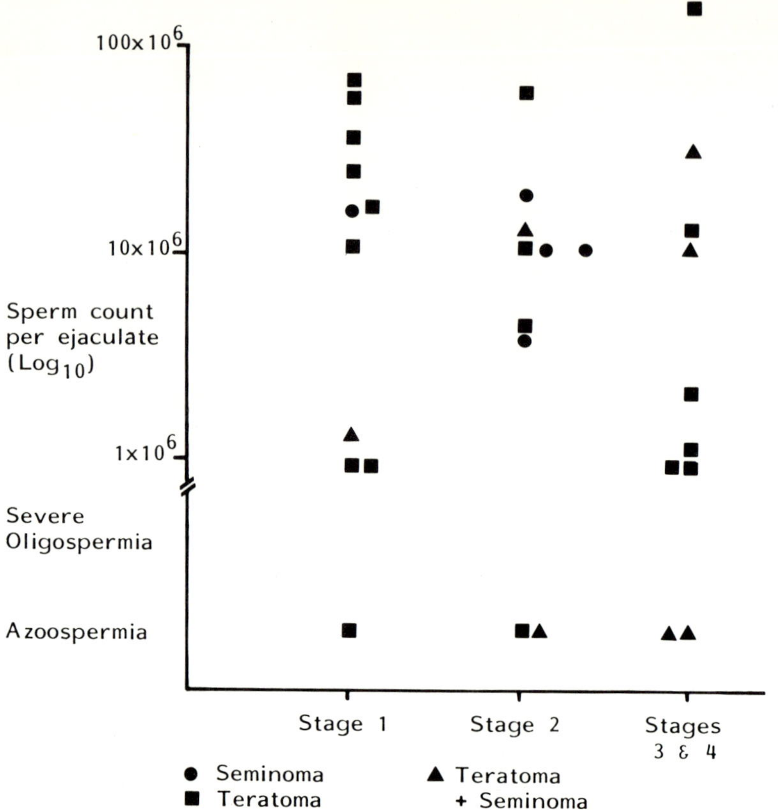

Fig. 12.1. *Pre-treatment sperm count in patients with testicular tumours.*

TABLE 12.1

Testis Tumours: Gonadal Function Pre-chemotherapy

Patient initials	Sperm count per ejaculate	FSH (u/litre)	LH (u/litre)	Prolactin (mu/litre)	Testo-sterone (nmol/litre)	Oestradiol (pmol/litre)
MS	88×10^6	5.5	7.3	—	—	290
IV	13×10^6	9.2	4.5	279	21	123
SR	81×10^6	7.4	12.0	—	—	—
DC	11×10^6	5.1	8.1	322	9	152
MB	32×10^6	6.9	5.9	276	22	145
CS	0	26.0	47.0	224	16	304
JW	0	3.3	26.0	706	20	—
JS	$< 0.2 \times 10^6$	9.8	12.8	368	21	186
JW	0	5.3	27.0	633	23	416

CONCERT IN AID OF THE ROYAL FREE HOSPITAL
BREAST CANCER APPEAL

NEW SANDLER PALM COURT TRIO

with

GRAHAM CLARK *tenor*

and

JOAN LAWRENCE *soprano*

at 7.30 p.m.

Saturday 12th January 1985

ST. JUDE'S CHURCH

Central Square, Hampstead Garden Suburb, London · N.W.11

1979). Fifty per cent of patients with the changes of *in situ* carcinoma have progressed to develop a germ cell tumour within five years (Berthelsen *et al.*, 1979).

The only other endocrinological factor of importance is the occurrence of gynaecomastia as an early clinical sign of testicular malignancy. This has been the presenting sign in nine of 120 patients treated by our department in the last four years, though its occurrence does not necessarily indicate metastases. Two of these patients had azoospermia, elevated gonado-trophins and elevated serum oestrogen, whilst the remaining seven had metastatic trophoblastic teratoma with elevated serum β-HCG. Four of these patients were grossly mismanaged, with a delay in diagnosis of up to two years. Though there are more frequently occurring benign causes of gynaecomastia, the prolonged delay in these cases indicates a need for better education of doctors of the seriousness of the condition and the need for the patient's testicles to be examined and the serum β-HCG level assessed.

Treatment

The success of modern chemotherapy today leads to more than 85% of patients presenting with germ cell tumours of the testis being free of disease at five years. Even for patients with established metastases, experience in handling the toxic chemotherapy regimens has led to improvement in survival rate from 60 to 80% (Einhorn, 1981; Oliver, 1982). Prior to the modern chemotherapy era there was one report on the use of medroxy-progesterone acetate to treat terminal patients with evidence of response in two cases (Bloom and Hendry, 1973), though other workers from the same centre were unable to confirm these observations (Smithers, 1972).

With this success, post-treatment assessment of normal tissue damage has become increasingly important. Though there has been no investigation of other endocrine organs it is clear that there are major effects on the testis. Spermatogenesis is non-existent early after treatment, but in a substantial proportion there is some recovery within two years (Fig. 12.2) (Drasaga *et al.*, 1983). This has been associated with the birth of normal children, though the endocrine profiles on these patients are far from normal (Table 12.2). In addition, about 5% develop gynaecomastia after treatment, associated with elevated FSH and LH, oestrogens, but normal HCG and no evidence of metastases. This can be controlled by giving androgen supplements.

Future Developments

The observation of testis tumours arising in infertile men, and the low sperm counts in patients with tumours at presentation, will be important areas for

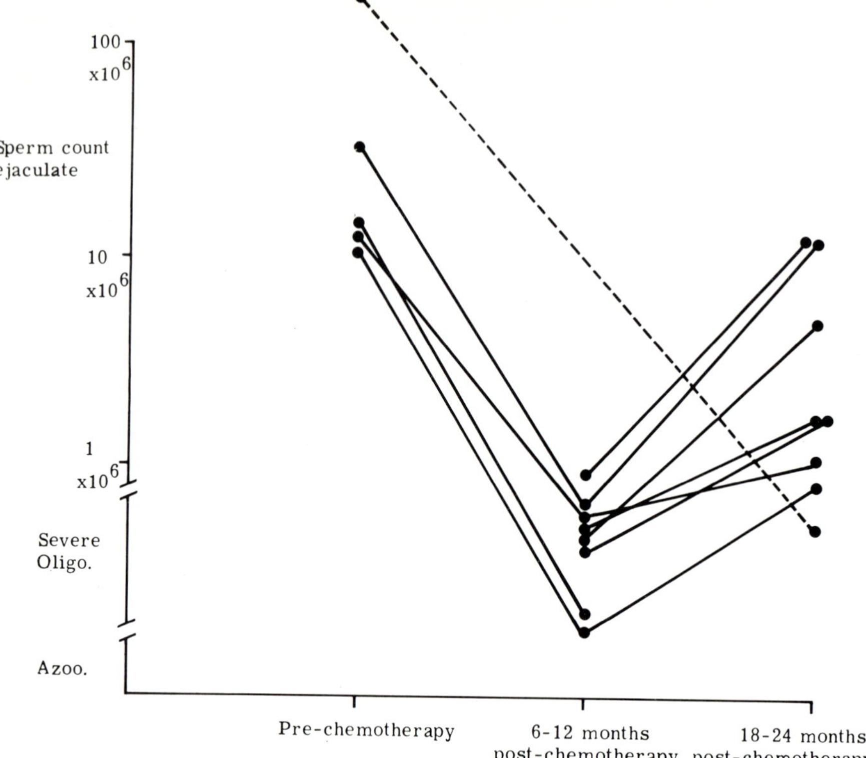

Fig. 12.2. *Sperm counts in patients on cisplatinum combination therapy.*

TABLE 12.2

Testis Tumours: Gonadal Function at Two Years Post-chemotherapy

Patient initials	Sperm count per ejaculate	FSH u/litre	LH u/litre	Prolactin mu/litre	Testosterone nmol/litre	Oestradiol pmol/litre
DK	3×10^6	16	29	322	20	414
JM	120×10^6	11	—	—	—	—
SK	32×10^6	11	7	212	20	—
DW	29×10^6	12	9	149	—	—
RM	8×10^6	17	15	582	—	—
BR	$< 0.2 \times 10^6$	22	39	—	26	161
BA	$< 0.2 \times 10^6$	17	7	146	18	152

future investigation, as they may provide important information on early factors in the cause of this disease. A small percentage of patients with testis tumours and low sperm counts at diagnosis have suppression of the contralateral gonad by a tumour product. There is some evidence that sperm counts return to a higher level in these patients post-treatment than in patients with normal counts prior to treatment (Hendry *et al.*, 1983). Currently, studies are in progress using gonadotrophin-releasing hormone analogues to switch off sperm production in patients with Hodgkin's disease to try to protect the gonad from damage by chemotherapy treatment, and this may be of benefit for patients with testis tumours undergoing chemotherapy.

RENAL PARENCHYMAL TUMOURS

Since the demonstration in hamsters (Bloom, 1972) that oestrogen can induce renal tumours and progesterone can suppress their growth, two decades of the use of medroxyprogesterone acetate as a relatively harmless though expensive placebo for patients with terminal metastatic disease have witnessed the response rate to this treatment falling from 17 to 3%, which is probably less than the chance of spontaneous remission (Oliver *et al.*, 1984). A recent publication of the use of this drug as an adjuvant has demonstrated worse survival than in a control population (Pizzocoro, 1983).

Ectopic Hormone Production and Genito-urinary Tumours

Polycythaemia in patients with renal tumours results from tumours of erythropoietin-producing cells. This is not commonly seen terminally, and it may either be that these tumours should not be regarded as very malignant or that erythropoietin production capability is lost as the tumour develops.

Symptomatic hypercalcaemia is frequent in renal cell cancer, and occurs more frequently than in bladder, prostate, or testis tumours (Table 12.3).

TABLE 12.3

Clinically Evident Endocrinopathies in Terminally Ill Patients with Metastatic Genito-urinary Tumours

Site	Number of patients	Hypercalcaemia	Gynaecomastia	Polycythaemia
Testis	23	1	4	0
Bladder	36	3	2	0
Prostate	12	0	0	0
Kidney	21	5	0	0

Though gynaecomastia has been reported anecdotally in patients with bladder cancer, the occurrence of two cases in 36, one of whom had an HCG of 1×10^6 iu/litre, suggests that it will be interesting to study HCG levels more frequently in such terminal patients.

CONCLUSIONS

This chapter has demonstrated important areas of interest for endocrinologists in all of the tumours discussed. The most important observation needing wider dissemination is the need for prompter investigations of young males in the 18 to 40 age group, who present with gynaecomastia as the first indication of an HCG-producing, trophoblastic, germ cell tumour of the testis. In addition, further evaluation of the endocrine treatment of patients with epithelial tumours of the ovary, and more detailed investigation of the mechanisms of response and relapse in patients with prostatic cancer is suggested.

REFERENCES

Athanasio A., Jendricke K., Bierich J.R. (1974). Clinical and hormonal effect of HCG in prepubertal cryptorchid boys. *J. Endocrinol*; **63**: 50.

Baker H.W.G., Burger H.G., de Kretser D.M., Hudson B., Stratton W.G. (1973). Effects of synthetic oral oestrogens in normal men and men with prostatic carcinoma. Lack of gonadotrophin suppression by chlorotrianisone. *Clin. Endocrinol*; **2**: 297–306.

Belchetz P.E., Plant T.M., Nakai Y., Keogh E.J., Knobil E. (1978). Hypophysial responses to continuous and intermittent delivery of hypothalamic gonadotrophin releasing hormone. *Science*; **202**: 631–2.

Bergquist C., Nilius S.J., Bergh T., Skarin G., Wide L. (1979). Inhibitory effects on gonadotrophin secretion and gonadal function in men during chronic treatment with a potent stimulatory LHRH analogue. *Acta Endocrinologia*; **91**: 601–608.

Berthelsen J.G., Skakkebaek N.E., Mogenson P., Sorenson B.L. (1979). Incidence of carcinoma *in situ* of germ cells. *Brit. Med. J*; **2**: 363–4.

Bhanalph T., Varkarakis M.J., Murphy G.P. (1974). Current status of bilateral adrenalectomy on advanced prostatic carcinoma. *Annals of Surgery*; **179**: 17–23.

Bloom H.J.G. (1972). Renal cancer. In *Endocrine Therapy in Malignant Disease* W.B. Saunders ed. pp. 339–67.

Bloom H.J.G., Hendry W.F. (1973). Possible role of hormones in treatment of metastatic testicular teratomas: Tumour regression with medroxyprogesterone acetate. *Brit. Med. J*; **3**: 563–7.

Bodey G.P. (1979). Current status of chemotherapy in metastatic renal carcinoma. In *Cancer of the Genitourinary Tract* (Johnson D.E., Samuels M.L., eds.) pp. 67–71. New York: Raven Press.

Bollen E.C.M., Lamers C.B.H.W., Jansen J.B.M., Larson L.I., Joosten H.M. (1981). Zollinger Ellison syndrome due to a gastrin producing ovarian cystadenocarcinoma. *Br. J. Surg*; **68**: 776–7.

Boyne A.R., Cole E.N., Phillips M.E.A., Hillier S.G., Cameron E.H.D. Griffiths K., Shamanesh M., Feneley R.C.L., Hartog M. (1974). Plasma prolactin growth hormone, luteinizing hormone, follicle stimulating hormone, thyroid stimulating hormone and testosterone during treatment of prostatic carcinoma with oestrogens. *Eur. J. Cancer*; 445–9.

Brendler H. (1973). Adrenalectomy and hypophysectomy for prostatic cancer. *Urology*; **2**: 99–102.

British Prostate Study Group (1979). Evaluation of plasma hormone concentrations in patients with prostatic cancer. *Br. J. Urology*; **51**: 382–9.

Brook C.G.D., Dombey S. (1979). Induction of puberty. Long term treatment with high dose LRH. *Clin. endocrinol*; **11**: 81–7.

Buell P., Dunn J.E. (1965). Cancer mortality among Japanese Issei and Nisei of California. *Cancer*; **18**: 656–64.

Cancer Statistics. (1980). Registrations. England & Wales 1974. MBI No. 4. HMSO.

Cancer Statistics. (1982). Registrations. England & Wales. MBI No. 6. HMSO.

Catalona W.J., Scott W.W. (1978). Carcinoma of the prostate: A review. *J. Urol*; **119**: 1–8.

Chase M.D., Geschwind I.I., Bern M.A. (1957). Synergistic role of prolactin in response of male rat accessories to androgen. *Proc. Soc. Exp. Biol. & Med*, **94**: 680.

Chassiri N., Pierrepoint C.G. (1979). Demonstration of differences in receptor site concentration for oestrogens in separated epithelial and stromal fractions of the canine prostate. *J. Endocrinol*; **81**: 147P.

Clark P., Houghton L. (1977). Subcapsular orchidectomy for carcinoma of the prostate. *Br. J. Urology*; **49**: 419–25.

Coy D.H., Schally A.V. (1978). Gonadotrophin releasing hormone analogues. *Ann. Clin. Res*; **10**: 139–44.

Darwish D.H. (1978). The effect of sex steroids on the *in vitro* synthesis of DNA by malignant ovarian tumours. *Br. J. Obst. & Gynaecol*; **85**: 627–33.

Davies J.M. (1981). Testicular cancer in England & Wales: Some epidemiological aspects. *Lancet*; **1**: 928.

Davy M., Torjesen P.A., Aakvaag A. (1977). Demonstration of an FSH receptor in a functioning granulosa cell tumour. *Acta Endocrinologica*; **85**: 615–23.

Drasga R.E., Einhorn L.H., Williams S.D., Patel D.N., Stevens E.E. (1983). Fertility after chemotherapy for testicular cancer. *J. Clin. Oncol*; **1**: 179–83.

Einhorn L.H. (1981). Testicular cancer as a model for a curable neoplasm. *Cancer Research*; **41**: 3275–80.

Ekman P., Snochwski M., Zetterberg A., Hogberg B., Gustafson J.A. (1979). Steroid receptor content in human prostatic carcinoma and response to endocrine therapy. *Cancer*; **44**: 1173–81.

Franchimont P. (1977). Pituitary gonadotrophins. *Clinics in Endocrinology & Metabolism*; **6**: 101–16.

Freeman D.A., Ascoli M. (1981). Desensitization to gonadotrophins in cultured Leydig tumour cells involves loss of gonadotrophin receptors and decreased capacity for steroidogenesis. *Proc. Nat. Acad. Sci. USA*; **78**: 6309–13.

Galloway D.A., McDougall J.K. (1983). The oncogenic potential of herpes simplex viruses: Evidence for a 'hit and run' mechanism. *Nature*; **303**: 21–4.

Givens J.R., Anderson R.N., Wiser W.L., Donelson A.J., Coleman S.A. (1975). A testosterone-secreting gonadotrophin responsive, pure thecoma and polycystic ovarian disease. *J. Clin. Endo. & Metab*; **41**: 845–53.

Glick J.H., Wein A., Padavic K., Negendark W., Harris D., Brodovsky H. (1980). Tamoxifen in refractory metastatic carcinoma of the prostate. *Cancer Treat. Rep*; **64**: 813–18.

Haenszel W., Kurihara M. (1967). Studies of Japanese migrants I. Mortality from cancer and other diseases among Japanese in the United States. *J. Natl. Canc. Inst*; **40**: 43–67.

Hamilton T.C., Davies P., Griffiths K. (1981). Androgen and oestrogen binding in cytosols of human ovarian tumours. *J. Endocrinol*; **90**: 421–31.

Happ J., Kollmann F., Draivehl C. (1978). Treatment of cryptorchidism with pernasal gonadotrophin-releasing hormone therapy. *Fertil. Steril*; **29**: 546.

Harrison R.G., Moreno de Marval M.J., Lewis-Jones D.I., Connolly R.C. (1981). Mechanism of damage to the contralateral testis in rats with ischaemic testis. *Lancet*; **2**: 723.

Hecker W., Heinz H.A. (1967). Cryptorchidism and fertility. *J. Paed. Surg*; **2**: 513.

Heinonen P.K., Tuimala R., Pyykko K., Pystynen P. (1982). Peripheral venous concentrations of oestrogens in postmenopausal women with ovarian cancer. *Br. J. Obst. & Gynaecol*; **89**: 84–6.

Henderson B.E., Benton B., Jing J. Yu M.C., Pike M.C. (1979). Risk factors for cancer of the testis in young men. *Int. J. Cancer*; **23**: 598–602.

Hendry W.F., Stedronska J., Jones C.R., Blackmore C.A., Barrett A., Peckham M.J. (1983). Semen analysis in testicular cancer and Hodgkin's disease: Pre and post treatment findings and implications for cryopreservation. *Br. J. Urol*; **55**: 769.

Holt J.A., Caputo T.A., Kelly K.M., Greenwald P., Chorost S. (1979). Estrogen and progestin binding in cytosols of ovarian adenocarcinoma. *Obs & Gynaecol*; **53**: 50–8.

Julian C.G., Woodruff J.D. (1969). The role of chemotherapy in the treatment of primary ovarian malignancy. *Obs & Gynae Surgery*; **24**: 1307–42.

Kammerman S., Demopoulos R.I., Raphael C., Ross J. (1981). Gonadotropic hormone binding to human ovarian tumours. *Human Pathology*; **12**: 886–90.

Krabbe S., Berthelsen J.G., Volsted P., Skakkebaek N.E., Eyben F.V., Mauritzen K., Niewen A.H. (1979). High incidence of undetected neoplasia in maldescended testes. *Lancet*; **1**: 999–1000.

Lamberts S.W.J., Timmers J.M., Oosterom R., Verleum T., Rommerts F.G., de Jong F.H. (1982). Testosterone secretion by cultured arrhenoblastoma cells: Suppression by a luteinizing hormone-releasing hormone agonist. *J. Clin. Endo. & Metab*; **54**: 450–4.

Lingeman C.H. (1974). Etiology of cancer of the human ovary: A review. *J. Nat. Canc. Inst*; **53**: 1603–18.

Long R.T.L., Evans A.M. (1963). Diethyl stilboestrol as a chemotherapeutic agent for ovarian carcinoma. *Missouri Medicine*; **60**: 1125–7.

Mandel F.P., Voet R.L., Weiland A.J., Judd H.L. (1981). Steroid secretion by masculinizing and feminizing hilus cell tumours. *J. Clin. Endo. & Metab*; **52**: 779–84.

Mangioni C., Franceschi S., Landoni F., La Vechhia C., Colombo E., Molina P. (1981). High dose progestin therapy for advanced ovarian cancer. An updated report. *Proceedings International Symposium on Medroxyprogesterone Acetate.* (Cavalli F., McGuire W.L., Pannuti F., Pellegrini A., Robustelli Della Cuna G. eds.) pp. 461–6. Excerpta Medica.

Mortality statistics: Cause. (1978). England & Wales. DH 2 No. 3. HMSO.

Mortality statistics: Cause. (1980). England & Wales. DH 2 No. 5. HMSO.

Myers A.M., Moore G.E., Major F.J. (1981). Advanced ovarian carcinoma: response to antiestrogen therapy. *Cancer*; **48**: 2368–70.

Neumann F. (1977). Pharmacology and potential use of cyproterone acetate. *Hormone & Metabolism Res*; **9**: 1–13.

Newhouse M.L., Pearson R.M., Fullerton J.M., Boesen E.A., Shannon H.S. (1977). A case control study of carcinoma of the ovary. *Br. J. Preventive & Social Med*; **31**: 148–53.

Oliver R.T.D. (1982). Progress in the management of testicular germ cell tumours. *Practitioner*; **226**: 1903–15.

Oliver R.T.D., Pancharatnam M.D. (1984). Relapsing herpes genitalis, testicular trauma and family history of malignancy as risk factors in causation of germ cell tumours of the testis. *Br. Med. J.*

Oliver R.T.D., Miller R.M., Barnett M.J. (1984). Impact of frequency of radiological investigations on frequency of spontaneous regression of metastases in patients with hypernephroma. (Submitted to *Eur. J. Urol*).

Pizzocoro G.L. (1983). Adjunctive medroxyprogesterone acetate for category Mo renal cell carcinoma. *Eur. J. Urol*; **9**: 202.

Prout G.R., Brewers W.R. (1967). Response of men with advanced prostatic carcinoma to exogenous administration of testosterone. *Cancer*; **20**: 1871–8.

Registrar General's Statistical Review of England & Wales: Supplement on Cancer 1968–1970.

Resnick M.I., Grayhack J.T. (1975). Treatment of stage IV carcinoma of the prostate. *Urol. Clinics of N. America*; **2**: 141–61.

Rome R.M., Fortune D.W., Quinn M.A., Brown J.B. (1981). Functioning ovarian tumors in postmenopausal women. *Obs & Gynae*; **57**: 705–10.

Sanford E.J., Drago J.R., Kohner T.J., Santen R., Lipton A. (1976). Aminoglutethimide medical adrenalectomy for advanced prostatic carcinoma. *J. Urol*; **115**: 170–4.

Santen R.J., Santner S., Davis B., Veldhuis J., Sanojlik E., Ruby E. (1978). Aminoglutethimide inhibits extraglandular estrogen production in post menopausal women with breast cancer. *J. Clin. Endo. & Metab*; **47**: 1257–65.

Shteri P., Wilson J.D., Mayfield J.A. (1970). Dihydrotestosterone in prostatic hypertrophy I. The formation and content of dihydrotestosterone in the hypertrophic prostate of man. *J. Clin. Invest*; **49**: 1737–45.

Silverberg G.D. (1977). Hypophysectomy in the treatment of disseminated prostatic cancer. *Cancer*; **39**: 1727–31.

Slayton R.E., Pagano M., Creech R.H. (1981). Progestin therapy for advanced ovarian carcinoma: A Phase II Eastern Co-operative Oncology Group Trial. *Cancer Treat. Rep*; **65**: 895–6.

Smith A.D., Crighton D.B. (1978). Relative activity, elimination and hypothalamic and pituitary degradation of synthetic luteinizing hormone releasing hormone and certain of its analogues. *J. Endocrinol*; **77**: 35P.

Smithers D.W. (1972). Chemotherapy for metastatic teratoma of the testis. *Br. J. Urol*; **44**: 217–28.

Tcholakian R.T., de la Cruz A., Chowdhury M., Sternberger A., Coy D., Schally A.V. (1978). Unusual anti-reproductive properties of the analog LHRH Ethylamide in male rats. *Fertility & Sterility*; **30**: 600–603.

Tobias J.S., Griffiths C.T. (1976). Management of ovarian cancer. *N. Engl. J. Med*; **294**: 877–82.

Tunn U.W., Graff J., Senge T.H. (1983). Treatment of inoperable prostatic cancer with cyproterone acetate. In *Androgens and Anti Androgens* (Schroder F.H., ed.) pp. 149–59. Shering Nederland.

Veterans Administration Co-operative Urological Research Group. (1967). Treatment and survival of patients with cancer of the prostate. *Surgery, Gynaecol & Obst*; **124**: 1011–17.

Walsh P.C., Wilson J.D. (1976). The induction of prostatic hypertrophy in the dog with androstenedione. *J. Clin. Invest*; **57**: 1093–7.

Waxman J.H., Wass J.A.H., Hendry W.F., Whitfield H.N., Besser G.M., Malpas J.S., Oliver R.T.D. (1983). Treatment with gonadotrophin releasing hormone analogue in advanced prostatic cancer. *Brit. Med. J*; **286**: 1309–12.

Weiss N.S., Lyon J.L., Krishnamurthy S., Dietert S.E., Liff J.M., Daling J.R. (1982). Non-contraceptive estrogen use and the occurrence of ovarian cancer. *J. Nat. Canc. Inst*; **68**: 95–8.

Whitaker R. (1980). The undescended testis. *Hospital Update*; 1115–23.

Worgul T.J., Santen R.J., Sanojlik E., Velduis J.D., Lipton A., Harvey H.A., Drago J.R., Rohner T.J. (1983). Clinical and biochemical effect of aminoglutethimide in the treatment of advanced prostatic carcinoma. *J. Urol*; **129**: 51–4.

Ylikorkala O., Kauppila A., Rajala T. (1979). Pituitary gonadotrophins and prolactin in patients with endometrial cancer, fibroids or ovarian tumours. *Br. J. Obs. & Gynaecol*; **86**: 901–904.

Chapter 13

Piers N. Plowman

Endocrine Effects of Therapy

INTRODUCTION

Some consider that too critical scrutiny of late side effects in cancer therapy is a luxury; that these late effects represent the 'pathology of survival'. However, given equally curative treatment schemes for any malignancy, the physician of tomorrow will hopefully pick the least morbid. Although perturbations of the hypothalamic–pituitary axis may have far reaching secondary consequences, primary end organ disturbances under separate headings will be discussed first, then the complexities of the orchestral conductor.

TESTIS

Cytotoxic Chemotherapy

Testicular biopsy, with calculation of the tubular fertility index (TFI; Lendon *et al.*, 1978), semen analysis and endocrine assessment (circulating blood levels of testosterone and gonadotrophins in particular) have been employed to study the effects of cytotoxic drugs on the testis. Whilst it is clear that some drugs may have profound effects on the testis, there are many variables at work. The pre-pubertal versus post-pubertal status of the patients under treatment may be relevant, the toxicity towards the germinal epithelium must be distinguished from Leydig cell function and the individual identities of the cytotoxic drugs administered, together with the total doses administered (and possibly the duration of administration too), need all to be known to reach conclusions useful to other patients. Further, the function of the testis in certain malignant diseases is not necessarily normal prior to therapy. The majority of the little data available on this topic derive mainly from single agent data in a few conditions and in the long term, survivors of acute lymphoblastic leukaemia (ALL) and Hodgkin's disease—both treated with combination chemotherapy.

Reviewing the single agent data first, there has been wide recognition of the testicular damage caused by alkylating agents (best documented for

cyclophosphamide and chlorambucil). Low dose oral continual cyclophosphamide (1–3 mg/kg daily) for six months or more, as used in glomerulonephritis, was found to result in germinal epithelial atrophy in all patients. In
a minority of patients studied off therapy for periods exceeding a year, some
evidence of tubular regeneration was apparent, and some mature sperma-
tozoa could be found in the semen (Fairly *et al.*, 1972; Kumar *et al.*, 1972);
overall, it can be concluded that this 'immunosuppressive' dose regimen of
cyclophosphamide caused prolonged and profound changes in the germinal
epithelium, often irreversible. A similar story has been built up around
studies of chlorambucil, and Richter *et al.* (1970) concluded that azoospermia was dose related, the minimal total dose associated with this being
400 mg. Busulphan and other alkylating agents may be expected to have
similar actions. Animal studies make it likely that procarbazine and cytosine
arabinoside will influence the activity of the germinal epithelium in man,
although it is not known that extrapolation to man is valid. Whilst high dose
methotrexate may cause temporary oligospermia during treatment, testicular function may be expected to return rapidly to normal soon after
cessation of this antimetabolite (Shamberger *et al.*, 1981). The same authors
were able to confirm for man the animal studies showing that vincristine
only mildly and reversibly affects the sperm count in conventional
therapeutic dosage. The difference between the effects on the pre-pubertal
versus post-pubertal testis is not known and the influence of these drugs, as
single agents, on Leydig cell function is also unclear, although as a general
conclusion it seems that Leydig cell function is very much more refractory to
damage.

Acute lymphoblastic leukaemia is now a highly curable malignancy, due
to the exquisite sensitivity of the lymphoblast to vincristine and pred-
nisoline. To these agents are added third, or third and fourth drugs
which differ in the induction schemes of different centres. Blatt *et al.* (1981)
concluded that when methotrexate (2 g cumulative dose (CD)) and 6-
mercaptopurine (60 g CD) were added to vincristine (80 mg CD) and
prednisolone (40 g CD) in pre-pubertal and post-pubertal males, Leydig
function (as assessed by physical examination and serum gonadotrophin and
testosterone levels) and germinal epithelial activity (as assessed by seminal
analysis where possible) were not meaningfully different from normal.
However, Lendon *et al.* (1978) had found that in patients in whom either
cyclophosphamide or cytosine arabinoside had been included in the
induction scheme at more than 1 g per square metre of body surface area,
impaired spermatogenesis was obvious. There was no identifiable relationship between the TFI and age at induction therapy, but the authors
did comment that they had observed improvement in the TFI with time in
some (but not all) cases. The hormone monitoring in these patients
suggested that Leydig cell dysfunction was rare following this combination
chemotherapy, and that puberty would be normal (Shalet *et al.*, 1981*a*).

That FSH levels were not found to be regularly raised in these boys with tubular atrophy, only complicates our current concept of a putative negative feedback of the germinal epithelium on the hypothalamic–pituitary axis (the 'inhibin–gonadocrinin' axis).

Advanced Hodgkin's disease is fairly universally treated by a four drug combination comprising nitrogen mustard (an alkylating agent), a vinca alkaloid (vincristine or vinblastine), procarbazine and prednisolone—as pulsed courses at intervals of four to six weeks for a minimum of six courses. This regimen can be predicted to be more toxic to the testis than chemotherapy for acute leukaemia. Sherins *et al.* (1978) studied 19 children so treated and made the following observations: nine of 13 post-pubertal children had germinal aplasia, gynaecomastia, a ten-fold increase in serum follicle stimulating hormone (FSH), a three-fold increase in luteinising hormone (LH), reduced testosterone and normal oestradiol and prolactin levels. Six pre-pubertal boys demonstrated no change in serum gonado-trophin levels and no gynaecomastia following chemotherapy, and this prompted the conclusion that the circulating serum gonadotrophin levels of pre-pubertal boys are not regulated by inhibin. Whitehead *et al.* (1982*b*) found similar results. Green *et al.* (1981) documented three pre-pubertal boys whose FSH levels remained normal after Hodgkin's chemotherapy until puberty; after puberty, FSH levels rose abnormally.

Chapman *et al.* (1979) studied the effects of this chemotherapy regimen in 74 post-pubertal males suffering advanced Hodgkin's disease. All patients were azoospermic after therapy and with a median follow-up period of 27 months, only four patients had regained spermatogenesis. Testicular biopsy showed an absence of germinal epithelium without other gross architectural changes. Follicle stimulating hormone levels were consistently raised for as long off therapy as the patients were studied; LH levels were high normal or slightly elevated, and testosterone levels were normal. The data suggested that the raised FSH reflected damaged germinal epithelium and the slightly elevated LH reflected compensated Leydig cell failure, although this may be too facile. Very interesting also was the observation by these authors of hyperprolactinaemia in 42% of these patients (an observation not found in a parallel study of similarly treated females). The incidence of gynaecomastia was not documented. Chapman *et al.* (1979) observed a reduction in libido during treatment and noted that, with the normal testosterone levels in their patients, androgen administration was not indicated. Most authors would now recommend sperm banking prior to such chemotherapy. However, it has recently been appreciated that many patients with Hodgkin's disease have low sperm counts prior to treatment, and this may have augmented the abnormal results of all authors studying the effects of this chemotherapy on the testis. The reduced libido during and following this chemotherapy, the persistently low sperm count, and the gonadotrophin and testosterone data were confirmed in the adult male study of Whitehead *et al.* (1982*b*), but

these authors did not confirm the hyperprolactinaemia although document-
ing gynaecomastia in a minority (seven of 93) of patients.

Is there a way that the testis can be protected? The study of Linde *et al.*
(1981) examined the administration of the decapeptide: gonadotrophin
releasing hormone (GnRH) on testicular function. Persistent high levels of
this agonist 'down regulate' pituitary receptors, causing low blood gonadotrophin levels and 'testicular sleep'. The study was designed to provide a male
contraceptive, but the associated decline in Leydig function with associated
fall in libido vitiated this aspect of study. However, the possible usefulness
of GnRH in patients on cytotoxic chemotherapy is currently under
investigation, although it has not been convincingly shown that the pre-
pubertal or sleeping testis is more resistant to chemotoxicity. The mutagenic
effects of cytotoxic chemotherapy on the testis are thought to be stochastic
phenomena (as with radiation). Thus, the documented anecdotal reports of
normal children being born to parents after chemotherapy, whilst very
gratifying and useful for us to quote to our patients, nevertheless do not
justify the conclusions of some authors that the mutagenic risk is not
increased.

Radiotherapy

When analysing the effects of radiation on the testis, there are several
variables that should be considered. The pubertal status of the patient, the
dose equivalent received by the testis, the dose equivalent rate, fractionation
scheme and total elapsed time, together with length of follow-up could all be
relevant.

In a censurable human experiment, employing single radiation fractions
to the testes and the monitoring of sperm counts, sperm morphology and
testicular histology, Rowley *et al.* (1974) observed that (as in animal
experiments) the type B spermatogonium was the most radiosensitive cell in
the sperm cell lineage. Probably on account of this, it was found that with
lower doses of radiation the time for the sperm count to drop to azoospermia
was longer (and incidentally the time to recovery shorter), than with higher
dose single fractions. It was found that with doses as high as 6 Gray (Gy),
recovery could still occur but might take up to five years. The germinal
epithelium began recovery significantly prior to any increase of sperm
count.

The single fraction situation is unusual in cancer patients (male and
female) receiving radiotherapy, whose gonads usually receive a low scattered total dose in a multifractionated and protracted administration (albeit
at high dose rate during each fraction). Ash (1980) has collated the published
data on the effects of fractionated testicular radiation. In summary, doses up
to 40 centiGray (cGy) fractionated over two to seven weeks will produce
graded and temporary degrees of oligospermia. Doses from 35–150 cGy,

received in a conventionally fractionated scheme over two (lower doses) or three to seven weeks, will result in temporary azoospermia, with some recovery noted (at least on testicular biopsy) within one year. Doses in excess of this may still lead only to a temporary azoospermia, but more than one year may need to elapse before recovery of the germinal epithelium occurs.

To set these testicular doses in clinical perspective, the scatter dose to the testes during standard radiotherapy to the bed of a Wilms' tumour will be up to 70 cGy week daily fractionation over two weeks, during 'dog-leg' radiotherapy in testicular tumours 50–100 cGy week daily fractionation over three to four weeks, and during inverted-Y radiotherapy in infra-diaphragmatic Hodgkin's disease 150–200 cGy week daily fractionation over four weeks (despite testicular lead cup shields). It may now be predicted that the germinal epithelium will recover after doses of this order, and Smithers *et al.* (1973) noted that of 74 men who had been treated by unilateral orchidectomy and 'dog-leg' radiotherapy for testicular tumours, 34 had fathered 52 children.

However, higher doses are permanently sterilising. Our own data, and others, show that after a testicular dose of 24 Gy in 12 fractions in 19 days (x-rays), permanent sterility will result. This prescription is delivered to testes infiltrated by acute leukaemia, in which situation it is mandatory to treat both testes. In childhood paratesticular rhabdomyosarcoma, however, the contralateral testis may not be at risk and would not be intentionally irradiated were it not for its proximity to the primary tumour. In this high dose radiation situation, we would attempt to transpose the contralateral testis for the duration of radiotherapy and so strive to preserve fertility.

Due to the absent shoulder on the Elkind survival curve for spermatogonia, it might be predicted that fractionated radiotherapy would be as damaging to the germinal epithelium as single dose radiation. Lushbaugh and Casaret (1976) have marshalled animal and human data to suggest that it may be more harmful. All this is quite consistent with the UNSCEAR report (1977), and may explain the famous, historic work of Regaud on the concept and radiobiological basis for fractionation in radiotherapy, as a means of enhancing the therapeutic ratio and protecting normal tissues—until now ironic observations, as they were made entirely on normal tissues (viz. normal skin and normal testis).

Shalet (1982) has added to our knowledge of radiation effects on Leydig cell function. The Manchester workers studied ten patients aged 17–36 years who had received wide field abdominal radiotherapy in childhood for Wilms' tumour. The scatter dose to the testes was approximately 270–1000 cGy in 20 fractions over four weeks. Eight of ten patients had oligo- or azoospermia and seven of eight of these had elevated FSH but there were no consistent changes in LH or testosterone. However, when they studied six boys who had received testicular radiation for leukaemia (24 Gy in 15 fractions over 21 days), Leydig cell dysfunction was apparent and there was no testosterone response to human chorionic gonadotrophin. Shalet concluded that up to 10 Gy (1000 cGy) testicular radiation, fractionated over four weeks, can be tolerated by Leydig cells, but above this dose Leydig cell failure will manifest. Once again, the mutagenic (and carcinogenic) effects of radiation are stochastic phenomena, the frequency of which is as yet only approximately quantified (UNSCEAR, 1977).

OVARY

Of the many obvious differences between male and female gonads, the most important to this discussion are first that the ovary contains its full complement of germinal cells at birth, and second that it is situated within the abdomen. Resting oocytes (in prophase) comprise the vast majority of the gametogenic cell population at all times. That the number of oocytes decreases with advancing years to a large part explains the age-related ovarian susceptibility to insults. Although it is not possible to routinely biopsy the ovaries, primary ovarian failure is relatively easy to diagnose by menopausal symptoms, vaginal and uterine atrophy, elevated FSH and LH and a fall in serum oestradiol.

Chemotherapy

Of the single agents, the alkylating agents are the best recognised group of drugs to cause primary ovarian failure. Koyama *et al.* (1977) studied the effect of cyclophosphamide (100 mg/day) on ovarian function following surgery for breast cancer. Fifteen of 18 premenopausal women who received 8.4–40 g CD cyclophosphamide developed permanent amenorrhoea with menopausal serum results; in all three patients coming to surgery, the ovaries lacked follicles. The authors found that higher doses of cyclophosphamide were needed to cause amenorrhoea in young women than in the late premenopausal age group. This study's findings were echoed in the NSABP report of adjuvant melphalan in breast cancer patients (Fisher *et al.*, 1979). With the standard dose of this agent, amenorrhoea occurred in three-quarters of patients in the fifth decade of life, but in only one-quarter of younger patients. Belohorsky *et al.* (1960) found that busulphan in continual dosage for chronic myeloid leukaemia for six months caused amenorrhoea in all ten premenopausal women studied. Shalet (1982) reviewed literature reports, finding no menstrual dysfunction amongst women who, in childhood, had received low dose oral cyclophosphamide for glomerulonephritis; this raises the possibility of increased resistance of the pre-pubertal ovary to toxic effects, although this concept is certainly not well substantiated at present (*see* below). High dose methotrexate has not been found to cause primary ovarian failure (Shamberger *et al.*, 1981).

Single agent therapy with the anti-oestrogen tamoxifen will induce the menopause in only one-third of premenopausal women. If one accepts that menses represent a good *in vivo* bioassay of oestrogen function, then it is difficult to foresee that this drug will substitute oophorectomy as the first endocrine manoeuvre in relapsed, young breast cancer patients. Whilst on this subject, cyclical oestrogen and progesterone therapy should not be used to palliate ovarian failure in this group of patients, although flushing can often be controlled by oral clonidine.

Siris *et al.* (1976) studied pubertal development and reproductive function in 35 girls and women on a combination chemotherapy protocol for ALL, containing vincristine, prednisolone, 6-mercaptopurine and methotrexate and noted primary ovarian failure in only three patients. One of 17 pre-pubertal girls suffered altered pubertal progression although six of 18 patients at or after puberty did experience some irregularities. With a cyclophosphamide containing ALL regimen, Shalet (1982) found evidence of primary ovarian failure in four of 12 pre-pubertal girls, although three have subsequently gone through puberty with the FSH falling to normal—indicating ovarian recovery. However, there are also preliminary data to suggest that, as in the male, severe damage to the pre-pubertal gonad may occur without a rise in FSH. Pizzuto *et al.* (1980) reported nine pregnant patients who at different trimesters of pregnancy received various ALL chemotherapy regimens; eight babies were born alive and six survived as apparently healthy children. Once again, these are interesting anecdotes that are not of themselves reassuring with regard to the late effects in F_1 or subsequent generations, nor are they sufficient to dismiss the teratogenic risk as small.

Chapman *et al.* (1979) studied the effects of MVPP chemotherapy in 41 adult women with Hodgkin's disease, who, unlike their male counterparts, appeared to have normal fertility pre-therapy. Half the women suffered primary ovarian failure and a further one-third had evidence of ovarian dysfunction; ovarian failure occurred after fewer cycles of MVPP (mustine, vinblastine, procarbazine, prednisolone) in older women. The authors recommended palliative cyclical oestrogen–progestogen therapy in amenorrhoeic patients. The high incidence of unexplained hyperprolactinaemia noted in their parallel male study was not encountered amongst the females. Overall, Chapman *et al.* (1979) found that gonadal function in women was less severely affected by MVPP chemotherapy than in men. Whitehead *et al.* (1982*b*) reported two children treated by MOPP without evidence of ovarian failure.

Is there a way in which the ovary can be protected? Chapman and Sutcliffe (1981) provided some preliminary and, as yet, largely unsubstantiated data that when women took combination oral contraceptives throught the course of MVPP therapy, some ovarian protection occurred. The effects of GnRH in this situation are not known.

Radiotherapy

It should be widely appreciated that routine curative, external beam radiotherapy for carcinoma of cervix and other pelvic cancer always causes irreversible, primary ovarian failure. More pertinent are the following considerations. Is the combination of radiotherapy and chemotherapy more likely to ablate the ovaries than either modality alone? Is the pre-pubertal ovary more resistant? What is the minimum radiation dose required to cause ovarian ablation?

The first two questions can be quickly dismissed, as the data suggest that chemotherapeutic and radiotherapeutic insults act additively against the ovary and the pre-pubertal variable has not been dissected out from age itself. The minimum radiation dose required to produce irreversible ovarian ablation is inversely related to a woman's age or, more precisely, inversely related to the number of oocytes remaining. The effect of the fractionation scheme by which the ovarian dose is received is poorly understood, but the differences between single dose effects and fractionated dose effects do not seem large. In general, Ash (1980) found that for humans, doses up to 150 cGy were tolerated without menstrual disturbances by most women. Total doses of 500–600 cGy led to ovarian failure in a variable number of patients depending on age, whereas total doses of the order of 800–1000 cGy are permanently sterilising in almost all. Unlike the testis, the dose to cause temporary ovarian ablation is close to that required to cause permanent ablation, and later recovery of ovarian function is uncommon. The author's routine mid-plane dose prescription of 12 Gy in three fractions in four days (MeV photons) has invariably caused the artificial menopause in patients requiring this.

Is there a way that the ovaries can be protected? In infradiaphragmatic Hodgkin's disease for example, the close proximity of the ovaries to the iliac lymph nodes leaves no alternative but to take this region to the curative radiation dose. Sterilisation may often be avoided, however, by a midline oophoropexy (the ovaries are brought together behind the uterus) performed at the time of diagnostic or staging laparotomy. Kaplan (1980) claimed 70% success in retaining normal periods after such a procedure in Hodgkin's, although Thomas *et al.* (1976) were less successful at reducing the ovarian dose. Nahhas *et al.* (1971) have used a lateral transposition technique in which the ovaries are swung laterally (retaining their vascular pedicle) and sutured to the anterior abdominal wall near the anterior superior iliac spine. This has the advantage in Hodgkin's radiotherapy, that the ovaries only receive scattered radiation from one direction, but the method has not been widely adopted. The mutagenic (and carcinogenic) effects of radiation on the ovary are stochastic phenomena only approximately quantified to date (UNSCEAR, 1977).

THYROID, ADRENAL, PANCREAS

Patients receiving the commonly used cytotoxic drugs remain clinically euthyroid with normal serum TSH; the adrenals and pancreas also seem relatively resistant. Although the head of the pancreas (bearing 20% of the β-cells) is encompassed by an inverted Y-portal, there have been no reports of increased incidences of diabetes mellitus in the large number of patients treated by this radiotherapy technique to 'Hodgkin's-cidal doses'. It is very rare that both adrenals are irradiated.

In 1964, Koulumies *et al.* reported a fall in the serum protein-bound iodine in 50% of patients radically irradiated for carcinoma of larynx. With current methods of thyroid function assessment, the Stanford and Baltimore groups find that following conventionally fractionated MeV photon mantle radiotherapy to 40–44 Gy, two-thirds of patients will develop a raised TSH and between one-fifth and one-quarter developed overt hypothyroidism by six years (Kaplan, 1980; Schimpff *et al.*, 1980). Following similar radiotherapy to lower doses (35–36 Gy), the Dartmouth group and our own data suggest a lower incidence of overt hypothyroidism—not more than 6% (Smith *et al.*, 1978). Glatstein *et al.* (1971) reported that the iodine load contribution from lymphography could be a co-factor in the genesis of later radiation-induced myxoedema, and this seems to have been confirmed. In laboratory animals, thyroid radiation followed by chronic high circulating TSH levels, leads to a higher incidence of thyroid cancer than radiation alone (i.e. with suppressed TSH). Acting from this datum, many recommend thyroxine administration long term to all patients who, post-neck irradiation develop high TSH levels; the author has not done this to date. Chronic thyroid hormone replacement (as following near total thyroidectomy and radioiodine ablation for follicular cell origin carcinoma) for several years may blunt the normal endogenous TSH response to thyroid hormone withdrawal (a point of importance to radioiodine screening programmes). That thyroid radiation may later lead to thyroid carcinoma is well-known (UNSCEAR, 1977).

CENTRAL NERVOUS SYSTEM (CNS)

There is much confusion over the radiation tolerance of the nervous system, and for simplicity only sparsely ionising radiation (x-rays and γ-rays) given by external beams will be discussed here. Early attempts to extrapolate the dose, time, fraction size isoeffect formulae (derived for the early radiation tolerance of pig skin), to that easily quantifiable late nervous system end point viz. brain necrosis, are now known to be invalid. Isoeffect formulae, giving a much heavier weighting to the fractional exponent, and much lighter weighting to the time exponent, do seem valid for this particular end point (van der Kogel and Barendsen, 1974; Wara *et al.*, 1975; Sheline, 1980). Whether the cause of this late brain damage is vascular, with secondary neural or primary damage to neural parenchyma, is still controversial, and both probably contribute (Hopewell, 1979); the enhanced importance of fraction size to the tolerance dose probably applies to both these phenomena. Late brain necrosis appears to be a non-stochastic effect of radiation; other factors may contribute to the risk of this event (Aristizabal *et al.*, 1979).

Despite the mistakes of the past, many authors have extrapolated from data such as those just cited to predict the likelihood of other end points/sequelae of CNS radiation following various dose, time, fraction size radiotherapy prescriptions; for example, the neuropsychological sequelae of whole brain radiotherapy in children and pituitary endocrine dysfunction. These sequelae are not known to have a threshold radiation dose equivalent, and may be consequent upon phenomena other than those contributing to brain necrosis. Their prediction based on the partial tolerance mathematics of the amended isoeffect formulae for late brain tolerance may well be bogus—although the greater significance of fraction size may remain true.

Other end points/sequelae of CNS radiation are more probably related to damage to the vasculoconnective tissue—for example, optic chiasmal damage and hypothalamic damage, and so may better accord with isoeffect formulae derived from the animal work for late brain damage. It must be remembered that the vascular supply to the nervous system is a highly specialised labyrinth of *vasa nervorum*, frequently at histological variance with other visceral blood vessels and often end-arteries. The unusual dual capillary plexus of the hypothalamic–pituitary portal system is also worthy of comment as a fragile vascular network.

In the discussion that follows, low, moderate and high radiotherapy dose equivalents will be referred to, without an attempt to refine the estimates further. The low dose equivalents would be of the order prescribed for cranial prophylaxis in acute leukaemia, moderate dose equivalents of the order prescribed for pituitary adenoma, and high dose equivalents of the order prescribed for glioma.

Growth

The most obvious examples of growth stunting following CNS radiation occur in children in whom the whole neuraxis has been irradiated (usually to low or moderate dose equivalents)—the radiation portals encompassing the growth centres of the axial skeleton (Figs. 13.1 and 13.2). The standing height is low and the ratio of arm span to sitting height is raised in all these children on follow-up, and they do not respond to exogenous growth hormone (GH).

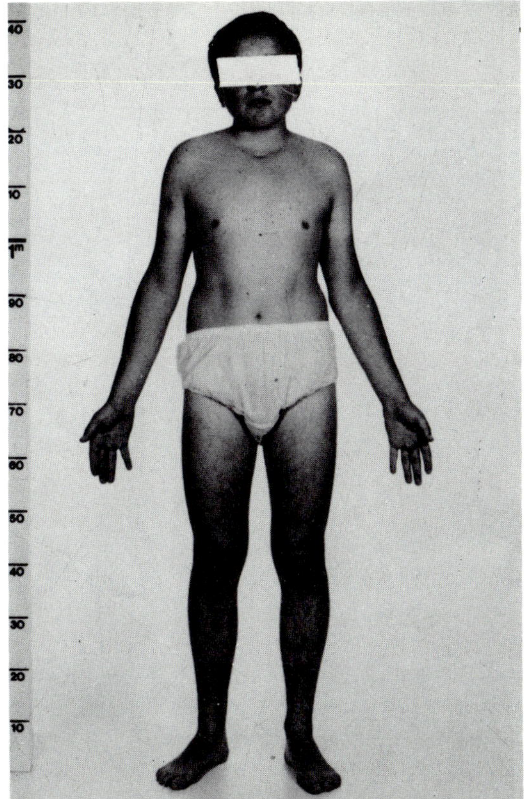

Fig. 13.1. *Twelve-year-old boy who received megavoltage photon, neuraxis radiotherapy for medulloblastoma in early childhood. Growth stunting of the neck and trunk is apparent.*

Early animal studies demonstrated that the acidophils (somatotrophes) were the most sensitive cell type in the anterior pituitary to radiation, and that the severity of the cell loss was related to the dose of radiation (Lawrence *et al.*, 1937; Simpson *et al.*, 1959). Human data have demonstrated that low dose equivalent radiation may produce late abnormalities in GH reserve, that GH hyporesponsiveness to stress/dynamic testing is more severe with increasing dose equivalents, and the significance of fraction size and/or time elapsed during the radiotherapy prescription has been established (Shalet *et al.*, 1976*a,b*). The St. Bartholomew's data showed that following low dose equivalents to the child's cranium (together with antileukaemic therapy including prednisolone) a small impairment in linear growth occurred within the first year and 'catch-up' growth did not occur later (Griffin and Wadsworth, 1980). Radiation-induced, endocrine-related growth stunting is more likely following higher radiation dose

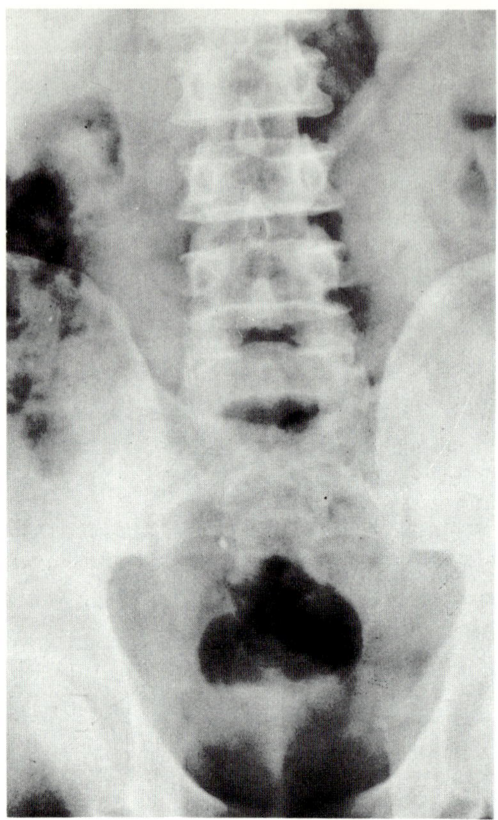

Fig. 13.2. *Lumbosacral spine x-ray of a 40-year-old man who received orthovoltage neuraxis radiotherapy for medulloblastoma in childhood. Marked growth stunting is apparent in the height of the lumbar vertebrae and width of sacrum. N.B. Bone absorption from orthovoltage radiotherapy is greater than from megavoltage radiotherapy. Photograph submitted by courtesy of Professor A.E. Jones, St. Bartholomew's Hospital.*

equivalents. Shalet *et al.* (1977) tested pituitary function in 20 adults who had received such radiotherapy in childhood. Nine patients had impaired GH responsiveness to hypoglycaemia (a pituitary stress test thought to be mediated through hypothalamic receptors), eight were below the third centile for height and a further four between the third and tenth centiles. Although there are no long-term studies of the effects of therapy in children with radiation-induced GH deficiency, nevertheless the early data from Manchester suggest that such children will respond to therapeutic exogenous GH (Shalet *et al.*, 1981*b*; Shalet, 1982).

Fuks *et al.* (1976) regarded the pituitary as a slow renewal tissue and cell killing with late expression of GH deficit as the reason for the observed radiation effect. This is likely to be the explanation for the GH response in acromegaly/gigantism, but it is less certain that this mechanism is entirely responsible for the decline in GH responsiveness or absolute levels in patients without acidophil adenomas. Reduced secretion by irradiated but surviving somatotrophes is another possible explanation, as is hypothalamic damage. The significantly greater impairment of the GH response to insulin (hypoglycaemic stress) than to arginine (a dynamic hypophyseal test that may act directly at the pituitary level) could be interpreted as supporting this last notion (Shalet *et al.*, 1979*a*). There are some experimental data, which need extending, that suggest that pituitary-region radiation can lead to growth stunting not due to any known anterior pituitary hormone deficit, nor responsive to exogenous GH therapy (Mosier and Jansons, 1968, 1970). Some human data may support these observations (Shalet *et al.*, 1978; Griffin and Wadsworth, 1980).

In conclusion, all children receiving radiotherapy to the pituitary region should, thereafter, be serially graphed for growth and more extensively investigated if the clinical parameters merit this.

Drug-induced growth retardation may be multifactorial and depends on the drug administered (e.g. prednisolone versus a conventional cytotoxic agent). Following cessation of therapy, a variable 'catch-up' growth spurt has been observed in some children.

Prolactin

Whilst there is now little doubt that moderate dose equivalent radiotherapy reduced the growth risk of macroscopic 'chromophobe' adenoma (Sheline, 1973), and that the normal lactotrophes are probably radioresponsive, nevertheless it has been observed that moderate to high dose equivalent pituitary radiation may lead to hyperprolactinaemia (Samaan *et al.*, 1975; Shalet *et al.*, 1979*b*). This interesting paradox has been attributed to radiation-induced damage to the hypothalamus, which normally keeps the pituitary lactotrophe under inhibitory control. Unfortunately, there is no reproducible dynamic endocrine test to verify this conclusion, and our own data do not entirely accord with those of others. The situation remains unclear.

Gonadotrophins

The data from three reports in particular suggest that following high dose equivalent hypothalamo–hypophyseal region radiotherapy there is a late risk of impaired gonadotrophin secretion (Samaan *et al.*, 1975; Huang, 1979; Rappaport *et al.*, 1982). Rappaport *et al.* (1982) reported the follow-up of 45 children whose pituitary region had received moderate to high dose equivalents over a mean period of five years earlier. Puberty was complete or progressing normally in 31 cases but was abnormal in 14 cases. Severe gonadotrophin deficiency, with impaired pubertal changes and gonadotrophin response to GnRH, was observed in five cases (two of whom had hyperprolactinaemia). Secondary amenorrhoea or lack of pubertal progression was found in five other cases. The findings of this study suggested a latency of four to five years between radiotherapy and hormonal deficit, and the authors predicted that with longer follow-up the prevalence of abnormalities would increase. (All gonadotrophin-deficient patients except one, were also GH deficient.) Any influence of pubertal status at the time of radiation is quite unknown at present.

Multiple Hypothalamo–Pituitary Hormonal Disturbances

Samaan *et al.* (1975) found hypothalamo–hypophyseal dysfunction following high dose equivalent therapy to this region in 13 of 15 patients studied. Thirteen patients seemed to show hypothalamic dysfunction; they all had hyperprolactinaemia. Eleven patients demonstrated impaired GH responsiveness and six had reduced cortisol responses to hypoglycaemia. Seven patients seemed to show pituitary dysfunction; five of these were hypothyroid, with low circulating thyrotrophin (TSH) levels and TSH hyporesponsiveness to thyrotrophin releasing hormone (TRH). Four patients were hyporeactive to GnRH. Richards *et al.* (1976) reported four children of short stature following high dose equivalent radiation to the pituitary region. One of the four children had a low plasma thyroxine and basal TSH, but a normal pituitary reserve on TRH testing. In addition, this child had an impaired ACTH response to hypoglycaemia and impaired gonadotrophin response to GnRH. Basal prolactin was normal. As this child's tumour was in the middle ear, the incrimination of radiation seemed valid. The datum purporting to show a threshold dose equivalent for multiple pituitary hormone deficiencies is not at present convincing.

In conclusion, radiation damage to both hypothalamus and pituitary may contribute to abnormal endocrine responsiveness. Multiple pituitary hormonal deficiencies are more likely to occur following higher radiation dose equivalents. Where possible, radiotherapy field shrinking techniques or lead screening of the pituitary region is recommended. Radiation damage to the function of the posterior pituitary does not seem a common or serious problem.

Drug Effects

Both vincristine and cyclophosphamide can induce antidiuretic hormone early after their administration and this interesting acute drug effect may have clinically obvious consequences (Bode *et al.*, 1980). Of the plethora of other possible drug–CNS effects with endocrine sequelae, space only permits mention of methotrexate (MTX). The late sequelae of intrathecal or even higher dosage intravenous MTX on the CNS include the widely recognised leucoencephalopathy and the computerised tomographic appearance of dystrophic cerebral calcification. The important clinical sequelae are heterogenous and are well described by Bleyer (1981). There is no doubt that MTX is toxic to the CNS, and that MTX and CNS radiation are additively or synergistically toxic. There are neuropsychological data demonstrating mild intellectual deficits following low dose equivalent cranial radiation in childhood (Eiser, 1980). It is difficult to know if concomitant MTX contributes to this—a point of great importance due to the widespread use of both modalities in the treatment of childhood ALL, and the substitution by some workers of MTX for cranial radiation prophylaxis in this disease. We have seen two children previously treated elsewhere with excessive amounts of intrathecal MTX and both are severely retarded intellectually as well as demonstrating motor signs. The neuro-endocrine effects have yet to be fully elucidated.

CONCLUSION

In conclusion, recent experimental studies and clinical analyses have led to the compilation of much additional knowledge concerning the late effects of cancer therapy. Rarely should these data cause us to reduce the intensity of effective therapy in otherwise fatal cancer, but they may allow us to perform precautionary and protectice procedures prior to radiotherapy or chemotherapy and should allow us to pick the least morbid of equally effective treatment schemes in the future.

REFERENCES

Aristizabal S., Boone M.L., Laguna J.E. (1979). Endocrine factors influencing radiation injury to central nervous tissue. *Int. J. Radiat. Oncol. Biol. Phys*; **5**: 349–53.

Ash P. (1980). The influence of radiation on fertility in man. *Br. J. Radiol*; **53**: 271–8.

Belohorsky B., Siracky J., Sandor L., Klauber E. (1960). Comments on the development of amenorrhoea caused by myleran in cases of chronic myelosis. *Neoplasma*; **4**: 397–402.

Blatt J., Poplack D.G., Sherins R.J. (1981). Testicular function in boys after chemotherapy for acute lymphoblastic leukaemia. *New Eng. J. Med*; **304**: 1121–4.

Bleyer A. (1981). Neurologic sequelae of methotrexate and ionising radiation: A new classification. *Cancer Treat. Rep*; **65** (suppl. 1): 89–98.

Bode U., Seif S.M., Levine A.S. (1980). Studies on the antidiuretic effect of cyclophosphamide: Vasopressin release and sodium excretion. *Med. Pediatr. Oncol*; **8**: 295–303.

Chapman R., Sutcliffe S.B. (1981). Protection of ovarian function by oral contraceptives in women receiving chemotherapy for Hodgkin's disease. *Blood*; **58**: 849–51.

Chapman R.M., Sutcliffe S.B., Malpas J.S. (1979). Cytotoxic induced ovarian failure in women with Hodgkin's disease. *J. Am. Med. Ass*; **242**: 1877–81.

Chapman R.M., Sutcliffe S.B., Rees L.H., Edwards C.R.W., Malpas J.S. (1979). Cyclical combination chemotherapy and gonadal function. *Lancet*; **1**: 285–9.

Eiser C. (1980). Effects of chronic illness on intellectual development. *Arch. Dis. Childh*; **55**: 766–70.

Fairley K.F., Barrie J.U., Johnson W. (1972). Sterility and testicular atrophy related to cyclophosphamide therapy. *Lancet*; **1**: 568–9.

Fisher B., Sherman B., Rockette H., Redmond C., Margolese R., Fisher E.R. (1979). L-phenylalanine mustard in the management of premenopausal patients with primary breast cancer. *Cancer*; **44**: 847–57.

Fuks Z., Glatstein E., Marsa G.W., Bagshaw M.A., Kaplan H.S. (1976). Long term effects of external radiation on the pituitary and thyroid glands. *Cancer*; **37**: 1152–61.

Glatstein E., McHardy-Young S., Brast N., Eltringham J.R., Kriss J.P. (1971). Alterations in serum thyrotrophin (TSH) and thyroid function following radiotherapy in patients with malignant lymphoma. *J. Clin. Endocrinol. Metab*; **32**: 833–47.

Green D.M., Brecher M.L., Lindsay A.N., Yakar D., Voorhese M.L., MacGillivray M.H., Freeman A.I. (1981). Gonadal function in pediatric patients following treatment for Hodgkin's disease. *Med. and Ped. Oncol*; **9**: 235–44.

Griffin N.K., Wadsworth J. (1980). Effect of treatment of malignant disease on growth in children. *Arch. Dis. Childh*; **55**: 600–603.

Hopewell J.W. (1979). Late radiation damage to the central nervous system: A radiobiological interpretation. *Neuropathol. and Applied Neurobiol*; **5**: 329–43.

Huang K. (1979). Assessment of hypothalamic–pituitary function in women after external head irradiation. *J. Clin. Endocrinol. Metab*; **46**: 623–9.

Kaplan H.S. (1980). *Hodgkin's Disease*, 2nd edn. Harvard University Press.

Koulumies M., Voultilaine A., Koulumies R. (1964). Effect of x-ray irradiation on laryngeal cancer on the function of the thyroid gland. *Ann. Med. Intern. Fenn*; **53**: 89–96.

Koyama H., Wada T., Nishizawa Y., Iwanaga T., Aoki Y., Terasawa T., Kosaki G., Yamamoto T., Wada A. (1977). Cyclophosphamide induced ovarian failure and its therapeutic significance in patients with breast cancer. *Cancer*; **39**: 1403–9.

Kumar R., Biggart J.D., McEvoy J., McGeown M.G. (1972). Cyclophosphamide and reproductive function. *Lancet*; **1**: 1212–14.

Lawrence J.H., Nelson W.O., Wilson H. (1937). Roentgen irradiation of the hypophysis. *Radiology*; **29**: 446–50.

Lendon M., Hann I.M., Palmer M.K., Shalet S.M., Morris Jones P.H. (1978). Testicular histology after combination chemotherapy in childhood acute lymphoblastic leukaemia. *Lancet*; **2**: 439–41.

Linde R., Doelle G.C., Alexander N., Kirchner F., Vale W., Rivier J., Rabin D. (1981). Reversible inhibition of testicular steroidogenesis and spermatogenesis by a potent gonadotrophin releasing hormone agonist in normal men. *New Engl. J. Med*; **305**: 663–7.

Lushbaugh C.C., Casaret G.W. (1976). The effects of gonadal irradiation in clinical radiation therapy: A review. *Cancer*; **37**: 1111–20.

Mosier H.D., Jansons R.A. (1967). Stunted growth in rats following X-irradiation to the head. *Growth*; **31**: 139–45.

Mosier H.D., Jansons R.A. (1970). Effect of X-irradiation of selected areas of the head of the newborn rat on growth. *Radiat. Res*; **43**: 92–8.

Nahhas W.A., Nisce L.A., D'Angio G.J., Lewis J.L. (1971). Lateral ovarian transposition. Ovarian relocation in patients with Hodgkin's disease. *Obstet. Gynecol*; **38**: 785–8.

Pizzuto J., Aviles A., Noriega L., Niz J., Morales M., Romero F. (1980). Treatment of acute leukaemia during pregnancy: presentation of nine cases. *Cancer Treat. Rep*; **64**: 679–83.

Rappaport R., Brauner R., Czernichow P., Thibaud E., Renier D., Zucker J.M., Lemerle J. (1982). Effect of hypothalamic and pituitary irradiation on pubertal development in children with cranial tumours. *J. Clin. Endocrinol. Metab*; **54**: 1164–8.

Richards G.E., Wara W.M., Grumbach M.M., Kaplan S.L., Sheline G.L., Conte F.A. (1976). Delayed onset of hypopituitarism: Sequelae of therapeutic irradiation of central nervous system, eye and middle ear tumours. *J. Pediatr*; **89**: 553–9.

Richter P., Calamera J.C., Morganfeld M.C. *et al.* (1970). Effect of chlorambucil on spermatogenesis in the human with malignant lymphoma. *Cancer*; **25**: 1026–30.

Rowley M., Leach D.R., Warner G.A., Heller C.G. (1974). Effect of graded doses of ionising radiation on the human testis. *Radiation Res*; **59**: 665–78.

Samaan N.A., Bakdash M.M., Caderao J.B., Cangir A., Jesse R.H., Ballantyne A.J. (1975). Hypopituitarism after external irradiation. Evidence for both hypothalamic and pituitary origin. *Am. Intern. Med*; **83**: 771–7.

Schimpff S.C., Diggs C.H., Wiswell J.G., Salvatore P.C., Wiernich P.H. (1980). Radiation related thyroid dysfunction: Implications for the treatment of Hodgkin's disease. *Ann. Int. Med*; **92**: 91–8.

Shalet S.M. (1982). Abnormalities of growth and gonadal function in children treated for malignant disease: A review. *J. Roy. Soc. Med*; **75**: 641–7.

Shalet S.M., Beardwell C.G., Morris Jones P.H., Bamford F.N., Ribeiro G.G., Pearson D. (1976*a*). Growth hormone deficiency in children with brain tumours. *Cancer*; **37**: 1144–8.

Shalet S.M., Beardwell C.G., Morris Jones P.H., Pearson D. (1976*b*). Growth hormone deficiency after treatment of acute leukaemia in children. *Arch. Dis. Childh*; **51**: 489–93.

Shalet S.M., Beardwell C.G., MacFarlane I.A., Morris Jones P.H., Pearson D. (1977). Endocrine morbidity in adults treated with cerebral irradiation for brain tumours during childhood. *Acta Endocrinologica*; **84**: 673–80.

Shalet S.M., Beardwell C.G., Aarons B.H., Pearson D., Morris Jones P.H. (1978). Growth impairment in children treated for brain tumours. *Arch. Dis. Childh*; **53**: 491–4.

Shalet S.M., Price D.A., Beardwell C.G., Morris Jones P.H., Pearson D. (1979*a*). Normal growth despite abnormalities of growth hormone secretion in children treated for acute leukaemia. *J. Paedriatr*; **94**: 719–22.

Shalet S.M., MacFarlane I.A., Beardwell C.G. (1979*b*). Radiation induced hyperprolactinaemia in a treated acromegalic. *Clin. Endocrinol*; **11**: 169–71.

Shalet S.M., Hann I.M., Lendon M., Morris Jones P.H., Beardwell C.G. (1981*a*). Testicular function after combination chemotherapy in childhood for acute lymphoblastic leukaemia. *Arch. Dis. Child*; **56**: 275–8.

Shalet S.M., Whitehead E., Chapman A.J., Beardwell C.G. (1981*b*). The effects of growth hromone therapy in children with radiation induced growth hormone deficiency. *Acta. Paediatr. Scand*; **70**: 81–6.

Shamberger R.C., Rosenberg S.A., Seipp C.A., Sherins R.J. (1981). Effects of high dose methotrexate and vincristine on ovarian and testicular functions in patients undergoing postoperative adjuvant treatment of osteosarcoma. *Cancer Treat. Rep*; **65**: 739–46.

Sheline G.E. (1973). Treatment of chromophobe adenomas of the pituitary gland and acromegaly. In *Diagnosis and Treatment of Pituitary Tumours* (Kohler P.O., Ross G.F., eds.) pp. 201–16. New York, Amsterdam, London: Elsevier.

Sheline G.E. (1980). Irradiation injury of the human brain: A review of clinical experience. In *Radiation Damage to the Nervous System* (Gilbert H.A., Kagan A.R., eds.) pp. 39–58. New York: Raven Press.

Sherins R.J., Olweny C.L.M., Ziegler J.L. (1978). Gynecomastia and gonadal dysfunction in adolescent boys treated with combination chemotherapy for Hodgkin's disease. *New Eng. J. Med*; **299**: 12–16.

Simpson M.E., Van Wagenen G., Van Dyke D.C., Koneff A.A., Tobias C.A. (1959). Deuteron irradiation of the monkey pituitary. *Endocrinology*; **65**: 831–6.

Siris E., Leventhal B.G., Vaitukaitis J.L. (1976). Effects of childhood leukaemia and chemotherapy on puberty and reproductive function in girls. *New Eng. J. Med*; **294**: 1143–6.

Smith R.E., Adler R.A., Mulherin P., Brinck-Johnson T., Tulloh M.E., Colton T. (1978). Thyroid function following mantle irradiation in Hodgkin's disease. *Proc. Am. Soc. Clin. Oncol*; **C-91**: 329.

Smithers D.W., Wallace D.M., Austin D.E. (1973). Fertility after unilateral orchidectomy and radiotherapy for patients with malignant tumours of the testis. *Brit. Med. J*; **4**: 77–9.

Thomas P.R.M., Winstanly D., Peckham M.J., Austin D.E., Murray M.A.F., Jacobs H.S. (1976). Reproductive and endocrine function in patients with Hodgkin's disease: Effects of oophorpexy and irradiation. *B.J. Cancer*; **33**: 226–31.

UNSCEAR Report. (1977). Sources and effects of ionising radiation. In *United Nations Scientific Committee on the Effects of Atomic Radiation 1977 Report to the General Assembly*. pp. 478–85.

Van der Kogel A.J., Barendsen G.W. (1974). Late effects of spinal cord irradiation with 300 KV x-rays and 15 MeV neutrons. *Br. J. Radiol*; **47**: 393–8.

Wara W.M., Phillips T.L., Sheline G.E., Schwade J.G. (1975). Radiation tolerance of the spinal cord. *Cancer*; **35**: 1558–62.

Whitehead E., Shalet S.M., Blackedge G., Todd I., Crowther D., Beardwell C.G. (1982*a*). The effects of Hodgkin's disease and combination chemotherapy on gonadal function in the adult male. *Cancer*; **49**: 418–22.

Whitehead E., Shalet S.M., Morris Jones P.H., Beardwell C.G., Deakin D.P. (1982*b*). Gonadal function after combination chemotherapy for Hodgkin's disease in childhood. *Arch. Dis. Child*; **47**: 287–91.

Chapter 14

John A. Lynn

The Clinical Management of Multiple Endocrine Adenomatosis

INTRODUCTION

The association of endocrine abnormalities within a family was known as early as the time of Harvey Cushing (Cushing, 1932). It remained for Wermer to propose in 1954 the term 'adenomatosis' of the endocrine glands, when investigating a family with multiple endocrine abnormalities (Wermer, 1954). Recent studies of a variety of families have shown that, in addition to the syndrome described by Wermer, now called 'multiple endocrine adenomatosis' (MEA type I), two other types of multiple endocrine abnormality exist, these being MEA type II and MEA type III. Multiple endocrine adenomatosis type II was first recognised when Sipple (1961) made the observation that there was an unusual association between phaeochromocytoma and thyroid cancer. Some workers regard MEA type III as a minor subdivision of MEA type II, and therefore label the syndromes MEA type IIA and MEA type IIB, respectively. Throughout this discussion the terms MEA types, I, II and III will be used.

Multiple endocrine adenomatosis type I or Wermer's syndrome is now known to be a familial disorder involving the pituitary, pancreas and the parathyroid glands (*see* Table 14.1). The entity is a genetic defect which is autosomal dominant in character with a high penetrance, but with variable expressibility. It is important to note that clinical involvement of any of the endocrine organs which may be affected can be synchronous or metachronous. Multiple endocrine adenomatosis type II as described by Sipple (1961) consists of a thyroid cancer arising not from the follicular cells of the thyroid but from the parafollicular cells. These cells, known as the 'C-cells', have the unique characteristic of secreting a specific hormone called 'calcitonin' which when the cells become hyperplastic or malignant, acts as a tumour marker. Steiner and co-workers (1968) recognised the association of the specific C-cell tumour which is now called medullary carcinoma of the thyroid, with hyperparathyroidism as well as phaeochromocytoma.

Multiple endocrine adenomatosis type III is very similar to MEA type II. In the MEA type III there is an aggressive form of medullary carcinoma of the thyroid, phaeochromocytoma of the adrenal glands, but interestingly

TABLE 14.1

Multiple Endocrine Adenomatosis Types I, II and III

Type I	Type II	Type III
Parathyroid adenomas and/or hyperplasia	Bilateral medullary carcinoma of the thyroid gland	Bilateral medullary carcinoma of the thyroid gland
Pancreatic islet adenomas (B or non-B cells)	Phaeochromocytoma (bilateral or extra-adrenal)	Phaeochromocytoma(s)
Pituitary adenomas (functioning or non-functioning)	Parathyroid hyperplasia	Parathyroids normal
Adrenocortical adenomas	No specific phenotype	Specific phenotype (mucosal neuromas)
Thyroid adenomas	Familial inheritance autosomal dominant	Infrequently familial
	Medullary carcinoma of thyroid relatively 'benign'	Medullary carcinoma of thyroid 'aggressive'
		Rare survivors aged 30

hyperparathyroidism is almost always absent. Patients with MEA type III have a characteristic phenotype consisting of Marfanoid features, rather prominent mandibles and puffy lips, with associated mucosal neuromas involving the eyelids, tongue and other mucous membranes. Other features include medullated corneal nerves, pes cavus and gastrointestinal abnormalities consisting of diverticulosis and ganglioneuromatosis. In MEA type III the physical appearances of the patient suggest the diagnosis. The disease of the thyroid is far more aggressive, and there is less tendency for there to be familial involvement, and patients frequently dying young.

The multiple endocrine adenomatosis syndromes have given us insight as to embryological tissue of origin of many endocrine cells and their associated tumours. These cells belong to the APUD group. The name APUD refers to a series of endocrine cells with specific characteristics. The APUD cells derive their name from their main histochemical features described by Pearse (1968). 'A' denotes a high amine content; 'PU' refers to their capacity for amine precursor uptake; and 'D' indicates the presence of the enzyme decarboxylase, which converts the precursors which are amino acids, into amines. The reason why patients develop a single or a combination of defects in these syndromes is unknown. It is also unknown why there is the presence of a parathyroid abnormality in multiple endocrine adenopathy types I and II, since the cells of the parathyroid are not derived from the neural crests and do not have features of the APUD cells.

MEA TYPE I SYNDROME

Multiple endocrine adenomatosis type I or Wermer's syndrome is now a term used to describe the inherited endocrine disorder consisting of tumours of the parathyroids, pancreatic islets and pituitary gland. On occasion, tumours also arise in the adrenals and the thyroid, although these are rare. The disease has been shown to be inherited and caused by an autosomal dominant gene, which as stated earlier, has a high degree of penetrance.

When the adrenal glands are involved, it may be secondary either to the pituitary involvement and consist of hyperplasia, or rarely be due to ectopic ACTH secretion either from carcinoid of the gastrointestinal tract or a carcinoid of the bronchus. On rare occasions, primary adrenocortical tumours may occur. In some families, multiple lipomas occur as seen in Dercum's disease. The one invariable aspect of the syndrome is the presence of primary hyperparathyroidism, usually due to hyperplasia of the four glands, although on occasion asymmetric hyperplasia may occur and even rarely a single parathyroid adenoma. The histology of the parathyroids usually shows a chief cell hyperplasia. In MEA type I the parathyroid abnormality is usually the presenting aspect of the disease. The symptoms of MEA type I, due to the parathyroid abnormality, are the same as those in uncomplicated primary hyperparathyroidism. These consist of polyuria, polydipsia, fatigue, gastrointestinal symptoms and renal stones. Despite the fact that the parathyroid element is the common presentation of MEA type I, in the general population of patients with parathyroid disease MEA type I syndrome is rare. Following routine screening of gastrin levels in all patients with primary hyperparathyroidism in our unit, the pick-up rate of MEA type I is small. The pick-up rate is increased after surgery, when patients with primary hyperparathyroidism are found to have chief cell hyperplasia and not the common single gland adenoma.

In patients with Zollinger–Ellison syndrome, it is essential to screen them for parathyroid abnormalities as they are so common. The management of the parathyroid glands in these patients is total parathyroidectomy, with auto-transplantation and possible cryo-preservation of the parathyroids. This technique is discussed in detail under MEA type II, and its rationale is similar to the MEA type II situation. It must be emphasised that the gastrinomas are usually malignant, whilst the insulinomas, which are producing the inappropriate secretion of insulin, are benign. As has been mentioned by Thompson (1982), in MEA type I syndrome the pancreas is always involved. This involvement may be either a gastrinoma resulting in the Zollinger–Ellison syndrome, or an insulinoma associated with hypogly-caemic attacks due to the inappropriate secretion of insulin. Pancreatic polypeptide has been shown by Friesen *et al.* (1979) to be a common secretory product of islet cell hyperplasia, microadenoma or frank pancreatic tumours in MEA type I. The production of pancreatic polypeptide on its own does not appear to produce any specific syndrome.

Zollinger-Ellison Syndrome

There are three facets to this entity. Most clinicians are familiar with the ulcerogenic form, more subtle though is the diarrhoeal type, with its resulting fluid and electrolyte imbalance. The third facet is as a component of the MEA type I syndrome. Each can occur singly or in combination.

The clinical presentation is that of intractable peptic ulcer diathesis or of recurrent ulceration after curative surgery. Particular attention should be paid to the patient who presents with recurrence and bleeding in the immediate post-operative period.

Radiological evidence of gastric dilatation and hypersensitivity, alongside duodenal or jejunal ulceration in the absence of gastric outlet obstruction, is highly suggestive of Zollinger–Ellison syndrome, although this picture may also be seen in antral G-cell hyperplasia. Selective arteriography is of little or no help. Ultrasonography or CAT scan can detect parapancreatic tumour nodules or hepatic metastatic lesions. Gastric acid hypersecretion and elevated serum gastrin levels are a veritable pointer to this disease; the confirmation should be based on the results of more than one sample.

Other causes of hypergastrinaemia, such as gastric outlet obstruction and retained antral mucosa, can be differentiated biochemically from the Zollinger–Ellison syndrome by the secretin stimulation test. Secretin infusion induces a rise in serum gastrin levels in the latter, but is unaffected or decreased in the former two conditions. If hypercalcaemia is superimposed on gastric acid hypersecretion, MEA I should be suspected.

The management of the gastrinoma element in MEA type I syndrome has been radically changed with the advent of the H_2-antagonist cimetidine. Prior to the advent of cimetidine, the only logical treatment for Zollinger–Ellison syndrome was total gastrectomy ablating completely the target organ with a small chance of pancreatic tumour resection. Prior to the advent of cimetidine the chance of cure was dictated by the nature of the disease, because only 5% of cases of Zollinger–Ellison syndrome were due to a single adenoma which was easily resectable. Cimetidine has allowed us to control the ulcer diathesis, and a change in policy has developed with its use. In the elderly, the gastric symptoms may be controlled by cimetidine, with no attempt to resect the pancreas. In the young, the ulcer diathesis may be controlled by cimetidine, the general nutritional status of the patient improved, and then a radical approach to attempt a cure by total pancreatectomy may be considered. It must be emphasised that the chance of pancreatic cure is less than 5% in both age groups. In the case of a solitary gastrinoma which has been successfully removed, further surgery in the form of total pancreatic resection may be necessary at a later date to deal with the islet cell hypertrophy, or multiple insulinomas.

It is important to restate that on all occasions it is essential to deal with the parathyroid element first, because it may be possible to control the gastrointestinal symptoms more easily with cimetidine once the hypercalcaemia has resolved. Pancreatic surgery may therefore not be necessary. Subtotal gastrectomy and vagotomy is a very poor alternative to total gastrectomy and necessitates long-term cimetidine therapy.

Insulinoma

Inappropriate insulin secretion (hyperinsulinism) is usually due to either an adenoma or a diffuse hyperplasia of the B-cells of pancreatic islets. These B-cells synthesise proinsulin, which undergoes proteolytic division into active insulin and a connective peptide (C-peptide). Both rise together during pancreatic islet stimulation, but the C-peptide does not appear to produce any specific syndrome.

To diagnose an insulinoma from other forms of fasting hypoglycaemia, such as dumping syndrome, alcoholic cirrhosis or Addison's disease, an autonomous insulin release must be proven. Blood samples are taken at intervals during a prolonged fasting period, and both blood glucose and insulin levels are assayed to determine the ratio of glucose to immunoreactive insulin. An inappropriately high insulin level during hypoglycaemia is diagnostic. Exogenous insulin administration does not suppress the endogenous insulin production by an insulinoma. In such a case, the C-peptide blood levels remain inappropriately high. Intravenous diazoxide injection normally depresses insulin release in the hypoglycaemic patient, but fails to do so in a case of insulinoma. There are also provocative tests by administration of substances such as tolbutamide, glucagon or L-leucine, which stimulate insulin release and produce diagnostic hyperinsulinism during hypoglycaemia. These tests can be dangerous and must be used only for hospitalised patients.

Once the autonomous hyperinsulinism has been proven, the next important step is the tumour localisation. This is quite difficult, since insulinomas are usually small. The CAT scan and sonogram are of little help. The best study is the selective pancreatic arteriogram. The pancreatic islets are quite vascular and the insulinoma may show up as a tumour blush. A very interesting technique is percutaneous and transhepatic cannulation of the portal vein and selective sampling along the course of the splenic vein. Finally, digital subtraction angiography may prove to be useful in such tumour localisation in the near future.

When hyperinsulinism occurs in the MEA type I syndrome it is rarely due to malignant disease, and is most likely to be associated with an insulinoma which on occasions may be multiple. The surgical management of hyperinsulinism in MEA type I syndrome is different from the management of a gastrinoma. Unlike the gastrinoma the insulinoma can often be completely removed and a permanent cure of the problem will result. When the insulinoma is localised to the pancreas, then either simple enucleation or partial resection of the pancreas may be performed. If there is diffuse disease, then a subtotal pancreatectomy may cure the patient, or may allow the patient's symptoms to be controlled by diazoxide. If diazoxide and subtotal resection does not control the symptoms, total pancreatectomy must be considered. Because the patient has had an insulinoma removed, there is still a chance of his developing a further islet cell tumour either an insulinoma or a gastrinoma. Therefore, patients should be followed-up for life. When there are metastases outside the pancreas, such as solitary lesions in the liver, then treatment with local resection or arterial embolisation of the tumour may be considered.

As regards management with chemotherapy, the best single agent for pancreatic tumours is streptozotocin, and regression has been obtained in approximately 50% of insulinomas and 25% in gastrinomas, and if this is not effective cyclophosphamide and 5-fluorouracil may be used. There is some suggestion that combined streptozotocin and 5-fluorouracil may give better results (Wood *et al.*, 1983).

Pituitary tumours in the MEA type I syndrome occur in approximately 65% of patients. Their effects can be due to local pressure or to endocrine changes due to specific hormone secretions. Acromegaly will occur due to growth hormone excess, galactorrhoea may be a presenting feature of a prolactinoma in men, whilst in women non-puerperal galactorrhoea or amenorrhoea may occur. Adrenocorticotrophin hormone hypersecretion will result in Cushing's syndrome, whilst on rare occasions excess production of TSH can produce thyrotoxicosis. The management of the pituitary tumour depends very much on the expertise available in the centre concerned. Trans-sphenoidal selective microdissection of pituitary tumours is particularly advantageous for the small hyperfunctioning adenoma seen in MEA type I syndrome. If the tumours are large or extra-sellar, it may be necessary to consider craniotomy or supervoltage irradiation, or in special centres proton beam irradiation.

MEA TYPE II SYNDROME

Multiple endocrine adenomatosis type II consists of abnormalities of the thyroid, the adrenal medulla and the parathyroid, and these abnormalities are listed in Table 14.1. As already stated, the association of abnormalities of the thyroid, adrenal medulla and parathyroid were first reported by Sipple in 1961 (the so-called Sipple syndrome). Attention was drawn to the syndrome by the presence of phaeochromocytomas, which if left untreated could be rapidly fatal. It was also noted that the condition could be hereditary. An important problem in MEA type II is whether or not the disease is sporadic or familial. Many authors have suggested that the sporadic form of the disease is most common. The recognition of the familial disease which is inherited as mendelian autosomal dominant, and the screening of relatives of patients with MEA type II has resulted at our own clinic in a much higher incidence of the familial form of the disease than the sporadic.

The management of MEA type II is complex, since it may present initially because of its thyroid, adrenal or parathyroid element, singly, synchronously or even metachronously.

The common form of presentation is in the thyroid component of the syndrome. This may be as a single nodule in the thyroid, associated with a raised calcitonin in a patient known to have a family history of MEA type II. Alternatively, it may be made at frozen section during a thyroid operation or as a pathological diagnosis after a thyroid mass has been removed. Medullary carcinoma in the MEA type II syndrome which arises from the C-cells, is identical histologically to that arising sporadically. The important point to be borne in mind is that in the MEA type II syndrome the tumour is almost always bilateral and tends to arise in the superior lateral part of the thyroid lobe, and may be multiple throughout the lobe. The neoplasm itself is a whitish-tan nodule and is histologically composed of sheets or cords of round- or spindle-shaped cells, separated by a variable amount of amorphous stromal material. If the patient is old, the medullary carcinoma of the thyroid may be primarily composed of fibrous tissue with very little cellular element. Congo red staining of the thyroid of a patient with medullary carcinoma will usually show amyloid-like material with a typical apple-green birefringence which is scattered among the amorphous stromal area. It is important to state that, although this is a common finding, its presence is not necessary to diagnose medullary carcinoma of the thyroid, because this substance is on occasion not seen in patients with primary or metastatic tumour foci. Specific antibodies with immunofluorescence to calcitonin will demonstrate the presence of calcitonin granules in these tumours.

The situation is complicated since it is now known that in many instances medullary carcinoma of the thyroid is preceded by hyperplasia of the C-cells. C-cell hyperplasia undoubtedly occurs in the familial form of the disease, but its incidence in the sporadic form, in which tumours may well be unilateral, is not known.

It cannot be emphasised too strongly that in any patient with medullary carcinoma of the thyroid, the status of the adrenals must be assessed prior to any surgical exploration of the neck, or any interventional radiological assessment which needs a general anaesthetic. Operating on the neck of a patient with an undiagnosed phaeochromocytoma may well prove to be fatal.

Bearing in mind that in all subjects the surgeon will have assessed the status of the adrenals and ruled out a phaeochromocytoma before subjecting the patient to a general anaesthetic or neck exploration, the surgeon then has to decide in which order to deal with the abnormalities of the syndrome, and how much tissue to remove from each of the organs involved. It is obvious that a phaeochromocytoma must be dealt with prior to any other procedure on the patient. Because the disease is usually bilateral in the thyroid, the only logical approach to a patient with disease localised in this organ, is the procedure of total thyroidectomy. There is no place for subtotal resection. This is a safe procedure with a low morbidity and virtually zero mortality, and in expert hands will result, if the parathyroids are normal, with an incidence of permanent hypoparathyroidism of less than 1%. It is essential when performing a total thyroidectomy to remember that the thyroid may extend upwards into the midline from the isthmus of the thyroid right up to the larynx, since if such thyroid tissue is not removed recurrence can easily occur in the remaining thyroid tissue. At neck exploration many of the thyroid tumours, particularly in familial cases, will not be obvious on the outside of the thyroid. (Such patients will have been diagnosed by their high calcitonin levels in association with their strong family history.)

On other occasions on exploring the neck, the typical nodules will be visible on the surface of the thyroid, with their typical whitish-brown hue. If the thyroid only is involved with medullary carcinoma, the procedure is quite simple and only a total thyroidectomy should be performed.

There is no evidence that radical removal of lymph nodes draining the thyroid, which are not involved with medullary carcinoma of the thyroid, in any way improves the prognosis. It is the author's policy, however, at the time of surgery, to subject several draining lymph nodes to frozen section, so that their status can be assessed. If the lymph nodes are positive either macroscopically or microscopically for medullary carcinoma, they should then be removed. Particular attention must be paid to the area around the recurrent laryngeal nerves where the local lymph nodes are often involved. The removal of the thymus will often facilitate the excision of the pre-tracheal lymph nodes, when they are extending down into the mediastinum. On occasions it may be necessary to split the sternum so as to remove the pre-tracheal lymph nodes which can often be removed on block with the thyroid. Unless the lateral lymph nodes in the neck are infiltrating the muscle, a modified form of neck dissection preserving the internal jugular vein and the major muscles of the neck, as well as the accessory nerve, should be performed. If there is direct infiltration into the muscle by the lymph nodes in the neck, then a standard radical neck dissection should be performed, with sacrifice of the accessory nerve and internal jugular vein. The question of tracheal involvement is a difficult problem. In an elderly patient, tracheostomy, with possible total laryngectomy, must be avoided if possible, because the fact that unless there is definite airways obstruction there is the possibility that the tumour is slow growing and the patient may die of an unrelated cause.

In MEA type II, at the time of exploration of the neck, it is essential that the status of all four parathyroids is assessed in detail. If the serum calcium is normal and the parathyroid element of the syndrome has not presented itself, then all four glands should be identified and one biopsied to see if there is any abnormality. If, however, the serum calcium is raised, then each parathyroid should be identified and a minute biopsy taken from each and these biopsies subjected to intra-operative frozen section. The common parathyroid abnormality is hyperplasia of all four glands. On occasions, asymmetrical hyperplasia may occur or more rarely a single parathyroid adenoma.

The management of hyperplasia of the parathyroids is difficult, and one has the choice of three possible techniques. The first technique is that of a subtotal parathyroidectomy, leaving behind in the neck approximately 120 mg of parathyroid tissue. This entails removing three parathyroids which are hyperplastic, and the majority of the fourth. This technique was widely used for several years in our own department, and has now been shown to have an unacceptable incidence of recurrence of the hypercalcaemic state. Other workers have confirmed our own findings. Clark *et al.* (1976) found recurrent post-operative hypercalcaemia in 33% of 22 patients undergoing surgery for familial hyperparathyroidism, whilst Lamers and Froeling (1979) reported a hypercalcaemic rate of 38% in patients with hyperplasia, which admittedly however was in the MEA type I situation. It is, therefore, the author's opinion that the second technique of total parathyroidectomy and transplantation of the parathyroids into the forearm muscle is the most satisfactory (Prinz *et al.*, 1981).

The third possibility of total parathyroidectomy and maintenance of normocalcaemia with vitamin D and calcium substitution alone would not seem a good alternative, unless the long-term results of a parathyroid transplantation are, at a later date, shown to be poor.

The great advantage of parathyroid transplantation is that if further surgery is needed to reduce the bulk of parathyroid tissue, it can be done under local anaesthetic with minimal morbidity. This is a minor procedure compared to a re-exploration of the neck. In patients on renal dialysis, in whom the MEA type II syndrome has resulted in renal failure, it is a good idea not to transplant the parathyroid tissue into the arm or leg but into the pectoralis muscle, since local surgery in the limbs may interfere with vascular access for haemodialysis at a later date.

Parathyroid transplantation may be performed immediately or as a delayed procedure. In the latter technique the parathyroid is cryo-preserved. The technique of parathyroid transplantation itself is quite simple; once the parathyroids have been removed and their nature confirmed by frozen section, the parathyroids are placed in chilled saline. The chilling not only reduces the metabolic activity of the tissue but has the advantage of making it firm and easy to cut. The parathyroids are sliced into pieces approximately $1 \times 1 \times 3$ mm in size, and usually 20 pieces are implanted into the donor site. The site is marked with metal clips so that the parathyroid tissue can be easily identified at a later date, if there is a need to re-explore the area. It is ideal where possible to cryo-preserve some of the parathyroid tissue. This has the advantage that if the parathyroid graft fails, there is further tissue available. This technique has been extensively used by Wells and his co-workers (1978). The tissue is preserved in a solution containing 10% dimethylsulphoxide, 10% autologous serum and 80% tissue culture medium. It has been shown by Romanus *et al.* (1982) that the use of dimethylsulphoxide in the freezing medium increases the yield of viable tissue in the cryo-preservation process.

Once the parathyroid tissue has been rapidly thawed, the technique of delayed parathyroid grafting is similar to that of the immediate graft method. The use of parathyroid grafting is not without its problems. The grafted tissue does not function immediately and support will be needed with vitamin D and calcium in the immediate post-operative period. By about eight weeks the graft will have taken, and calcium and vitamin D therapy can be discontinued. In some patients however the graft will fail, and then either a regraft should be performed using the cryo-preservation technique, or if this is not possible, long-term therapy with vitamin D and calcium will be necessary.

The other side of the coin is graft-dependent hyperparathyroidism. Under no circumstances should a parathyroid adenoma be grafted, since a severe form of hyperparathyroidism may result which is very difficult to treat due to very aggressive disease in the forearm (Brennan *et al.*, 1978). On occasions, recurrent hyperparathyroidism will occur because the transplanted material which is known to be hyperfunctional is producing far more parathyroid hormone than the body requires. In the circumstances it is quite simple to re-operate under local anaesthesia, and remove a small percentage of the parathyroid transplant. This technique may need to be repeated on several occasions until the right amount of parathyroid tissue is present in the forearm.

The screening for phaeochromocytoma consists of the usual techniques of urinary VMA, plasma noradrenaline and adrenaline and also CAT scanning of the adrenal.

The phaeochromocytomas that occur in MEA type II syndrome have a tendency to be multiple and also extra-adrenal. Pre-operative management prior to dealing with a phaeochromocytoma should consist of a two week preparation with the alpha-receptor blocker phenoxybenzamine. It is not routine in the author's experience to regularly use a beta-adrenergic receptor blocker unless a tachycardia or an irregular rhythm occurs with the phenoxybenzamine. The phaeochromocytomas in the MEA type II syndrome always appear to be benign, and this concurs with the experience of Farndon's group (Farndon *et al.*, 1982) in America. Weiland and his group (Weiland *et al.*, 1980; Sisson *et al.*, 1982) have developed imaging of the phaeochromocytoma by the use of a specific radionuclide in the catecholamine precursors of the adrenal medulla (I) metaiodobenzylguanidine—MIBG. This technique which has recently been evaluated by Sisson and his co-workers (Sisson *et al.*, 1981), will undoubtedly be of great value in the future, not only for localisation of the tumour but also possibly for screening. Allison *et al.* (1983) have shown the value in difficult diagnostic cases of selective venous sampling from the adrenal veins of adrenaline and noradrenaline. Also in difficult diagnostic cases Brown *et al.* (1981) have used a pentolinium suppression technique for increasing the pick-up rate of phaeochromocytomas.

Exploration of the abdomen for phaeochromocytomas should be performed from an anterior approach searching on both sides of the abdomen with meticulous inspection of the adrenals, and a careful search from the crura of the diaphragm down to the bladder for sites of para-aortic ectopic tumours arising from the chromaffin chain.

It must also be emphasised that, even though a single phaeochromocytoma has been removed in the past, this does not prevent the patient developing a further phaeochromocytoma in another site at a later date. Therefore, following excision of their phaeochromocytomas, patients who may at a later date need surgery on either their parathyroids or thyroid, must always be re-evaluated to exclude a second or even a third phaeochromocytoma.

Carney *et al.* (1975) have emphasised that the adrenal pathology in the MEA type II syndrome is not limited to phaeochromocytomas, but there may be an element of adrenal medullary hyperplasia. This finding has caused some workers to routinely remove apparently normal tissue, since it is felt that there is a high risk of local recurrence of the phaeochromocytoma syndrome if microscopic hyperplastic medullary tissue is left *in situ*. This is a highly aggressive approach, which is not policy in the author's department, where intra-operative frozen section of the apparently normal adrenal is used. Total adrenalectomy would commit the patient to lifelong corticosteroid replacement, and since the patients are being carefully followed up, a less aggressive approach would seem a reasonable compromise.

The management of metastatic medullary carcinoma of the thyroid is a difficult problem. Management of the metastases of the local lymph nodes has already been discussed and when they are removable should be treated by surgery. When disease is irremovable, radiotherapy should be used. Metastases may also arise in the lungs, liver or bone and may be associated with severe diarrhoea, the exact cause of which is not known. The diarrhoea which has been treated by a variety of agents, from simple measures such as codeine phosphate to resins such as cholestyramine, is often intractable and is debilitating for the patient. It has been the author's experience that simple measures such as codeine phosphate offers the best palliation. More exotic agents have been of little value. Metastases of the liver when solitary should be considered either for local resection or for embolisation of the hepatic artery. Unfortunately, most liver metastases are multiple and the results of total hepatic arterial embolisation have not proved as encouraging as when used in the carcinoid syndrome.

Solitary lung metastases are rare but may on occasion be amenable to segmental resection. A solitary bone metastasis may respond well to local radiotherapy. Unlike other forms of thyroid cancer, there is no role for radio-active iodine, because the lesions do not arise from the follicular cells and therefore do not concentrate iodine.

Following surgery for medullary carcinoma of the thyroid the calcitonin level may return to normal, particularly if it is an early lesion and there is a good chance of cure. It is the experience of most workers that in extensive disease treated by apparent curative surgery, it is rare for the calcitonin in the blood to become undetectable. This has been the author's and his colleagues experience, and also the experience of the group at the Royal Marsden Hospital, London (Palmer *et al.*, 1982). Despite the fact that patients following apparent successful surgery have a raised calcitonin level in their blood, many of these patients remain remarkably well for anything up to 20 years and are asymptomatic. Groups in the USA have studied patients who have raised calcitonin levels in their blood by selective venous sampling of areas in the neck, and have shown 'hot spots' for calcitonin in the neck, even though there is no palpable disease. Such patients have been subjected to radical neck dissection and the calcitonin level in their blood has become undetectable. This unfortunately has not been the experience in the author's department, since we have found it difficult to find metastatic medullary carcinoma in the neck without a palpable lump.

The results of chemotherapy in medullary carcinoma are poor. There is little data at the moment on chemotherapeutic agents, although Adriamycin has been used by some workers with some response (Gottlieb and Hill, 1974).

The decision as to whether a new case of medullary carcinoma of the thyroid which is part of the MEA type II syndrome is sporadic or familial, can be extremely difficult. If there is a family history of phaeochromocytoma or thyroid lumps, often it is likely that one is dealing with an MEA type II familial case. This raises the problem of screening relatives of patients with MEA type II syndrome. It is our policy to screen all the near relatives for basal and stimulated calcitonin levels in the blood whenever we pick up a new case of medullary carcinoma of the thyroid. The technique used at the Royal Postgraduate Medical School, London, is to stimulate the patients with oral ethanol and then take samples at five and ten minutes. The use of pentagastrin and calcium, although possibly more sensitive, is not an easy technique in mass screening. Melvin *et al.* (1971) have emphasised that the early diagnosis of medullary carcinoma of the thyroid by means of the calcitonin assay in patients with no clinical manifestation of neoplasm, either by palpation of the neck or thyroid scan, will result in a higher cure rate than leaving them to develop a lump. Some patients picked up in this way will not even have a tumour but C-cell hyperplasia, which is supposedly indicative of the pre-malignant phase of medullary carcinoma of the thyroid.

The decision whether to operate on patients with minimally raised calcitonins is complicated by the fact that in the author's experience, several patients whose calcitonin levels have been minimally raised have not been found to have either hyperplasia or tumours of their thyroid glands. This may mean that the calcitonin in these patients is being secreted from sites other than the thyroid or that, despite meticulous histology, small areas of C-cell hyperplasia have not been detected. This complication has resulted in us operating on patients whose calcitonin levels are minimally raised only if the family history is particularly aggressive, or when regular tests have shown a progressive rise in the calcitonin level. This experience is contrary to the American experience, but one has evidence from several other surgical centres in the UK that this problem is more widespread.

MEA TYPE III SYNDROME

Multiple endocrine adenomatosis type III is very similar to MEA type II but is rarely familial, almost never has parathyroid elements to it, and is highly aggressive. The phaeochromocytomas found in the MEA type III are very similar to those found in MEA type II. The medullary carcinoma of the thyroid element however is very aggressive, and there is much to be said for prophylactic total thyroidectomy, irrespective of the calcitonin level.

CONCLUSION

The MEA syndromes types I, II and III provide challenging problems for the geneticist, biochemist, oncologist, endocrinologist and finally the surgeon. The golden rule when dealing with these abnormalities is to be aware that other facets of the syndromes may occur synchronously or metachronously, and having found one abnormality within the syndrome to follow the patient for life, always being aware that another facet may arise. In the MEA type II and III syndromes the presence of a phaeochromocytoma must always be suspected at all stages of the disease, particularly when surgery is considered for some unrelated condition.

Screening of the families may be difficult logistically and patients will often refuse to co-operate, so it needs great tact and understanding on the part of the doctor. There are often psychological problems, since patients feel guilty about the condition of their children, and sympathetic genetic counselling should be advised to such families.

REFERENCES

Allison D.J., Brown M.J., Jones D.H., Timmis J.B. (1983). Role of venous sampling in locating a phaeochromocytoma. *Br. Med. J*; **286**: 1122–4.

Brennan M.F., Brown E.M., Marx S.J. *et al.* (1978). Recurrent hyperparathyroidism from an autotransplanted parathyroid adenoma. *New Engl. J. Med*; **299**: 1057–9.

Brown M.J., Allison D.J., Jenner D.A., Lewis P.J., Dollery C.T. (1981). Increased sensitivity and accuracy of phaeochromocytoma. Diagnosis achieved by plasma-adrenaline estimations and a pentolinium suppression test. *Lancet*; **2**: 174–7.

Carney J.A., Sizemore G.W., Tyce G.M. (1975). Bilateral adrenal medullary hyperplasia in multiple endocrine neoplasia, Type 2. *Mayo Clin. Proc.*, **50**: 3.

Clark O.M., Way L.W., Hunt T.K. (1976). Recurrent hyperparathyroidism. *Ann. Surg*; **184**: 391–9.

Cushing H. (1932). The basophil adenomas of the pituitary body and their clinical manifestations (pituitary basophilism). *Bull. John Hopkins Hosp*; **50**: 137–195.

Farndon J.R., Fagraeus L., Wells S.A. (1982). Recent development in the management of phaeochromocytoma. *Surgery 2, Endocrine Surgery* (Johnston I.D.A., Thompson N.W., eds.) Ch. 12, pp. 189–202. Butterworths International Medical Reviews.

Friesen S.R., Kimmel J.R., Tomita T. (1979). Pancreatic polypeptide as a screening marker for pancreatic polypeptide apudomas in multiple endocrinopathies. *Am. J. Surg*; **139**: 61–72.

Gottlieb J.A., Hill C.S. (1974). Chemotherapy of thyroid cancer with Adriamycin. *N. Engl. J. Med*; **290**: 193–7.

Lamers C.B.H.W., Froeling, P.G.A.M. (1979). Clinical significance of hyperparathyroidism in familial multiple endocrine adenomatosis Type I (MEA I). *Am. J. Med*; **66**: 422–4.

Melvin K.E.W., Miller H.H., Tashjian A.H. Jr. (1971). Early diagnosis of medullary carcinoma of the thyroid by means of calcitonin assay. *N. Engl. J. Med*; **285**: 1115–20.

Palmer B.V., Harmer C.L., Shaw H.J. (1982). Calcitonin and carcinoembryonic antigen in the follow up of patients with medullary carcinoma of the thyroid. Paper given at *British Association of Surgical Oncology*, 23rd Scientific Meeting.

Pearse A.G.E. (1968). Common cytochemical and ultrastructural characteristics of cells producing polypeptide hormones (the APUD series) and their relevance to thyroid and ultimoranchial C cells and calcitonin. *Proc. R. Soc. Lond. (Biol)*; **170**: 71–80.

Prinz R.A., Gamvros O.I., Sellu D., Lynn J.A. (1981). Subtotal parathyroidectomy for primary chief cell hyperplasia of the multiple endocrine neoplasia type I syndrome. *Ann. Surg*; **193**: 26–9.

Romanus M.E., Farndon J.R., Wells S.A. (1982). Transplantation of the parathyroid glands. *Surgery 2, Endocrine Surgery* (Johnston I.D.A., Thompson N.W., eds.) Ch. 3, pp. 25–40. Butterworths International Medical Reviews.

Sipple J.F. (1961) Association of phaeochromocytoma with carcinoma of thyroid gland. *Am. J. Med*; **31**: 163–6.

Sisson J.C., Frager M.S., Valk T.W. *et al.* (1981). Scintigraphic localisation of phaeochromocytoma. *New Engl. J. Med*; **305**: 12–17.

Steiner A.L., Goodman A.D., Powers S.R. (1968). Study of a kindred with phaeochromocytoma, medullary thyroid carcinoma, hyperparathyroidism and Cushing's disease. Multiple endocrine neoplasia, Type 2. *Medicine*; **47**: 371–409.

Thompson N.W. (1982). Surgical consideration in the MEN I syndrome. *Surgery 2, Endocrine Surgery* (Johnston I.D.A., Thompson N.W., eds.) Ch. 9, pp. 144–63. Butterworths International Medical Reviews.

Weiland D.M., Wu J., Brown L.E. *et al.* (1980). Radiolabelled adrenergic neuron-blocking agents: Andrenomedullary imaging with (^{131}I) iodobenzylguanidine. *J. Nucl. Med*; **21**: 349–53.

Weiland D.M., Brown L.E., Tobes M.C. *et al.* (1981). Imaging the primate adrenal medulla with (^{123}I) and (^{131}I) metaiodobenzylguanidine: Concise communication. *J. Nucl. Med*; **22**: 358–64.

Wells S.A., Stirman J.A., Bolman R.M., Gunnells J.C. (1978). Transplantation of the parathyroid glands. Clinical and experimental results. *Surg. Clin. North Am*; **58**: 391–402.

Wermer P. (1954) Genetic aspects of adenomatosis of endocrine glands. *Am. J. Med*; **16**: 363–71.

Wood S.M., Polak J.M., Bloom S.R. (1983). Gut hormone secreting tumours. *Scand. J. Gastroenterology* supplement (in press).

Chapter 15

Richard J. Pye

Skin Changes in Cancer

INTRODUCTION

Many imagine that the skin is a window, and if they gaze through it long enough the diagnosis will emerge. Sadly, this is not always the case for internal disease and all too often systemic malignancies have no cutaneous markers. Nevertheless, there are some markers which have remarkable specificity not only for malignancy but also for particular tumours. It is the purpose of this chapter to point out the possibilities and pitfalls of this aspect of dermatology. There are a number of well described clinical syndromes, many of which are very rare and thus of limited practical value in clinical diagnosis. Even those with a special interest in this subject may have to wait several years between cases. The mechanisms for most of the manifestations are quite unknown, and although there is much to suggest that humoral mediators are involved none have yet been identified. Detection of these mediators may in the future prove to be a useful means of early diagnosis of occult tumours.

There are a number of ways in which the skin may manifest either a high probability of, or the actual presence of internal malignancy. The skin may become directly invaded by malignant cells. These may be discrete metastases often involving the scalp and usually occurring late. More rarely these may be diffuse and present as lymphoedema, mimic cellulitis, or produce widespread erythema and oedema as in Sezary cell syndrome and chronic lymphocytic leukaemia. Paget's disease of the nipple is another well recognised and distinctive example of direct involvement of the skin.

There are a group of genetically determined syndromes with cutaneous signs which are associated with a high risk of internal malignancy. The list is long, but the better known examples include xeroderma pigmentosa, neurofibromatosis, Gardner's, and Peutz–Jegher's and Wiskott–Aldrich's syndromes. There are also a number of cutaneous markers of exposure to carcinogens such as arsenical pigmentation, ionising radiation damage and solar elastosis from extensive sunlight exposure. These may lead to a high incidence of skin tumours and occasionally internal malignancy.

The most intriguing group is the cutaneous reactions to neoplasia and this is the subject of the following section.

DERMATOMYOSITIS

This is a rare disorder affecting the skin, muscle and blood vessels, all to a variable degree. The clinical manifestations of this condition are well known and do not usually present a difficult diagnostic problem. Typically, patients develop aching and mild weakness of proximal muscles, oedema and reddish-purple or heliotrope discoloration around the eyes. Indurated erythema may be present over the dorsum of the hands, especially over the extensor tendons with vascular changes around the nail folds (Fig. 15.1). Occasionally, the typical cutaneous signs may be either absent and the patient presents with a polymyositis, or present as a non-specific dermatitis eventually leading to erythroderma. (This latter group can present enormous diagnostic problems).

Skin biopsy may help in difficult cases, although many of the histological changes are similar to lupus erythematosus and can be very subtle. Direct immunofluorescence often shows IgG, IgM and sometimes IgA high in the dermis. Creatine phosphokinase (CPK) is not always raised and, therefore, is not a good screening test for the disease. Muscle biopsy and EMG show changes of an acute polymyositis. In childhood the condition is rarely if ever associated with tumours although it may be in patients in the age group of 40–60 years. The precise incidence is not known, but the range in the

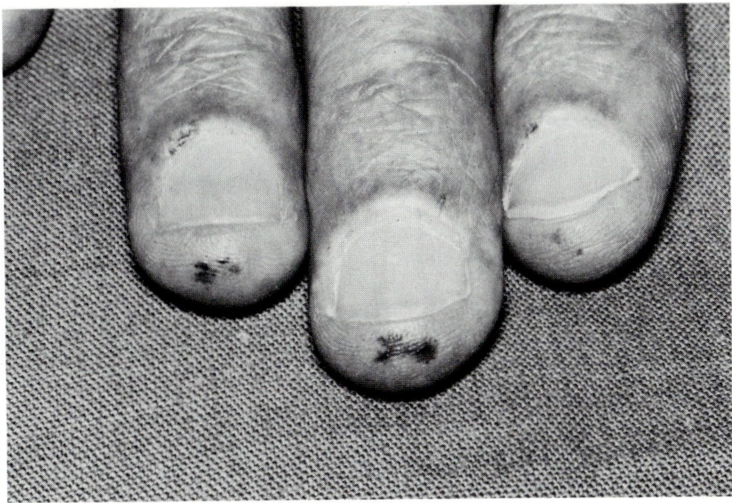

Fig. 15.1. *Dermatomyositis showing vascular changes around the nail fold and on the pulps of the fingers.*

published literature is from 6–50%. The association, however, is good enough to warrant quite detailed investigation, but it is probable that even these older patients represent a heterogeneous group. A wide range of tumours have been linked with dermatomyositis, interestingly so has penicillamine. Resection of the tumour does not always lead to resolution of symptoms especially the myositis, this possibly reflects inadequate tumour removal.

ERYTHEMAS

Annular Erythema (Erythema Annulare Centrifugum)

This condition starts as a pink papule often on the buttock, thigh or upper arm, which enlarges to form a ring of palpable erythema (Fig. 15.2). After a variable time, from a few days to weeks, it flattens and fades. The condition

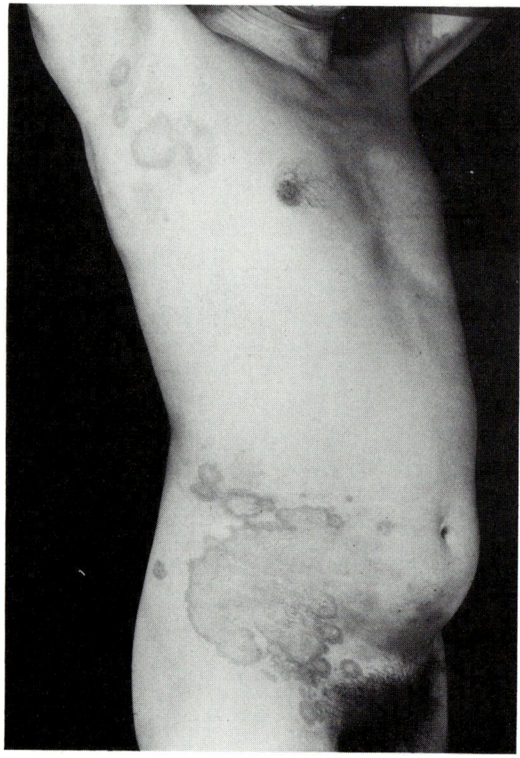

Fig. 15.2. *Annular erythema showing raised erythematous rings and central clearing with some post-inflammatory changes.*

runs a chronic course and although neoplasia may be associated, extensive investigation is not warranted as it usually appears to be idiopathic.

Erythema Gyratum Repens

This condition although very rare indeed has a quite distinctive clinical pattern. The annular erythema develops in waves and in the early stages may be similar to erythema annulare centrifugum. Later, however, rings within rings appear, giving a wood grain pattern (Fig. 15.3). It has an almost 100% association with malignancy and resection of the tumour leads to regression of the erythema.

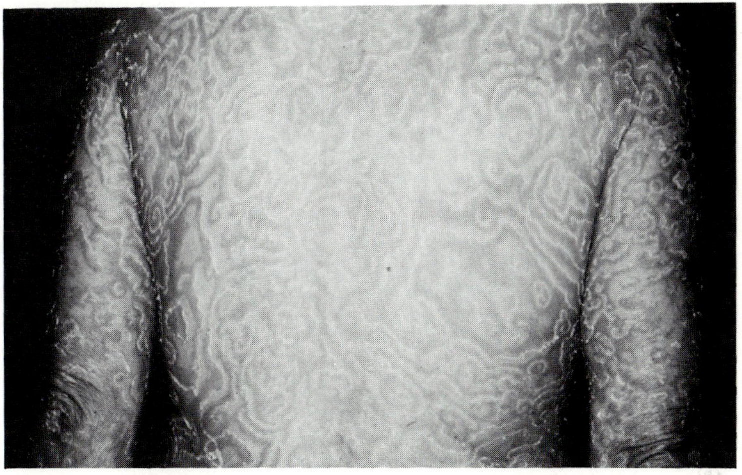

Fig. 15.3. *Erythema gyratum repens showing the distinctive wood grain pattern.*

Necrolytic Migratory Erythema (Glucagonoma Syndrome)

The eruption starts on the abdomen or groin, as an erythema. The central area rapidly becomes blistered and eroded. There is irregular centrifugal spread, with central healing giving an annular or figurate pattern. Glossitis with circumoral crusting usually features and, in addition, mild diabetes mellitus is often present. Originally, this syndrome was described in patients with glucagon-secreting pancreatic tumours, characterised by elevated levels of glucagon and low levels of amino acids. Successful resection of the tumour results in resolution of the eruption. More recently, patients have been reported with identical clinical signs but no tumour and normal levels of glucagon. This suggests the syndrome is not directly due to increased glucagon levels, although low levels of amino acid remain a possible aetiological factor.

PANNICULITIS

Mild panniculitis (inflammation of subcutaneous fat) may be present in a number of clinical syndromes, such as erythema nodosum. However, a more severe form is recognisable and is associated with pancreatic disease. Subcutaneous fat necrosis occurs and presents as crops of widespread numerous tender red nodules. It is associated with a polyarthritis, fever and eosinophilia. Elevated levels of serum lipase and amylase are usually present and are thought to be responsible for these signs. Many of these patients have a functioning acinar cell carcinoma of the pancreas, but an identical syndrome can develop with acute or chronic pancreatitis.

MIGRATORY THROMBOPHLEBITIS

Simple thrombophlebitis is not an uncommon condition and has no true association with neoplasia. However, if the thomboses are severe and migratory it may indicate the presence of pancreatic carcinoma, although the mechanism is not understood.

BULLOUS ERUPTIONS

Pemphigoid (Bullous Pemphigoid)

This disease is characterised by large tense blisters usually on an erythematous base and with subepidermal bulla formation (Fig. 15.4). There have been many case reports of an association between this disease and internal malignancy, but few have clearly demonstrated a parallel clinical course. It seems unlikely to be a common association and it must be remembered that pemphigoid is almost exclusively a disease of the elderly, a group with a high cancer risk.

Pemphigus

This group of disorders is characterised by flaccid and easily ruptured blisters, which often lead to erosions. Bulla formation is within the epidermis and associated with acantholysis (Figs. 15.5 and 15.6). An association with either benign or malignant thymoma, although rare, is well established. However, removal of the tumour does not alter the course of the

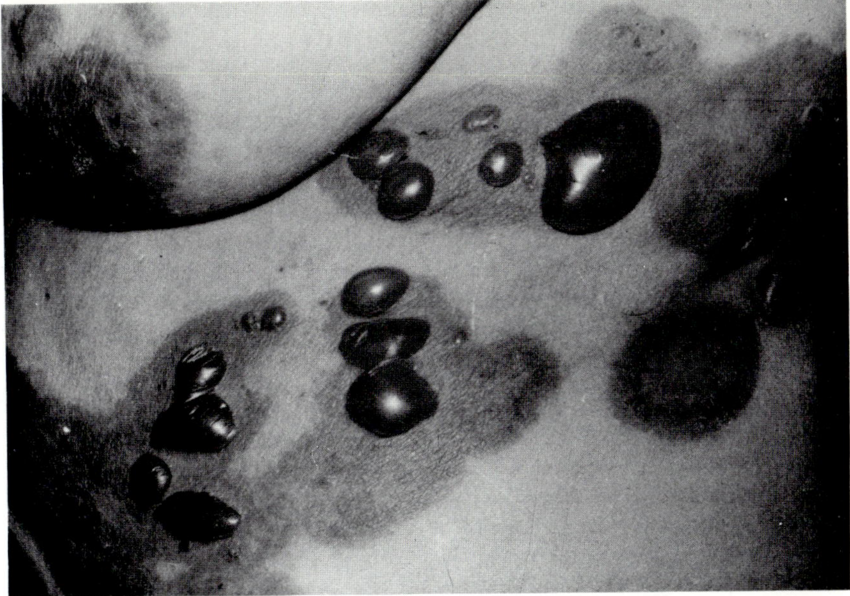

Fig. 15.4. *Pemphigoid showing large tense blisters on an erythematous base*

pemphigus. A number of other tumours have been reported with pemphigus but it seems doubtful if malignancy is more common than in a suitable control group.

Bullous Pyoderma

Although this is probably a variant of pyoderma gangrenosum it is sufficiently distinctive to warrant a different title. The condition often starts like pyoderma gangrenosum as a pustule or furuncle-like nodule, but as the lesion extends it is characterised by haemorrhagic bullae with central ulceration (Fig. 15.7). Moderate doses of oral steroids lead to rapid healing with surprisingly little scarring, unlike pyoderma gangrenosum. However, investigation is warranted since a high percentage, possibly half the patients, have acute myeloid leukaemia.

ACQUIRED HYPERTRICHOSIS LANUGINOSA

This rare condition is characterised by the appearance of long, fine, silky and unpigmented hair, particularly on normally hairless sites of the face. It is almost always associated with a tumour. The prognosis is gloomy since the

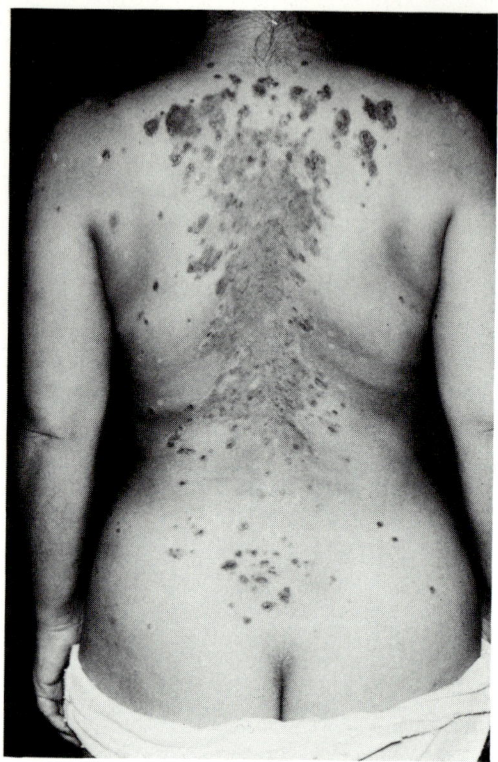

Fig. 15.5. *Pemphigus showing erosions in typical distribution over the back.*

condition is a late marker of malignancy and often indicates widespread disease. A number of drugs, especially diazoxide, minoxidil and diphenyl-hydantoin can cause hypertrichosis which may initially be fine and mimic acquired hypertrichosis lanuginosa.

ACQUIRED ICHTHYOSIS

Clinically this is characterised by dry scaly skin and is very similar to congenital ichthyosis vulgaris (Fig. 15.8). However, the development of ichthyosis after childhood requires investigation, since it has a strong association with lymphoma and more rarely with other malignancies. Ichthyosis may also occur in a number of other conditions such as leprosy, gross nutritional deficiency and panhypopituitarism.

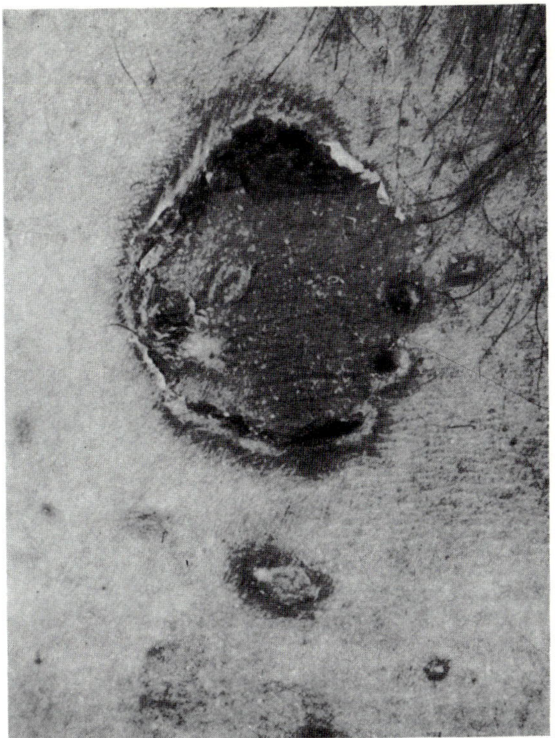

Fig. 15.6. *Pemphigus showing close up of lesion with blistered edge and eroded centre.*

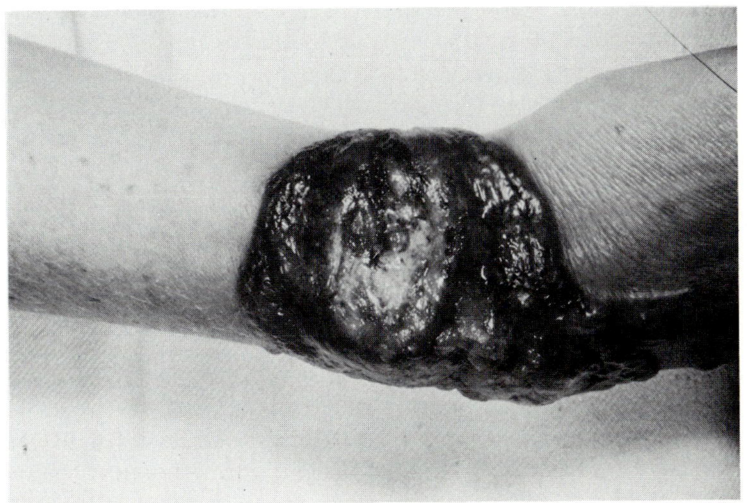

Fig. 15.7. *Bullous pyoderma showing haemorrhagic bullae and central ulceration.*

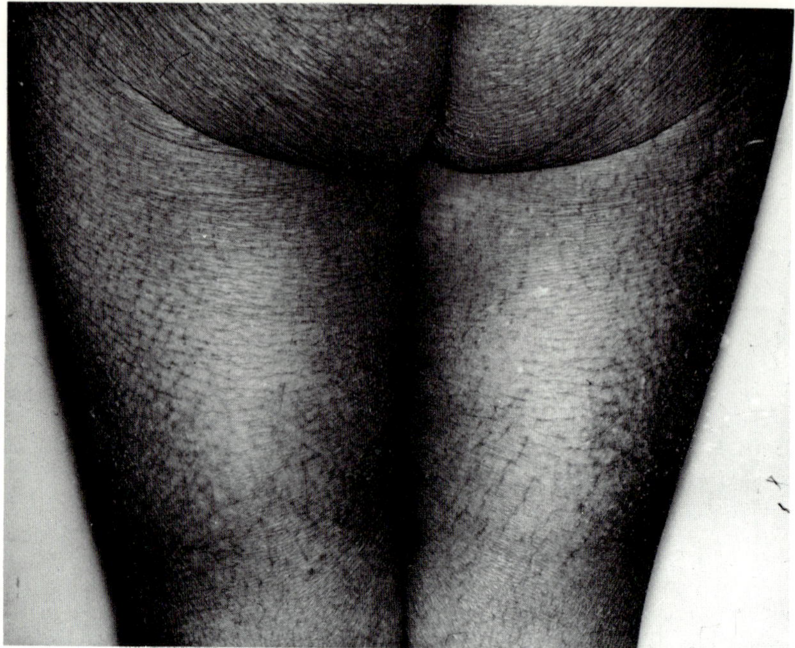

Fig. 15.8. *Acquired ichthyosis showing dryness and large scales surrounded by erythema.*

ACANTHOSIS NIGRICANS

This is a rare cutaneous disorder characterised by hyperkeratosis and hyperpigmentation. The earliest signs are roughness and dryness of the skin with hyperpigmentation. As the condition develops, the thickening increases and eventually may become warty. It usually involves flexures (Fig. 15.9) but may involve the entire skin. It can occur either as an isolated developmental defect or as a manifestation of other diseases. The malignant variant is usually severe and progresses rapidly. The pigmentation is more prominent and mucous membranes are involved in half the patients, resulting in warty papillomatous thickening around the lips (Fig. 15.10). Onset of the condition may precede evidence of a tumour by as much as five years and regression usually follows removal of the tumour.

PARANEOPLASTIC ACROKERATOSIS (BAZEX SYNDROME)

This condition is very rare indeed and is characterised by hyperkeratotic psoriasiform plaques which may affect feet, hands, nose or ears. The facial

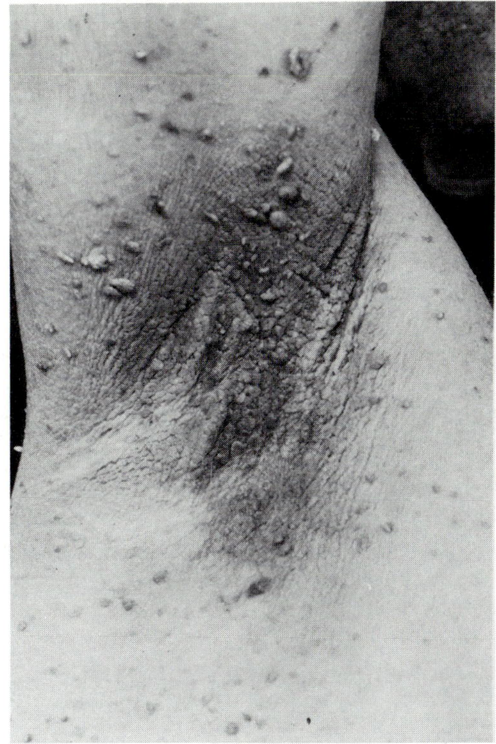

Fig. 15.9. *Acanthosis nigricans showing hyperkeratosis, hyperpigmentation and the beginning of warty changes.*

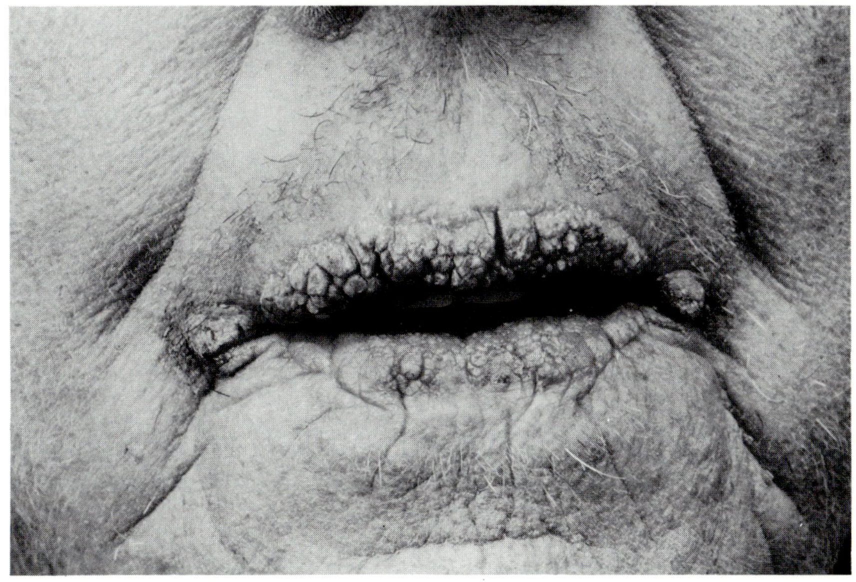

Fig. 15.10. *Acanthosis nigricans showing warty changes around the lips.*

                                    Endocrine Problems in Cancer

lesions may clinically resemble lupus erythematosus and the acrokeratosis
may suggest Reiter's syndrome. All the reported cases have been associated
with neoplasms of either the oropharynx or upper respiratory tract.

GENERALISED PRURITUS

This common symptom can be an uncommon presentation of a lymphoma,
particularly Hodgkin's. It is usually associated with minimal or absent skin
signs. Alcohol-induced pruritus has been reported but this is much rarer
than alcohol-induced pain.

CLUBBING AND HYPERTROPHIC OSTEOARTHROPATHY

Clubbing is well recognised as a manifestation of a number of diseases. The
underlying mechanism of subperiosteal bone formation may also involve
other long bones in hypertrophic osteoarthropathy. This process may
progress to give cutaneous thickening which can result in cylindrical limbs
and coarsening of the facial features known as pachydermoperiostosis.
When the underlying disease is neoplastic it is always intrathoracic, whether
primary or secondary and regardless of cell type.

ACKNOWLEDGEMENTS

Figures 15.2, 15.3, 15.9 and 15.10 were kindly supplied by The Department
of Medical Illustrations, Institute of Dermatology, London.

REFERENCES

Braverman I.M. (1981). Skin signs of systemic disease. *Cancer.* pp. 1–108.
  Philadelphia: W.B. Saunders.
Roberts S.O.B., Rook A.J. (1979). Cutaneous markers of internal malignancy. In
  Textbook of Dermatology. (Rook A.J., Wilkinson D.S., Ebling F.J.G., eds.) pp.
  2104–8. Oxford: Blackwell Scientific Publications.
Waldenstrom J.E. (1978). *Paraneoplasia, Biological Signals in the Diagnosis of
  Cancer.* New York: J. Wiley & Sons.

Chapter 16

John Rhodes

Effects of Tumours on the Immune System

PERTURBATIONS OF THE IMMUNE SYSTEM OCCURRING IN CANCER

Cell-mediated Immunity

Cell-mediated immunity (CMI) assayed by means of the delayed-type hypersensitivity reaction (DH reaction) is one of the oldest subjects for study in the field of immunology. Correctly used, the term embraces a number of phenomena which have the following characteristics in common. Antigen in the form of non-self or altered-self cells is specifically recognised by T-lymphocytes. The antigen may be in the form of foreign grafted cells, chemically modified host cells (as when a contact sensitising chemical is applied to the skin), or host cells infected with an intracellular virus, bacterium or protozoan. The foreign antigenic determinants in association with self-antigens encoded in the major histocompatibility complex (MHC) are recognised by certain T-cells, which are then stimulated to proliferate. One subset of the T-cell population, recognising the HLA-A, B and C products of the MHC, directly induce irreversible lytic changes in the antigenic target cell (cytotoxic T-cells). Another subset, recognising HLA-DR products of the MHC, respond to antigen by releasing mediators that attract and activate other cells (delayed-hypersensitivity T-cells). It is the signals released by these cells that lead to the accumulation of macrophages at the site of the reaction. There is a two-way interaction between T-cells and macrophages, both producing soluble signals (interleukins) that activate the other. Activated macrophages are then able to kill the target cells that provoked the reaction. It is the accumulation of macrophages, eosinophils and basophils and the inflammatory mediators which they subsequently release, that increase vascular permeability and produce the local inflammation characteristic of the delayed hypersensitivity reaction.

Experimental DH reactions that can be visualised and quantitated are secondary responses to antigens previously encountered by the host, and it is relatively easy to perform such tests on cancer patients. Antigens to which the majority of patients have been naturally exposed (e.g. purified protein derivative (PPD), mumps, candida) have been used, and so too have contact sensitising agents such as dinitrochlorobenzene (DNCB). In addition to DH skin tests the proliferative response of peripheral blood lymphocytes to antigen and, more commonly, polyclonal mitogens such as phytohaemagglutinin (PHA) has come to be considered as a test for CMI although the relationship between mitogenic responses and CMI as described above is not rigourously defined. On the basis of such tests a large number of studies have reported defective CMI in cancer patients (Catalona *et al.*, 1973; Dalbow *et al.*, 1977; Israel, 1976; Kopersztych *et al.*, 1976; Lichtenstein *et al.*, 1980; Adler *et al.*, 1980) and correlation between stage of disease, poor prognosis and defective CMI has been noted (Adler *et al.*, 1980; Barnes *et al.*, 1975; Dalbow *et al.*, 1977; Han and Takita, 1972; Bolton *et al.*, 1976; Liberati *et al.*, 1982). Whether such tests are of significant clinical or prognostic value, in comparison with the already well established tests of clinical performance status and disease extent is arguable (Liberati *et al.*, 1982; Barg *et al.*, 1981).

Studies of this kind do not, of course, measure specific anti-tumour immunity. Quite a number of laboratories claim to measure tumour-specific CMI in cancer patients in response to various extracts of tumour tissue (Hollinshead *et al.*, 1974; Stewart and Orizaga, 1971; Vose *et al.*, 1977; Sega *et al.*, 1980). However, it is difficult to put these demonstrations of specific CMI into a quantitative context, and their value is presently limited by the lack of well-defined tumour-specific antigens in man.

What is certainly occurring in patients with both lymphoproliferative and solid tumours is a general depression of cell-mediated immune responsiveness, which becomes more evident with advancing disease. It seems unlikely that defective immunity of this kind precedes (and by inference predisposes to) neoplastic disease (except in special cases; for example, Kaposi's sarcoma) but rather that progressing tumours exert suppressive effects on the immune system. The mechanisms by which they may do so are considered in the section starting on p. 303. For detailed reviews of defective CMI in cancer see Hersh *et al.* (1974), Burdick *et al.* (1975), and Nathanson (1977).

Monocyte and Macrophage Function

Cells of the monocyte–macrophage lineage are notable for the diversity of function ascribed to them by immunologists and pathologists. In addition to their role in first-line defence against bacteria and fungi and in tissue homeostasis, macrophages are involved in a number of crucial immunological functions. Thus, certain T-lymphocytes, proliferating in response to antigen, release lymphokines which both inhibit the migration of macrophages (MIF) and at the same time activate them (MAF). Activation of macrophages probably involves a quantitative increase in a number of cellular functions such as enzyme synthesis, membrane turnover, etc., and, as a consequence of these changes, activated macrophages can kill bacteria and other target cells that resting macrophages cannot. Macrophages possess receptors for the Fc portion of IgG antibody and for the C3 component of complement which facilitate phagocytosis, so that the fate of antigen that has provoked an antibody response is often phagocytosis by the cells of this system. Macrophages and/or specialised cells of the same lineage play a crucial role in presenting antigen to specific lymphocytes which recognise the foreign determinants in association with products of the HLA-DR region (Ia region in mouse) of the MHC expressed in the macrophage membrane. The lymphocyte is apparently unable to respond to antigen unless it is presented in this context. Macrophages fulfilling this role also release a soluble mediator that activates T-cells (interleukin I). One of the most important characteristics of macrophages is their capacity to migrate into inflammatory sites (as described in the previous section), and it is now well established that this function, and its *in vitro* correlate of macrophage migration and polarisation in response to chemoattractants, is defective in patients with cancer (Dizon and Southam, 1963; Lacour *et al.*, 1977; Boetcher and Leonard, 1974; Hausman *et al.*, 1975; Snyderman *et al.*, 1975; Rubin *et al.*, 1976; Snyderman *et al.*, 1978). Defective migration is not due to a reduced availability of peripheral blood monocytes, since monocytosis commonly occurs in cancer patients (Barret, 1970; Rhodes, 1977). *In vitro* studies show an increased scatter of migration values in response to chemoattractants, with around half the values falling below the lower limit of normal as defined by healthy donors and by donors with non-malignant diseases (Snyderman *et al.*, 1975). Normal responses correlate with delayed appearance of nodal metastases in malignant melanoma (Boetcher and Leonard, 1974), while depressed responses correlate with a poor prognosis (Rubin *et al.*, 1976). Resection of breast tumours results in a return to normal chemotactic responsiveness, indicating a tumour-mediated defect (Snyderman *et al.*, 1978). A recent study suggests that the human tumour-derived signal mediating this effect may be similar to a structural protein of type C-retroviruses (Cianciolo *et al.*, 1981).

In contrast to the depression of chemotactic function, certain other aspects of peripheral blood monocyte function are elevated in cancer patients. These include Fc receptor expression (Rhodes, 1977; Ruco *et al.*, 1980), antibody dependent cytotoxicity (Nyholm and Currie, 1978), and cytostasis of tumour cell lines (Mytar *et al.*, 1982; Jerrells *et al.*, 1979).

However, monocyte maturation *in vitro* may be defective (Dent and Cole, 1981). In spite of systemic activation as judged by Fc receptor expression, there is a local depression of macrophage function in the vicinity of primary lung carcinomas (Rhodes *et al.*, 1981). The mechanisms whereby tumours influence macrophage function are considered later in this chapter.

Natural Cell-mediated Cytotoxicity (NCMC)

Unlike specific T-cell cytotoxicity which requires recognition of antigen in association with self-MHC products on the target cell, and which is adaptive in that T-cell clones specific for a given target are expanded, NCMC does not require antigen, is not MHC restricted, and is not adaptive. Natural killer (NK) cells effect this type of cytotoxicity. They spontaneously kill a variety of tumour cell-lines and may recognise altered carbohydrate moieties. Their activity is enhanced by interferon. The significance of NCMC is yet to be determined but many authorities believe it may represent an anti-tumour surveillance mechanism.

In general, studies of natural cell-mediated cytotoxicity in cancer patients have revealed a significant reduction in this function in comparison with peripheral blood lymphocytes of normal donors (Vose *et al.*, 1977; Pross and Baines, 1976; DeBoer *et al.*, 1982). In one study of patients with lung cancer or malignant melanoma NCMC levels were lower than in normal age-matched controls, but the levels of NCMC were positively correlated with the extent of disease (Forbes *et al.*, 1981). The question of systemic versus local changes was addressed in a study of carcinomatous pleural effusions in patients with primary or secondary lung cancer (Uchida and Micksche, 1981). In this population, NK activity was reduced still further or absent in comparison with peripheral blood of the same patient, although mitogenic responsiveness was elevated compared to that of blood lymphocytes. Significant NK activity was detectable in non-malignant pleural effusions.

Antibody Dependent Cellular Cytotoxicity (K-cell activity)

Antibody dependent cellular cytotoxicity (ADCC) occurs when lymphocytes (K-cells), with receptors of the Fc portion of IgG, bind to target cells previously sensitised with specific antibody. Irreversible lytic changes follow this interaction. Antibody dependent cellular cytotoxicity and NK activity are probably mediated by the same or overlapping populations of lymphocytes. These are large, granular, non-adherent, non-phagocytic cells which have Fc receptors and which form low-affinity rosettes with sheep erythrocytes (i.e. not classical T- or B-cells). There is controversy over whether ADCC is decreased or not in patients with malignant disease. Some have found depressed function (Stratton *et al.*, 1977; Ting and Terasaki, 1974), returning to normal following treatment (Stratton *et al.*, 1977). Others have found no influence of cancer on ADCC (Peter *et al.*, 1975; DeBoer *et al.*, 1982), even where NK activity was decreased (DeBoer *et al.*, 1982). High levels of ADCC may be a favourable prognostic feature in bronchogenic carcinoma (Liberati *et al.*, 1982). Monocyte-mediated ADCC, as distinct from K-cell ADCC, is elevated in cancer patients (Nyholm and Currie, 1978; Hersh *et al.*, 1982).

Antibody

Relatively little attention has been given to humoral antibody production in cancer patients. An extensive study of antibody responses to flagellin in patients with non-lymphoid tumours revealed a depressed response directly related to the extent of disease (Lee *et al.*, 1970). Antibody responses depend upon a sequence of cellular events in which an antigen-presenting cell interacts with a lymphocyte recognising foreign determinants in association with self MHC antigens (HLA-DR). Helper T-cells activated in this way co-operate with B-cells, both cells recognising different determinants on the same immunogenic molecule or on different molecules in the same supramolecular structure (e.g. cell surface). As a consequence of this interaction B-cells differentiate into antibody-producing plasma cells. In patients with cancer, Umeda and colleagues (1982) have detected diminished helper T-cell function.

Where total immunoglobulin levels have been evaluated an increase in IgA levels has been noted in lung cancer. High levels were correlated with a longer time to progression but not with longer survival (Liberati *et al.*, 1982). A number of immunologic hormonal factors other than antibody may be altered in patients with cancer. These include tumour necrosis factor (a macrophage product), thymosin (a product of thymus cells), lymphotoxin (a partially characterised lymphokine) and interferon. For references see Evans (1982).

Lymphocyte Numbers and Lymphocyte Traffic

It is well known that lymphocytopenia occurs in advanced malignant disease and that monocytosis also occurs, possibly before lymphocytopenia becomes apparent. The consequential change in monocyte:lymphocyte ratios may exert effects on lymphocyte reactivity as discussed below. It seems likely that tumours infiltrating the lymphatics may affect the normal traffic of lymphocytes although few studies have been undertaken. In a recent study of lymphocytes defined by monoclonal antibodies, Harris and colleagues (1982) found T-cell subpopulations unchanged in cancer patients but confirmed that lymphocytopenia and monocytosis occur.

MECHANISMS BY WHICH TUMOURS MAY PERTURB THE IMMUNE SYSTEM

Suppressor Cells

Certain regimens of antigen administration result in specific non-responsiveness mediated by suppressor T-cells. As a result of interaction with antigen this population produces soluble antigen-specific factors bearing MHC determinants encoded in the I-J subregion. These factors act on a second set of T-cells, which in turn block helper T-cell collaboration with B-cells or cytotoxic T-cells in a non-specific manner. The function of this complex system is probably to regulate immune responses in the normal immunocompetent host. In addition to this potentially well-defined system the term suppressor cell has been applied to a variety of partially defined populations that inhibit lymphocyte responsiveness non-specifically. Experimentally it is possible to distinguish between these two kinds of suppression in the same murine tumour host (Howie and McBride, 1982). The necessary techniques are not so easily applied to human cancer. Nevertheless, the presence of tumour-specific suppressor cells has been demonstrated in patients with osteogenic sarcoma (Yu *et al.*, 1977). A large literature exists describing non-specific suppressor cells in cancer, and many authors agree that suppression of mitogen-induced lymphocyte proliferation in the peripheral blood of cancer patients is due to a glass-adherent population, presumably monocytes. There has been disagreement over whether this effect is merely due to the increased proportion of monocytes in the mononuclear cell population of cancer patients (Rhodes, 1977; Laughter and Twomey, 1977), or a qualitative tumour-induced change in monocyte function (Berlinger *et al.*, 1976; Jerrells *et al.*, 1978; Zembala *et al.*, 1977; Braun and Harris, 1981). Suppression mediated by adherent cells may be reversed by indomethacin (Braun and Harris, 1981; Murray *et al.*, 1981), indicating that prostaglandins produced by monocytes are responsible for suppression. However, others find that the immune modulating effects of indomethacin in melanoma patients are not related to prostaglandin-mediated suppression (Tilden and Balch, 1982). Mytar and colleagues found that monocytes from patients with gastrointestinal tract cancer are inhibitory towards mitogen-induced lymphoproliferation, but also exhibit increased cytostasis of tumour cell lines (Mytar *et al.*, 1982). Exactly how tumours directly or indirectly induce monocytes to become suppressive is not known. Glass adherent cells (probably monocytes) also suppress NK- and K-cell function in solid tumour patients by a mechanism that is not dependent on prostaglandin (DeBoer *et al.*, 1982).

Antigen Shedding, Antibody and Immune Complexes

Experiments with immunogenic animal tumours have identified a number of specific mechanisms whereby tumour antigens block cell-mediated anti-tumour responses. These include receptor blockade by shed antigens, specific (enhancing) antibody that inhibits CMI, and immune complexes that similarly block CMI. Whether such mechanisms are significant in human cancer is unknown, although there is some evidence for their occurrence (Baldwin *et al.*, 1973; Jose and Seshadri, 1974).

Partially Characterised Soluble Tumour-derived and Tumour-associated Factors

A good deal of work has been done on soluble tumour-derived factors in animal tumour systems (Nelson *et al.*, 1981). Less has been done on human tumour-derived signals that modulate the immune system. As in the animal systems a number of low-molecular-weight factors have been detected in the supernatants of various tumour cultures and shown to influence monocyte or lymphocyte function. Notable amongst recent studies are those of Cianciolo and colleagues (1981) who found that an inhibitor of monocyte chemotactic polarisation present in cancerous effusions is recognised by monoclonal antibodies to a structural protein of murine retroviruses. The inhibitory factor may thus be a cross-reacting human oncogene product. Studies of certain naturally occurring polypeptides in tissue fluids that have immunosuppressive properties, and that may be implicated in immune depression in cancer patients, have been going on for more than a decade (Cooperband *et al.*, 1976). Serum factors from patients with lung carcinoma promote macrophage activation, whereas a soluble tumour-derived signal isolated from carcinoma tissues *in vitro* inhibits macrophage activation. Thus, systemic factors in cancer patient's sera activate, whereas local tumour-derived factors inhibit human macrophage function *in vitro*; and this is consistent with the *ex vivo* picture of activated circulating monocytes, but suppressed tissue macrophages in the vicinity of lung tumours (Rhodes, 1977; Rhodes *et al.*, 1979; Rhodes *et al.*, 1981). Lipid-like agents from human carcinoma cells, characterised by enzyme susceptibility, ultrafiltration and solvent extraction, have been shown to inhibit macrophage tumouricidal function (Hakim, 1980) and this is consistent with recent findings in a murine system (Young *et al.*, 1982). Factors from human colonic carcinoma tissue have been shown to inhibit T-lymphocyte function *in vitro* (Remacle-Bonnet *et al.*, 1976; Whitehead and Kim, 1980).

Prostaglandins

Prostaglandins are in many ways attractive candidates for mediators of tumour-induced immunosuppression in man. Although prostaglandins promote vasodilation and the action of inflammatory mediators, they are inhibitory towards other immunological functions. Thus, PGE_2 inhibits mitogen-induced lymphocyte proliferation (Smith *et al.*, 1971), lymphokine production (Gordon *et al.*, 1976), cell-mediated cytotoxicity (Henney *et al.*, 1972), and antibody production (Bourne *et al.*, 1974). Moreover, prostaglandin levels are increased in the serum of patients with squamous cell carcinoma of the lung (Seyberth *et al.*, 1975), breast carcinoma (Powles *et al.*, 1977), renal cell carcinoma (Cummings and

Robertson, 1977), and various other human malignancies (Demers *et al.*, 1977; Levine, 1981). Resected carcinoma tissues have been found to contain more PGE_2 than normal tissues (Bennett *et al.*, 1977) and to synthesise large amounts *in vitro* (Bennett *et al.*, 1975). Further weight has been added to the case for prostaglandin-mediated, tumour-induced immuno-suppression by observations in animal systems showing that indomethacin (an inhibitor of PG synthesis) reverses immunosuppression in tumour hosts (reviewed by Goodwin *et al.*, 1980).

The source of immunosuppressive PGE in cancer patients need not be the tumour itself. The properties of glass-adherent suppressor cells synthesising PGE in peripheral blood of cancer patients have been described previously. Although the induction of suppressor cell activity seems to depend upon tumour growth, the mechanism of induction is unclear. The partially characterised tumour-derived signals discussed above may be involved.

It should be mentioned that conflicting evidence exists in that PGE and its analogues can also exert anti-tumour effects (Goodwin *et al.*, 1980), and in that the anti-tumour effects of indomethacin may not be due to its inhibitory action on prostaglandins (Tilden and Balch, 1982).

Acute Phase Reactant Proteins

Acute phase reactant proteins (APRPs) are elevated in the serum of cancer patients (Cooper *et al.*, 1976; Harris *et al.*, 1974; Mueller *et al.*, 1971) and the levels of these proteins appear to correlate with extent of disease. In an extensive study, Samak and colleagues (1982) found that haptoglobin and fibrinogen depressed both lymphocyte mitogenic responses and monocyte chemotactic responses at doses approximating those found in cancer patients but not at doses approximating levels found in normal serum. Another APRP, orosomucoid, depressed chemotaxis but not lymphoproliferation. The study did not formally distinguish between direct effects and the possible generation of suppressor cells by APRP.

Tumour Sequestered Retinoids

Retinol (vitamin A) and retinoic acid exert potent inhibitory effects on monocyte and macrophage function of the kind that occur in the vicinity of primary lung tumours *in vivo*, and *in vitro* in response to supernatants from explanted carcinoma tissue (Rhodes and Oliver, 1980). Retinoic acid also inhibits natural killer cell activity (Abb *et al.*, 1982). In its effects on both monocytes and NK-cells, retinoic acid is antagonistic to the effects of interferon (Rhodes and Stokes, 1982; Abb *et al.*, 1982). Since human carcinoma tissue contains binding proteins for retinoic acid that are not present in surrounding normal tissues (Ong *et al.*, 1975; Huber *et al.*, 1978;

Clamon *et al.*, 1981) retinoic acid may be preferentially sequestered in carcinoma tissue, where it may exert local inhibitory effects on macrophage and NK-cell-mediated anti-tumour host defence.

Other Mechanisms

Some authors believe that monocytes from patients with cancer become armed with cytophilic anti-tumour antibody and that when presented with antigenic extracts of tumours *in vitro* release, as a consequence of the antigen–antibody interaction, substances pharmacologically similar to leukotrienes which then modulate leukocyte behaviour. For an introduction to this literature see Thomson *et al.* (1982). In addition to those described above there are, no doubt, many other hormone-like signals directly or indirectly released as a consequence of progressive malignant disease, which have yet to be tested in the assays commonly deployed by tumour immunologists. The transforming growth factors released by human tumour cells and detectable in the urine of cancer patients (Twardzik *et al.*, 1982) are an example.

Most of our current understanding of immune mechanisms has depended upon studies made in animal systems. In the present brief account, however, specific reference to such studies is largely omitted. Neither has an attempt been made to assess the doubtless significant effects of chemotherapy, radiotherapy and surgery on immune function. No doubt further studies of immunity in cancer patients will be motivated by the notion that immune mechanisms are protective against tumour incidence and that successful tumours subvert or evade immunologic surveillance. For reviews in this area see Nelson *et al.* (1981), Serrou (1982) and Kumar and Penny (1982).

REFERENCES

Abb J., Abb H., Deinhardt F. (1982). Effect of retinoic acid on the spontaneous and interferon-induced activity of human natural killer cells. *Int. J. Cancer*; **30**: 307–10.

Adler A., Stein J.A., Ben-Efraim S. (1980). Immunocompetence immunosuppression, and human breast cancer. III Prognostic significance of initial level of immunocompetence in early and advanced disease. *Cancer*; **45**: 2074–83.

Baldwin R.W., Price M.R., Robins R.A. (1973). Inhibition of hepatoma-immune lymph node cell cytotoxicity by tumour-bearer serum and solubilised hepatoma antigen. *Int. J. Cancer*; **11**: 527–35.

Barg S., Levin M., Rezzonico R. (1981). Importance of the immunological study in the prognosis of a cancer patient. *Cell. Mol. Biol*; **27**: 563–9.

Barnes E.W., Farmer A., Penhale W.J., Irvine W.J., Roscoe P., Horne N.W. (1975). Phytohaemagglutinin-induced lymphocyte transformation in newly presenting patients with primary carcinoma of the lung. *Cancer*; **36**: 187–93.

Barret O'N. (1970). Monocytosis in malignant disease. *Ann. Intern. Med*; **73**:991–2.

Bennett A., Del Tacca M., Stamford I.F., Zebro T. (1977). Prostaglandins from tumours of human large bowel. *Brit. J. Cancer*; **35**: 881–4.

Bennett A., McDonald A.M., Simpson J.S., Stamford I.F. (1975). Breast cancer, prostaglandins, and bone metastases. *Lancet*; **1**: 1218–20.

Berlinger N.R., Lopez C., Good R.A. (1976). Facilitation or attenuation of mixed leukocyte culture responsiveness by adherent cells. *Nature*; **260**: 145–6.

Boetcher D.A., Leonard E.J. (1974). Abnormal monocyte chemotactic response in cancer patients. *J. Natl. Cancer Inst*; **52**: 1091–9.

Bolton P.M., Teasdale C., Mander A.M. *et al.* (1976). Immune competence in breast cancer: Relationship of pretreatment immunological tests to diagnosis and tumour stage. *Cancer Immunol. Immunother*; **1**: 251–8.

Bourne H.R., Lichtenstein L.M., Melmon K.L., Henney C.S., Weinstein Y., Sherer G.M. (1974). Modulation of inflammation and immunity by cyclic AMP. *Science*; **184**: 19–28.

Braun D.P., Harris J.E. (1981). Relationship of leukocyte numbers, immunoregulatory cell function and phytohaemagglutinin responsiveness in cancer patients. *J. Natl. Cancer Inst*; **67**: 809–14.

Burdick J.F., Wells S.A. Jr., Herberman R.B. (1975). Immunologic evaluation of patients with cancer by delayed hypersensitivity reactions. *Surg. Gynecol. Obstet*; **141**: 779–94.

Catalona W.J., Sample W.F., Chretien P.B. (1973). Lymphocyte reactivity in cancer patients: correlation with tumour histology and clinical stage. *Cancer*; **31**:65–71.

Cianciolo G., Hunter J., Silva J., Haskill J.S., Snyderman R. (1981). Inhibitors of monocyte responses to chemotaxins are present in human cancerous effusions and react with monoclonal antibodies to the P15(E) structural protein of retro viruses. *J. Clin. Invest*; **68**: 831–44.

Clamon G.H., Nugent K.M., Rossi N'P. (1981). Cellular retinoic acid-binding proteins in human lung carcinomas. *J. Natl. Cancer Inst*; **67**: 61–3.

Cooper E.H., Turner R., Greekie A., *et al.*, (1976). Alpha-globulins in the surveillance of colorectal carcinoma. *Biomedicine*; **24**: 171–8.

Cooperband S.R., Nimber R., Schmid K. *et al.*, (1976). Humoral immunosuppressive factors. *Transplant. Proc*; **8**: 225–42.

Cummings K.B., Robertson R.P. (1977). Prostaglandin: Increased production by renal cell carcinoma. *J. Urol*; **118**: 720–3.

Dalbow M.H., Concannon J.P., Eng C.P., Idfil C.S., Conway J., Nambinan P.T.N. (1977). Lymphocyte mitogen stimulation studies for patients with lung cancer: Evaluation of prognostic significance of pre-irradiation therapy studies. *J. Lab. Clin. Med*; **90**: 295–302.

DeBoer K., Braun D.P., Harris J.E. (1982). Natural cytotoxicity and antibody-dependent cytoxicity in solid tumour cancer patients: Regulation by adherent cells. *Clin. Immunol. Immunopathol*; **23**: 133–44.

Demers L.M., Allegra J.C., Harvey H.A., *et al.* (1977). Plasma prostaglandins in hypercalcemic patients with neoplastic diseases. *Cancer*; **39**: 1559–62.

Dent R.G., Cole P. (1981). *In vitro* monocyte maturation in squamous carcinoma of the lung. *Brit. J. Cancer*; **43**: 486–95.

Dizon Q.S., Southam C.M. (1963). Abnormal cellular responses to skin abrasions in cancer patients. *Cancer*; **16**: 1288–92.

Evans C.H. (1982). Lymphotoxin—An immunologic hormone with anticarcinogenic and anti-tumour activity. *Cancer Immunol. Immunother*; **12**: 181–90.

Forbes J.T., Greco F.A., Oldham R.K. (1981). Human natural cell-mediated cytotoxicity. ii. Levels in neoplastic disease. *Cancer Immunol. Immunother*; **11**: 147–53.

Goodwin J.S. Jr., Husby G., Williams R.C. (1980). Prostaglandin E and cancer growth. *Cancer Immunol. Immunother*; **18**: 3–7.

Gordon D., Bray M., Morley J. (1976). Control of lymphokine secretion by prostaglandins. *Nature*; **362**: 401–402.

Hakim A.A. (1980). Lipid-like agents from human neoplastic cells suppress cell-mediated immunity. *Cancer Immunol. Immunother*; **8**: 133–41.

Han T., Takita H. (1972). Impaired lymphocyte response to allogeneic cultured lymphoid cells in patients with lung cancer. *New Eng. J. Med*; **286**: 605–606.

Harris J.E., DeBoer K., Eabey A.L., Braun D.P. (1982). The measurement of leukocyte subsets in the peripheral blood of cancer patients with solid tumours using monoclonal antibody reagents. *Med. Ped. Oncol.*; **10**: 185–94.

Harris C.C., Primack A., Cohen M.H. (1974). Elevated αl-antitrypsin levels in lung cancer patients. *Cancer*; **34**: 280–1.

Hausman M.S., Brosman S., Snyderman R., Mickey M.R., Fahey J. (1975). Defective monocyte function in patients with genitourinary tract carcinoma. *J. Natl. Cancer Inst*; **55**: 1047–54.

Henney C.S., Bourne H.R., Lichtenstein L.M. (1972). The role of cyclic 3′5′ adenosine monophosphate in the specific cytolitic activity of lymphocytes. *J. Immunol*; **108**; 1526–34.

Hersh E.M., Freireich E.J., McCredie K.B. *et al.* (1974). Primary and secondary immune response in the evaluation of immunocompetence and prognosis in cancer patients. *Recent Results in Cancer Research*; **47**: 25–36.

Hersh E.M., Murphy S.G., Gutterman J.U. *et al.* (1982). Antibody-dependent cell-mediated cytotoxicity in human cancer: Characterisation of patients leukocyte activity and treatment effects. *Cancer*; **49**: 251–60.

Hollinshead C., Stewart T.H., Herberman R.B. (1974). Delayed hypersensitivity reactions to solube membrane antigens of human malignant lung cells. *J. Natl. Cancer Inst*; **52**: 327–38.

Howie S., McBride W.H. (1982). Tumour-specific T helper activity can be abrogated by two distinct suppressor cell mechanisms. *Eur. J. Immunol*; **12**: 671–5.

Huber P.R., Geyer E., Kung W., Matter A., Torhorst J., Eppenberger U. (1978). Retinoic acid—binding protein in human breast cancer and dysplasia. *J. Natl. Cancer Inst*; **61**: 1375–8.

Israel L. (1976). Nonspecific immunological alterations in patients with lung cancer. In *Lung Cancer Natural History Prognosis and Therapy* (Israel L., Chahinian A.P., eds.) pp. 141–50. New York: Academic Press.

Jerrells T.R., Dean J.H., McCoy J.L., Richardson G.L., Herberman R.B. (1978). Role of suppressor cells in depression of *in vitro* lymphoproliferative responses of lung and breast cancer patients. *J. Natl. Cancer Inst*; **61**: 1001–1009.

Jerrells T.R., Dean J.H., Richardson G., Cannon G.B., Herberman R.B. (1979). Increased monocyte mediated cytostasis of lymphoid cell lines in breast and lung cancer patients. *Int. J. Cancer*; **23**: 768–74.

Jose D.G., Seshadri R. (1974). Circulating immune complexes in human neuro-blastoma: Direct assay and role in blocking specific cellular immunity. *Int. J. Cancer*; **13**: 824–38.

Kopersztych S., Rezkallah M.T., Miki S.S., Naspitz C.K., Mendes N.F. (1976). Cell-mediated immunity in patients with carcinoma. *Cancer*; **38**: 1149–54.

Kumar R.K., Penny R. (1982). Escape of tumours from immunological destruction. *Pathology*; **14**: 173–9.

Lacour F., Delage G., Lacour J. (1977). Diminution du pourcentage de phagocytes mononuclees chez les malade atteintes de cancer du sein. *CR Acad. Sci. D (Paris)*; **284**: 2447–50.

Laughter A.H., Twomey J.J. (1977). Suppression of lymphoproliferation by high concentrations of normal human mononuclear phagocytes. *J. Immunol*; **119**: 173–9.

Lee A.K.Y., Rowley M., Mackay I.R. (1970). Antibody-producing capacity in human cancer. *Brit. J. Cancer*; **24**: 454–63.

Levine L. (1981). Arachidonic acid transformation and tumour production. *Advan. Cancer Res*; **35**: 49–79.

Liberati A.M., Voelkel J.G., Borden E.C., Coates A.S., Citrin D.L., Bryan G.T. (1982). Influence of non-specific immunologic factors on prognosis in advanced bronchogenic carcinoma. *Cancer Immunol. Immunother*; **13**: 140–4.

Lichtenstein A., Zighelboin J., Dorey F., Brossman S., Fahey J.L. (1980). Comparison of immune derangements in patient with different malignancies. *Cancer*; **45**: 2090–5.

Mueller W.K., Handschumacher R., Wade M.E. (1971). Serum haptoglobin in patients with ovarian malignancies. *Obstet. Gynaecol*; **38**: 427–35.

Murray J.L., Springle C., Ishmael R.D. *et al.* (1981). Adherent indomethacin-sensitive suppressor cells in malignant melanoma. *Cancer Immunol. Immunother*; **11**: 165–72.

Mytar B., Zembala M., Uracz W., Czupryna A. (1982). Cytostatic activity on tumour cells of monocytes from patients with gastrointestinal cancer. *Cancer Immunol. Immunother*; **13**: 190–3.

Nathanson L. (1977). Immunology and immunotherapy of human breast cancer. *Cancer Immunol. Immunother*; **2**: 209–24.

Nelson D.S., Nelson M., Farram E., Inoue Y. (1981). Cancer and subversion of host defences. *Austral. J. Exp. Biol. Med. Sci*; **59**: 229–62.

Nyholm R.E., Currie G.A. (1978). Monocytes and macrophages in malignant melanoma. II. Lysis of antibody-coated erythrocytes as an assay of monocyte function. *Brit. J. Cancer*; **37**: 337–44.

Ong D.E., Page D.T., Chytil T. (1975). Retinoic acid binding protein: Occurrence in human tumours. *Science*; **190**: 60–1.

Peter H.H., Pavie-Fischer T., Fridman W.H. *et al.* (1975). Cell-mediated cyto-toxicity *in vitro* of human lymphocytes against a tissue culture melanoma cell line (IGR3). *J. Immunol*; **115**: 539–48.

Powles T.J., Coombes R.C., Neville A.M., Ford H.T., Gazet J.C., Levine L. (1977). 15-keto-13,14, dihydro-prostaglandin E_2 concentrations in serum of patients with breast cancer. *Lancet*; **2**: 138–9.

Pross H.F., Baines M.G. (1976). Spontaneous human lymphocyte mediated cytotoxicity against tumour target cells. I. The effect of malignant disease. *Int. J. Cancer*; **18**: 593–604.

Remacle-Bonnet M.M., Pommier G.J., Kaplanski S., Rance R.J., Depieds R.C. (1976). Inhibition of normal-allogeneic lymphocyte mitogenesis by a soluble inhibitor extracted from human colonic carcinoma. *J. Immunol*; **117**; 1145–51.

Rhodes J. (1977). Altered expression of human monocyte Fc receptors in malignant disease. *Nature*; **265**: 253–5.

Rhodes J. (1978). Regulatory effects of normal human monocytes and monocytes activated in cancer on normal lymphocyte responses to mitogen. In *The Macrophage and Cancer* (James K., McBride W., Stuart A., eds.) pp. 390–402. Edinburgh: James McBride & Stuart.

Rhodes J., Bishop M., Benfield J. (1979). Tumour surveillance: How tumours may resist macrophage-mediated host defence. *Science*; **203**: 179–82.

Rhodes J., Oliver S. (1980). Retinoids as regulators of macrophage function. *Immunology*; **40**: 467–72.

Rhodes J., Plowman P., Bishop M., Lipscomb D. (1981). Human macrophage function in cancer: Systemic and local changes detected by an assay for Fc receptor expression. *J. Natl. Cancer Inst*; **66**: 423–9.

Rhodes J., Stokes P. (1982). Interferon-induced changes in the monocyte membrane: inhibition by retinol and retinoic acid. *Immunology*; **45**: 531–6.

Rubin R.A., Cosimi A.B., Goetzl E.J. (1976). Defective human mononuclear leukocyte chemotaxis as an index of host resistance to malignant melanoma. *Clin. Immunol. Immunopathol*; **6**: 376–88.

Ruco L.P., Procopio A., Uccini S., Baroni C.D. (1980). Increased monocyte phagocytosis in cancer patients. *Euro. J. Cancer*; **16**: 1315–20.

Samak R., Edelstein R., Israel L. (1982). Immunosuppressive effect of acute-phase reactant proteins *in vitro* and its relevance to cancer. *Cancer Immunol. Immunother*; **13**: 38–43.

Sega E., Mottolese M., Curcio C.G., Citro G. (1980). Specific blastogenic response of peripheral blood lymphocytes from lung cancer patients to a fetal lung antigen. *J. Natl. Cancer Inst*; **64**: 1001–6.

Serrou B. (1982). Immune imbalance and immune modulation in solid tumour patients: new insights. *Recent Results in Cancer Res*; **80**: 9–16.

Seyberth H.W., Segre G.V., Morgan J.L., Sweetman B.J., Potts J.T., Oates J.A. (1975). Prostaglandins as mediators of hypercalcemia associated with certain types of cancer. *New Eng. J. Med*; **293**: 1278–83.

Smith J.W., Steiner A.L., Parker C.W. (1971). Human lymphocyte metabolism: Effect of cyclic and non-cyclic nucleotides on stimulation by phytohaemagglutinin. *J. Clin. Invest*; **50**: 442–8.

Snyderman R., Meadows L., Holder W., Wells S. Jr. (1978). Abnormal monocyte chemotaxis in patients with breast cancer: Evidence for a tumour mediated effect. *J. Natl. Cancer Inst*; **60**: 737–40.

Snyderman R., Pike M.C., Altman L.C. (1975). Abnormalities of leukocyte chemostasis in human disease. *Ann. NY Acad. Sci*; **256**: 386–401.

Stewart T.H., Orizaga M. (1971). The presence of delayed hypersensitivity reactions in patients towards cellular extracts of their malignant tumours. *Cancer*; **28**: 1472–8.

Stratton M.L., Herz J., Loeffler R.A. *et al.* (1977). Antibody-dependent cell-mediated cytoxicity in treated and non-treated cancer patients. *Cancer*; **40**: 1045–51.

Thomson D.M.P., Phelan K., Morton D.G., Bach M.K. (1982). Armed human monocytes challenged with a sensitising cancer extract release substances pharmacologically similar to leukotrienes. *Int. J. Cancer;* **30**: 299–306.

Tilden A.B., Balch C.M. (1982). Immune modulating effects of indomethacin in melanoma patients are not related to prostaglandin E_2 mediated suppression. *Surgery*; **92**: 528–32.

Ting A., Terasaki P.I. (1974). Depressed lymphocyte-mediated killing of sensitized targets in cancer patients. *Cancer Res*; **34**: 2694–8.

Twardzik D.R., Shenoin S.A., Ranchalis J., Todaro G.J. (1982). Transforming growth factors in the urine of normal, pregnant and tumour bearing humans. *J. Natl. Cancer Inst*; **69**: 793–8.

Uchida A., Micksche M. (1981). Natural killer cells in carcinomatous pleural effusions. *Cancer Immunol. Immunother*; **11**: 131–8.

Umeda T., Hara T., Kosek K., Kobayashi K., Akaza H., Nijima T. (1982). Diminished helper T lymphocyte function in cancer patients. *Cell. Mol. Biol*; **28**: 67–71.

Vose B.M., Argov S., Klein E., Vanky F. (1977). Natural cytotoxicity in man: activity of lymph node and tumour infiltrating lymphocytes. *Europ. J. Immunol*; **7**: 353–7.

Vose B.M., Kimber I., Moore M. (1977). Leukocyte migration inhibition in human pulmonary neoplasia. *J. Natl. Cancer Inst*; **58**: 483–8.

Whitehead J.S., Kim Y.S. (1980). An inhibitor of lymphocyte proliferation produced by a human colonic adenocarcinoma cell line in culture. *Cancer Res*; **40**: 29–35.

Young R.M., Sundharadas G., Cantarow W.D., Kumar P.R. (1982). Purification and functional characterisation of a low-molecular-weight immune modulating factor produced by Lewis lung carcinoma. *Int. J. Cancer*; **30**: 517–24.

Yu A., Watts H., Jaffe N., Parkman R. (1977). Concomitant presence of tumour-specific cytotoxic and inhibitor lymphocytes in patients with osteogenic sarcoma. *New Eng. J. Med*; **297**: 121–7.

Zembala M., Mytar B., Popiela T., Asherson G.L. (1977). Depressed *in vitro* peripheral blood lymphocyte response to mitogens in cancer patients: The role of suppressor cells. *Int. J. Cancer*; **19**: 605–609.

Index